DATE DUE

DEMCO 38-296

The Physician's Perspective on Medical Law, Volume II

AANS Publications Committee
Howard H. Kaufman, MD, and
Jeff L. Lewin, JD, Editors

Neurosurgical Topics

The American Association of
Neurological Surgeons

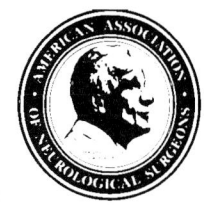

Library of Congress Catalog
ISBN: 1-879284-53-7

Neurosurgical Topics ISBN: 0-9624246-6-8

Warren R. Selman, MD, Chairman
AANS Publications Committee

Gay Palazzo, AANS Staff Editor

AANS1.4M897

Neurosurgical Topics SERIES

FORTHCOMING BOOKS

The Physician's Perspective on Medical Law, Volume I
Edited by Howard H. Kaufman, MD, and Jeff L. Lewin, JD

Advanced Techniques in Central Nervous System Metastases
Edited by Robert J. Maciunas, MD

Calvarial and Dural Reconstruction
Edited by Setti S. Rengachary, MD, and Edward C. Benzel, MD

DEDICATIONS

To Romaine Kaufman and my sons, Ezekiel and Zachary, at least one of whom may enter the legal profession.

H.H.K.

To Alison Williams Lewin and our children, Eleanor, Gregory, and Sylvia, for their tolerance during my immersion in this project and for the delightful exuberance with which they occasionally succeeded in distracting me from the task.

J.L.L.

To Joyce Herschberger whose hard work and persistence were essential to the completion of this project, and to Gay Palazzo for her patience while awaiting the manuscript and for her superb editorial refinements thereof.

H.H.K.
J.L.L.

CONTENTS

VOLUME II

PART III: THE PHYSICIAN AND PUBLIC HEALTH ISSUES

LIST OF CONTRIBUTORS

Volumes I and II

Alan M. Ducatman, MD, MS
Director
Institute of Occupational and
    Environmental Health
West Virginia School of Medicine
Morgantown, West Virginia

Mathis P. Frick, MD
Department of Radiology
Robert C. Byrd Health Sciences Center
West Virginia University
Morgantown, West Virginia

James L. Frost, MD
Deputy Chief Medical Examiner
Office of the Chief Medical Examiner
North Central Region
State of West Virginia
Morgantown, West Virginia

Mark Gibson, MD
Professor and Chairman
Department of Obstetrics and Gynecology
Robert C. Byrd Health Sciences Center
West Virginia University
Morgantown, West Virginia

Ellen E. Hrabovsky, MD
Professor and Chief
Section of Pediatric Surgery
Robert C. Byrd Health Sciences Center
West Virginia University
Morgantown, West Virginia

Howard H. Kaufman, MD
Department of Neurosurgery
Robert C. Byrd Health Sciences Center
West Virginia University
Morgantown, West Virginia

Robert W. Keefover, MD
Associate Professor
Departments of Neurology and
    BehavioralMedicine and Psychiatry
Robert C. Byrd Health Sciences Center
West Virginia University
Morgantown, West Virginia

Leroy J. Korb, MD
Department of Radiology
Robert C. Byrd Health Sciences Center
West Virginia University
Morgantown, West Virginia

Jeff L. Lewin, JD
Professor of Law
Widener University School of Law
Wilmington, Delaware

Joyce McConnell, JD, LLM
Associate Professor
College of Law
West Virginia University
Morgantown, West Virginia

Robert F. Munzner, PhD
Chief, Neurological Devices Branch,
Device Evaluation
US Food and Drug Administration
Center for Devices and Radiological Health
Rockville, Maryland

G. Robert Nugent, MD
Professor of Neurosurgery
Robert C. Byrd Health Sciences Center
West Virginia University
Morgantown, West Virginia

Perry Oxley, JD
Waters, Warren & Harris
Clarksburg, West Virginia

Conrad J. Pesyna, BS
Director of Medical Records
West Virginia Hospitals, Inc.
Morgantown, West Virginia

Sandra A. Price, JD
Risk Manager
Robert C. Byrd Health Sciences Center
West Virginia University
Morgantown, West Virginia

Mark A. Reynolds, MD
Interim Director,
Jon Michael Moore Trauma Center
Interim Chief, Section of Trauma and Surgery
Assistant Professor
Department of Surgery
West Virginia University
Morgantown, West Virginia

Carolyn B. Reynolds, MD
Department of Emergency Medicine
Preston Memorial Hospital
Kingwood, West Virginia

Cheng B. Saw, PhD
Division of Radiation Oncology
University of Iowa Hospital and Clinics
200 Hawkins Drive W189Z-GH
Iowa City, Iowa

Raymond A. Smego, Jr., MD, MPH, FACP, DTM&H
Professor of Medicine
Section of Infectious Diseases
Director, International Health Program
Robert C. Byrd Health Sciences Center
West Virginia University
Morgantown, West Virginia

James M. Stevenson, MD
Professor and Chairman
Behavioral Medicine and Psychiatry
West Virginia University
Morgantown, West Virginia

Daniel R. Sullivan, MD, JD
Adjunct Professor
Department of Anesthesiology
Robert C. Byrd Health Sciences Center
West Virginia University
Morgantown, West Virginia

Gregory A. Timberlake, MD, FACS
Director of Trauma Services
Department of Neurosurgery
Health Sciences Center
Morgantown, West Virginia

Janie R. Vale, MD, MSPH
Columbia Occupational Medicine
Columbia, Missouri

Grace J. Wigal, JD
Director of Legal Research and
    Writing Program
West Virginia University College of Law
Morgantown, West Virginia

Janet M. Williams, MD, FACEP
Assistant Professor
Department of Emergency Medicine
West Virginia University
Morgantown, West Virginia

AANS Publications Committee

Warren R. Selman, MD, *Chair*
Michael L.J. Apuzzo, MD
Julian E. Bailes, Jr., MD
Daniel L. Barrow, MD
Joshua B. Bederson, MD
Edward C. Benzel, MD
T. Forcht Dagi, MD

John G. Golfinos, MD
Howard H. Kaufman, MD
Christopher M. Loftus, MD
Robert J. Maciunas, MD
Ian E. McCutcheon, MD
Setti S. Rengachary, MD
John A. Jane, MD, *ex officio*

The American Association of Neurological Surgeons is accredited by the Accreditation Council for Continuing Medical Education (CME) to sponsor continuing medical education for physicians.

The American Association of Neurological Surgeons designates the continuing medical education activity as 15 credit hours in Category I of the Physician's Recognition Award of the American Medical Association.

PREFACE

The professional activities of most physicians lead to numerous contacts with the legal system, either in relation to patients or to public health issues about which physicians have unique experience and knowledge. In our experience many physicians feel that they are neither informed about nor comfortable with the legal rules that affect their relations with patients and with society. This monograph has been prepared to provide information about these rules and about the legal and social context in which they arise.

Physicians have an ethical and legal responsibility to participate in the legal system, both as advocates for patients and as good citizens. In order for physicians to carry out these responsibilities and comport themselves appropriately, they should become familiar with the legal system and the legal rules that govern their participation in judicial proceedings.

Physicians must understand the legal rules governing their relations with patients. In addition to familiarity with the general rules about the physician-patient relationship and the handling of confidential patient information, physicians face special problems in making medical decisions at the end of life, evaluating patients who may lack mental competence, and protecting vulnerable patients such as children, spouses, and the elderly.

Beyond caring for their patients, physicians as citizens ought to take an active role in public health issues that cause the greatest problems in our society, especially violence, accidents, firearms, alcohol, tobacco and infectious disease. They also should be aware of problems arising from exposure to such potential public health hazards as radiation, toxic substances, and regulated drugs and devices.

Physicians must also be prepared to protect both themselves and their patients in interactions with the health care system. For themselves, physicians need to negotiate their way through the systems that control their licensure and privileges. Physicians need to assist their patients and also protect their own monetary interests in relation to various private and public payors; the newly evolving systems encompassed in the term "managed care" pose special challenges. Physicians should understand their role in determining patient eligibility for public benefits from the federal Social Security program and state workers' compensation systems. Finally, physicians confront the risk of medical malpractice claims by their patients and the problems posed by this aspect of the law.

We note that a book on this subject necessarily must be considered a work in progress. Many of the chapters involve areas of law that are evolving rapidly in response to medical advances and emerging social developments. The issue of assisted suicide is being considered by the United States Supreme Court as this book is going to press. The proliferation of medical information transmission via the Internet has generated proposals for protecting confidentiality in computerized medical records. Turning to public health issues, there has been a recent decrease in the amount of violent crime, but the reason is not certain. Competing interest groups are seeking to tighten or ease restrictions on accessibility of guns. With regard to efforts to curtail the use of tobacco, the Food and Drug Administration has begun to institute new regulations of nicotine, while newspapers report important developments in lawsuits by states and individuals against tobacco companies. Responding to concern about abuses by managed care organizations in exacting large profits while limiting patient care, courts and legislatures are developing new rules to control these entities and protect patient rights. Accordingly, the editors and authors plan on regularly revising this book and possibly converting it to a looseleaf format to better accommodate anticipated changes in the law which are certain to occur at irregular and unpredictable intervals.

We hope this book will prove useful in presenting information that can help physicians, as well as lawyers and others, understand the legal aspects of physicians' activities. Although this book is primarily about law, most of the chapters are written by non-lawyers. Frequently, the authors convey physician perspectives on controversial medical and social issues. No consensus exists on many of these issues, either within the medical or legal professions or among the editors and authors of this book. The views expressed in any particular chapter are not necessarily shared by the editors or by authors of other chapters. We hope the book provides both a stimulus to and a foundation for informed debate on these important topics.

Howard H. Kaufman, M.D.
Morgantown, West Virginia

Jeff L. Lewin, J.D.
Wilmington, Delaware

June 1997

CHAPTER 13

GUNSHOT INJURIES AND GUN CONTROL

HOWARD H. KAUFMAN, MD

Attitudes about the ownership and use of guns in the United States date to the days of the early European settlers, when guns were indispensable for protection and hunting on the frontier. The defining historical event which required guns was the American Revolution, when the country was dependent on a citizen army and the establishment of a professional army was considered anathema.

Even today, many people want to own guns. There is now a huge pool of guns in the U.S., numbering over 250 million. There are guns in one-half of homes (half of these have handguns) and one-quarter of businesses. Nine million people carry guns, including 7.5 million private citizens.[32] Guns are more common in small town and rural settings, in the homes of whites, in the South and West, and in high-income households.[32] Almost 10 million guns are transferred to new owners each year (and 250,000 are stolen).[42] More guns are produced and imported annually than deteriorate or are destroyed, so the number of guns available is growing by millions each year.[32,44]

However, guns also represent a problem in the U.S., because of injury related to gunshot wounds. In 1985, gunshot wounds represented 268,000 (0.5%) of 56,859,000 injuries but cost $14.4 billion (9%) of the $157.6 billion spent to treat these injuries. Of the deaths from gunshot wounds in 1985, 56% were due to suicide, 39% to homicide, and 5% to accidents. In 1985, the average cost per patient was $54,831; per fatality, $373,520; per hospitalization, $33,159; and per non-hospitalized patient, $458.[46] In 1990, gunshot wounds caused 31,556 deaths (22% of all injury deaths) and 65,129 nonfatal hospitalizations (3%). The estimated cost was $20.4 billion.[36] Other cost estimates have been 10-fold higher. In 1991, there were 38,317 deaths from firearms, including 18,507 suicides and 17,971 homicides. Firearm deaths caused 1,072,565 years of potential life lost for people aged less than 65 years (YPLL-65), up 14% in a decade. Firearm deaths were the etiology in 60% of suicides and 68% of homicides, accounting for the increases in both these categories in the prior decade (Figures 1 and 2).[11] By 1992-93 there were estimated to be 99,025 gunshot injuries in the U.S.[1] There are now 40,000 people killed by gunshot wounds a year and 150,000 seriously injured.[8]

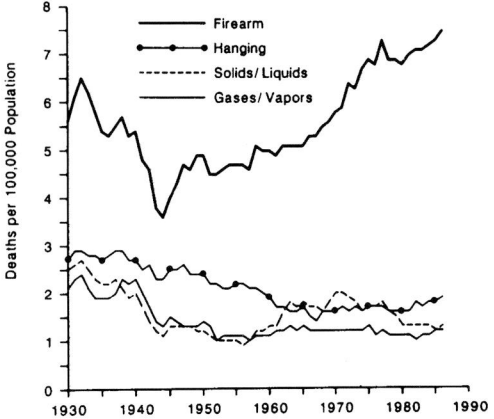

Figure 1: Death rates from suicide by year and method, 1930-1986. (Reproduced from *The Injury Fact Book.* 2nd ed.[2])

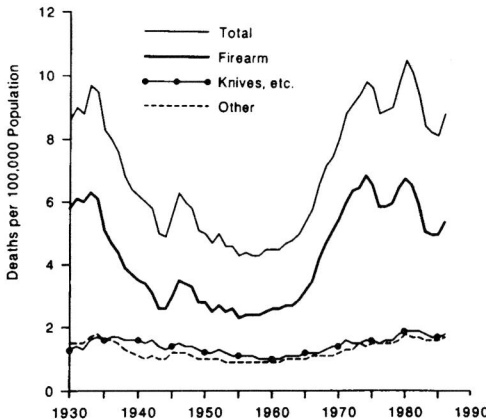

Figure 2: Death rates from homicide by year and method, 1930-1986. (Reproduced from *The Injury Fact Book.* 2nd ed.[2])

Guns play an important role in crime. There are many guns in the hands of criminals, and most guns used in crimes are not obtained through legal channels.[44,65] In 1993, of 43.6 million criminal victimizations, 4.4 million were violent crimes (rape and sexual assault, robbery, and aggravated assault). In violent crimes, 1.3 million perpetrators had a gun (86% a handgun). In addition, 70% of the 24,526 murders in 1993 were committed with firearms (81% of these with handguns).[66] The risk of homicide from a gunshot wound is highest for adolescent and young adult black males in central cities. The risk of suicide is highest for older white males.[2,5]

Our young are at particular risk. Guns are easy to obtain, even for high school students.[7] Indeed, weapons violations by teenagers are growing, especially in cities, with the worst offenders being 18-year-old males who are involved in a growing share of violent crimes.[19] This problem is highlighted by the increased rates of murder arrests of nonwhite males, with a peak for those who are 18 years old.[4]

As an etiology of traumatic death, gunshot wounds have been second only to motor-vehicle accidents (MVA). In several states, they have surpassed MVA and it is anticipated that they will be the first cause of traumatic death by about the year 2000.[46,47] Since 1990, gunshot wounds have been the largest cause of deaths from brain injury nationwide.[51]

Victims of gunshot injury include more than those subjected to self-inflicted injuries, crimes, and accidents. Other victims include their families and friends, society, which uses resources to care for them and loses their services, and the health care workers who must expend their energies to treat them.

The assassinations of President John Kennedy in 1963 and Robert Kennedy and Martin Luther King in 1968, the injury to Ronald Reagan in 1991, the growing numbers of homicides in inner cities, and numerous multiple random shootings, sometimes involving assault weapons, have brought the problem of gunshot-related violence to the public attention.

In *Healthy People 2000* (the outline of the federal public health aims for the decade 1990-2000), the homicide and suicide rates for 1987, including firearm death rates, were noted and targets were set for improvement by 2000.[56] Unfortunately, data for 1992 revealed increasing homicides (particularly of children, adolescents/young adults, and especially blacks, mainly due to handguns), as well as increased suicides of adolescents/young adults and especially blacks (again due to firearms), although suicides of adults decreased.[39] In 1995, more assaultive injuries and homicides were reported, although there were fewer suicides.[38] Drug-related violence and gangs in inner cities are thought to be the primary factor in these increases.[44]

Certain statistics have suggested a major factor in these injuries is the accessibility of guns. It is well known that homicide, including firearm-related homicide, occurs with far less frequency in other developed nations, so the situation in the U.S. is clearly not inevitable.[47] Because the disparity in violent crimes is not so great and because the major difference between the U.S. and most other advanced countries is the availability of guns here, it has been suggested there is a *causal* relationship between the availability of guns and the number of gun-related injuries and deaths. Therefore, restricting access to guns, so-called "gun control," should decrease the number of such injuries and deaths. The complexity of this issue, however, is exemplified by Switzerland and Israel; in both countries there is a high level of gun ownership (related to military duties), although few crimes are committed using guns.[6]

Persons using handguns represent the worst offenders. Although handguns constitute only one-third of the guns in the United States, they are involved in a far larger proportion of gun-related suicides and homicides. One-third of new handguns will be used in a crime.[44,65] It has been argued that because handguns are such a problem, they should be regulated more strictly than long guns.

In order to prevent this violence, it is first necessary to understand in detail what is known about suicide, homicide, and accidents.

EPIDEMIOLOGY

Suicide and Gunshot Wounds

The methods of suicide have been graded according to availability, lethality, painlessness, quickness, ease, expertise required, and lack of disfigurement. From the victim's perspectives, carbon monoxide poisoning has been judged as better than gunshot wounds and hanging is rated as equivalent. Other methods are almost as sure, and gunshot wounds are more disfiguring than most other methods, although this may not be appreciated.[32]

It has been thought that suicide via shooting is favored because it allows maximum control over the final act, it is a symbolically masculine act (most suicides are men), and men are "so-cialized" into gun use. A great proportion of suicides are from gunshot wounds to the head, of which 98% are fatal.[24] It appears that handguns are used more often than long guns in urban settings, but this may not hold true in rural settings where long guns are more common.

Guns in the home are a risk factor for suicide.[5,29,31,35] If guns were not immediately available, it appears that in some cases people would not substitute another method, then or ever. It has been reported that only 5%-10% of guns used in suicides are bought especially for this purpose, apparently because there are already so many readily available. A review of studies of locales with stricter gun laws has turned up contradictory findings about this issue,[32] but some of the findings indicating that gun controls are salutary are striking.[31] Although unknown, the true effect of restrictive gun laws depends on how many people commit suicide impulsively.

Interpersonal Violence and Gunshot Wounds

In 1985, there were about 650,000 crimes committed with guns, including 407,600 aggravated assaults, 12,100 rapes, 210,000 robberies, and 9,200 murders.[20] Today, the number of crimes committed with guns is thought to approach one million.[63] Comparing these numbers with the total numbers of such crimes, it would appear that guns are used in about 25% of aggravated assaults, 9% of rapes, 18% of robberies, and 39% of murders,[44] although these figures may be inaccurate by a factor of two to three.

The effectiveness of gun control depends on the nature of the acts, that is on which acts are spur-of-the-moment and thus are facilitated by easy access to guns. Presumably, many crimes are related to acute emotions and are facilitated by the presence of handguns. In 1992, murderers included relatives (12%), acquaintances (35%), and strangers (14%), while for 39% the relationship was not known. In 1993, between one-half and two-thirds of homicides were committed by relatives or acquaintances.[52] Most murders among family members and acquaintances are crimes of passion carried out on the spur of the moment, and these might not have occurred if a lethal weapon were not present.[30] In addition, many people who go on to murder have a history of violent behavior,[23] which could indicate that their access to guns should be eliminated. However, it may only be after a crime has been committed that a pattern of violent behavior can be detected.

In terms of gunshot wounds related to other crimes, criminals can be classified as casual or professional, and this may determine if general or targeted limitations of access would prevent injuries and deaths. There are "casual" criminals for whom the psychological and physical support of guns increases their propensity to crime. Decreased access of guns could diminish their activities, particularly after their first crime,[44] although some have suggested that they would substitute other weapons and attack more vulnerable targets, which might cancel out the effects of gun control.[32] Professional criminals and assassins, on the other hand, would find ways to obtain guns, at least until nationwide licensing, registration, and confiscation had been in place and enforced for several years.

It is known that assaults are more likely to result in death to the victim but less likely to result in injury if a gun is used. In robberies of commercial businesses, where the act is planned, the gun is the weapon of choice, while in assaults on a vulnerable victim, other weapons such as knives are often used. Hospitalization of a victim is more common when a knife is used than a gun, although death is less frequent. On balance, to avoid death, elimination of the use of guns should be helpful.

One disturbing trend is the use of more dangerous guns (and a concomitant increase in the severity of injuries). Semiautomatic pistols with larger ammunition capacity, ranging from large and expensive to small and inexpensive, have increasingly replaced revolvers in both fatal and nonfatal violence since the mid-1980s. Many guns are relatively small and easily concealable. They have been made more efficient by adding accessories such as recoil compensation or larger aiming devices.[64]

Accidents and Gunshot Wounds

There are perhaps 1,400 fatal accidents involving gunshot wounds each year and 17,000 injuries. Almost 40% of the nonfatal accidents require hospitalization. One-half of all accidents involve ingestion of alcohol.[32] About one-half of "accidental" deaths occur in the home and one-half occur elsewhere. About 10% of accidental deaths are actually suicides, while 8% of deaths classified as suicides are probably accidents. Accidents are most frequently self-inflicted and involve an extremity. These accidents are most common in males, persons aged 15 to 24 years, and blacks. The factors involved in accidents include accessibility, carelessness, aggressiveness, and lack of supervision.[32,49] In general, unintentional injury from firearms is declining.

Somewhere between 50 and 300 fatal accidents each year involve children younger than 15 years old who shoot themselves or are shot by another while playing with loaded guns.[22,32] Here the problem is accessibility, ease of operation, and lack of supervision. A person who leaves a loaded gun within the reach of children generally tends to be careless in other respects.[22] Improved safety features in guns might protect at least some children.[32]

Hunting accidents cause more than one-sixth (over 250) of the 1,400 fatal accidents each year. These range from truly unavoidable accidents to careless or even reckless behavior; 60%-80% involve members of the same hunting party.

It is believed that safety training would not reach or influence the majority of those involved in accidents. Laws assigning responsibility for accidents to owners who do not safely store or use guns should result in fewer accidents occurring.

USEFULNESS OF GUNS AND RISKS INVOLVED

People want to own guns for a variety of reasons. One of the most important reasons is for protection of self and property from animal pests and for hunting game to obtain food. Some people enjoy target practice, hunting for sport, or collecting guns.

Perhaps the most compelling reason to own a gun is the desire for defense from crime. However, the usefulness of guns in self-defense is controversial. Kleck[32] has estimated that guns are used in self-defense between 700,000 and 1,000,000 times a year, although several reinterpretations of Kleck's data have decreased the number to 329,000 and other figures suggest the number is 82,000 or possibly even fewer,[37] of which 20,000 are by law enforcement officers.[63] It has been estimated that 40% of defensive gun uses are at home, although if one counts defense in interpersonal violence, the frequency of use for protection may be greater. Victims of crimes apparently do not defend themselves frequently with firearms (1.2% robberies, 1.4% assaults, 3.1% burglaries, and <1% rapes).[44] One study indicated that guns were used defensively in 0.18% of all crimes and 0.85% of violent offenses.[37] When a gun is used for defense, it is fired only one-half to one-quarter of the time, and in less than 2% of the instances is the criminal wounded (10,000-20,000/year) or killed (1,500-2,800/year),[32] but these estimated figures may be much higher than is actually the case. In several instances in which gun laws have been liberalized or citizens were encouraged to obtain guns or trained to use them, crime rates dropped,[32] although the changes did not persist and the situations were complex. When guns are used, the crime victim has a decreased risk of injury; however, if he suffers an injury, it is more likely to be serious or fatal. On the other hand, some have argued that guns enable women to protect themselves from spouse abuse and rape and that this use has not undergone adequate study.[21] The major risk of guns is that they convert spur-of-the-moment altercations and suicide attempts into lethal events. Firearm wounds are particularly lethal; more so, for instance, than knife wounds by a factor of five.[32,44] Indeed, gunshot wounds to the head lead to death in about 90% of cases.[25] The lethality is based on intent, and the ratio of nonfatal to fatal wounds is 14.5 for accidents, 5.25 for assaults, and 0.181 for suicides.[44]

Guns kept in the home for self-defense have been related to increased risks of accidents, homicide, and suicide. In one study,[29] for every episode of self-protection homicide, there were 1.3 unintentional deaths, 4.5 criminal homicides, and 37 suicides. It has been estimated that in about 1% of defensive uses, the criminal takes the gun from the victim.[32] This is more common than the use of a gun to deter a burglar.[27]

THE NEED FOR MORE DATA

As mentioned, despite the huge amount of information about guns and gun-related violence, much remains to be learned about the usefulness and the risks associated with ownership of guns. Most of the national health planning committees as well as private individuals have noted this need and recommended the collection of information in sufficient detail to permit understanding of the circumstances, of not only deaths but also injuries, and so to facilitate the planning of strategies to prevent gun-related violence.[44,53,55,67] Kellermann[26] has detailed the difficulties faced in order for such information to be acquired, including insufficient funding, too few trained researchers, inadequacies in tracking systems, methodological problems, fatalistic attitudes toward prevention, barriers to interdisciplinary research, and opposition from interest groups. Mark Rosenberg, Director of the Division of Injury Control of the Centers for Disease Control, has detailed three areas to evaluate with a view to preventing firearm injuries:[47]

1. monitoring morbidity and disability (which are not as well known as mortality) as well as behavioral risk factors;
2. determining the importance of firearm possession; and
3. evaluating regulations and other interventions that might affect the risk of firearm injury.

SOLUTIONS

Strategies to control violence include changes in the social environment and changes in individuals, as well as changes in the physical environment (including instituting gun control) (Table 1).[41] The Panel on the Understanding and Control of Violent Behavior has suggested a variety of legal, public education, and technological strategies but noted that it was not possible to predict their effects without testing.[44] Intervention is possible at many points, and there are many models to conceptualize various approaches.

Several voluntary methods, such as education and training, have been tried. However, most

TABLE 1

STRATEGIES FOR PREVENTING VIOLENCE AND ITS CONSEQUENCES*

Strategy Type	Description	Intervention Examples
Change individual knowledge, skills, or attitudes	Deliver information to individuals to develop prosocial attitudes and beliefs	Conflict resolution education
	Increase knowledge	Social skills training
	Impart social, marketable, or professional skills	Job skills training
	Deter criminal actions	Public information and education campaigns
	Parenting education	Training of health care professionals in identification and referral of family violence
	Mandatory sentences for crimes committed using guns	
Change social environment	Alter the way people interact by improving their social or economic circumstances	Adult mentoring of youth
		Job creation programs
		Respite day care
		Battered-women's shelters
		Economic incentives for family stability
		Antidiscrimination laws enforced
		Deconcentrated lower-income housing
Change physical environment	Modify the design, use, or availability of dangerous commodities, structures, or space we move through	Restrictive licensing of handguns
		Prohibition or control of alcohol sales at events
		Increased visibility of high-risk areas
		Disruption of illegal gun markets
		Metal detectors in schools

* Reprinted by permission of Project HOPE, Public health policy for preventing violence, *Health Affairs*, Vol 12, p 14, Copyright 1993, *The People-to-People Health Foundation*.

voluntary methods do not influence the people who represent the greatest problem (namely those who are careless, emotionally unstable, or violent) and efforts aimed at these people have not been successful.[15,32] One very promising change would be to decrease exposure to violence, particularly on television.[41]

One alternative is to try to limit access to guns for those who would misuse them, while preserving access to guns for those who want or need to own them and have not demonstrated misuse. Several considerations need to be addressed in the creation of gun control laws, including whether they would be effective and whether they would be favored by the citizenry.

Gun Control

Federal laws addressing the problem of violence due to guns might range from complete elimination of guns to a *laissez faire* approach with almost no regulation except perhaps to prohibit possession of the most dangerous weapons by violent criminals and by psychiatric patients such as those with paranoid schizophrenia.[54] Because of the high value placed on freedom of choice and the reasonable desire and even need of many people to own guns and do so safely, it is apparent that it would not be practical or appropriate to eliminate gun ownership completely. However, some control, especially if proven effective in decreasing the number of injuries and deaths, would seem to be acceptable to the majority of people in the U.S.

Controlling firearm-related violence would require a national coordinated comprehensive effort ranging from data gathering to education to regulation.[58] It is important to consider both supply and demand.[8] One model of control strategies uses the 10 categories of corrective activities that Haddon developed as a comprehensive approach to dealing with motor-vehicle accidents.[28] Another model involves categorizing gun laws depending on when in the life of a gun they apply (Table 2).[54] These include the manufacture and importation, transfer (sale and purchase or gift), storage, carrying, and use.[32,44,60]

Limitations might be set on the types of guns (and ammunition) that could be manufactured and imported. There are several kinds of guns to be considered. Machine guns are already prohibited. Assault weapons are another class. For military use, these weapons are often fully automatic, but they are sold to civilians in semiautomatic versions. The danger is that they can be fired rapidly, they have large magazines (which can be changed quickly) and can be used to fire many shots in rapid succession, and they can be converted back to an automatic weapon. Assault weapons can be divided into assault pistols and assault rifles. Assault pistols are certainly more concealable and convenient. They are becoming more favored by criminals, especially violent ones and psychotics, and are perceived by most citizens as a growing menace. Their use has also been associated with illegal narcotics activities and organized crime.[9] There has been some dispute on how to define assault weapons and whether their ban would be useful. It has been said that sport weapons have some of the same characteristics and, therefore, trying to define and ban such weapons is inappropriate.[32] It can be argued that weapons which can fire rapidly and that have large, exchangeable magazines are not needed for ordinary protection and sport, and therefore no weapons should be sold which have these characteristics. A federal law passed in 1994 banning certain assault weapons and other weapons of certain types has not proven comprehensive enough to be effective. On March 22, 1996 the U.S. House of Representatives voted 239-173 to repeal this ban, although the U.S. Senate is not expected to uphold this vote.

Even without regulations, civil liability may cause gun manufacturers to limit access to assault weapons. A recent ruling by a California Superior Court Judge permitted a suit against the maker of an assault weapon, which was used to kill a number of people, on the grounds that it was inherently "ultra hazardous" and that the maker should be aware of this.[40]

Another problematic class of weapons is those made without metal. These weapons are dangerous because they can be taken without detection into supposedly secure areas, such as airplanes. Their manufacture and importation could be banned.

Another class of objectionable guns is "Saturday night specials" (i.e., cheap handguns that are made without quality control). The risk is that they can be purchased so inexpensively that they can be obtained even by children and that their poor construction makes them dangerous. The argument against banning them is that persons without financial resources need access to them for personal protection, although it is hard to justify the availability of weapons that are poorly made. Federal laws could keep these guns out of the hands of those who should not possess them. Some have argued that no handgun is truly a necessity and that, since handguns are responsible for a disproportionate percentage of injuries and deaths because they are convenient and concealable, they should be banned completely. Whether this kind of ban would receive enough popular support is questionable.

In addition, guns could be made more safe for use by providing devices to indicate if they

TABLE 2
Nosology of Gun Policy*

1 Policy related to the manufacture of guns
  1.1 Ban the manufacture of guns
    1.1.1 All guns
    1.1.2 Certain guns
      1.1.2.1 All handguns
      1.1.2.2 Saturday night specials
      1.1.2.3 Assault weapons
      1.1.2.4 Automatic weapons
      1.1.2.5 Long guns
      1.1.2.6 Others
  1.2 Regulate the manufacture of guns
    1.2.1 Product design, safety regulations
      1.2.1.1 Personalization—require guns to be designed so that only authorized persons can operate them
      1.2.1.2 Childproofing—require guns to be designed so that they are inoperable by children
      1.2.1.3 Safety devices—require guns to incorporate such features as magazine interlocks or loaded chamber indicators
      1.2.1.4 Other safety criteria—require domestically manufactured guns to incorporate the same safety features required for inported guns
    1.2.2 Regulate the quantity of all or certain guns manufactured
  1.3 Impose strict liability on manufacturers—permit the transfer of the costs of gun injuries back to the manufacturer through litigation
  1.4 Tax manufacturers for each gun produced

2 Policy related to the sale of guns
  2.1 Ban the sale of guns
    2.1.1 All guns
    2.1.2 Certain guns (see 1.1.2)
  2.2 Ban the sale of guns to certain people
    2.2.1 By age
    2.2.2 By mental health status
    2.2.3 By criminal history
      2.2.3.1 By felony conviction
      2.2.3.2 By selected misdemeanor convictions
      2.2.3.3 By arrest record
    2.2.4 By citizenship
    2.2.5 By high-risk behavior, such as substance addiction
    2.2.6 By other means (for example, dishonorable discharge from the military)
  2.3 Limit the number of guns that can be sold to a person within a given time period
  2.4 Impose waiting periods
    2.4.1 Purpose for waiting period
      2.4.1.1 Background check
        2.4.1.1.1 Approval required before sale
      2.4.1.2 Cooling-off period
    2.4.2 Duration of waiting period (several days to several months)
    2.4.3 Guns to which waiting period applies
      2.4.3.1 All guns
      2.4.3.2 Certain guns (see 1.1.2)
    2.4.4 Sales to which waiting period applies
      2.4.4.1 All sales (including private sales)
      2.4.4.2 Only sales involving dealers
  2.5 Strengthen requirements for licensed sellers
    2.5.1 Stricter envorcement of federal firearm license provisions
      2.5.1.1 "Doing business" provisions (i.e., dealer must actually be in the same business of selling guns)
      2.5.1.2 Inspection and compliance monitoring

      2.5.1.3 Prosecution for "straw-man" sales
      2.5.1.4 Prosecution for direct sales to prohibited persons
   2.5.2 Higher license fee
  2.6 Impose strict liability on sellers
   2.6.1 On all sellers (including private sales)
   2.6.2 On dealer sales only
  2.7 Tax sales
  2.8 Require sales to include after-market safety devices

3 Regulate the marketing and advertising of guns by manufacturers and sellers
  3.1 Prohibit some venues of advertising (for example, television)
  3.2 Regulate content of advertising
   3.2.1 Prohibit false claims
   3.2.2 Prohibit advertising that appeals to children

4 Policy related to the possession of guns
  4.1 Ban possession
   4.1.1 Ban possession of all guns
   4.1.2 Ban possession of certain guns (see 1.1.2)
   4.1.3 Ban possession by certain people (see 2.2)
  4.2 Register possession
   4.2.1 Register all guns
   4.2.2 Register certain guns (see 1.1.2)
   4.2.3 Increase registration fees
  4.3 Restrict possession
   4.3.1 By location
      4.3.1.1 In public places
      4.3.1.2 In high-risk places
      4.3.1.3 In schools
   4.3.2 By requiring storage mode
      4.3.2.1 Childproof storage laws (including parental liability statutes)
   4.3.3 By requiring safety course to possess
  4.4 License the carrying of guns
   4.4.1 By type of gun
      4.4.1.1 All guns
      4.4.1.2 Handguns
      4.4.1.3 Other selected guns
   4.4.2 By location
      4.4.2.1 All locations
      4.4.2.2 Restricted areas
      4.4.2.3 Vehicles
   4.4.3 By carrying mode
      4.4.3.1 Concealed weapons
      4.4.3.2 Exposed weapons
  4.5 Enhance the detection of illegal possession
   4.5.1 Metal detector installation
      4.5.1.1 In public places
      4.5.1.2 In high-risk places
      4.5.1.3 In schools

5 Policy related to the use of guns
  5.1 Ban the discharge of guns
  5.2 Mandatory jail for crimes using guns
  5.3 Mandatory jail for illegal possession of guns
  5.4 Enhanced sentences for crimes using guns

6 Policy related to the regulation of importation of guns

7 Policy related to the regulation of ammunition (manufacture, sale, and possession)

---

* Reprinted by permission of Project HOPE, Policies to prevent firearm injuries, *Health Affairs,* Vol 12, pp 98-101, Copyright 1993, *The People-to-People Health Foundation.*

are loaded, better safety locks, triggers requiring more force, and other features. Some of these devices are very sophisticated and, of course, would result in increasing the cost of manufacture of these guns.

Weapons can be modified to make them more dangerous (e.g., sawing off the end of a shotgun so it is more concealable, and converting a semi-automatic to automatic firing). Laws can be created to forbid such modification of a gun.

High-powered and/or deformable ammunition which can pierce flak jackets and walls is another concern. Hunters may argue that they want access to ammunition that gives them the ability to bring down game at a distance. Deformable ammunition, which can be extremely injurious, would definitely seem inappropriate. It can be argued that guns and ammunition can be produced by individuals,[32] but laws can be created to control this.

The next point of control might be transfer of guns from one owner to another. Since perhaps 80% of the firearms used to commit crimes are obtained via theft or through illegal or unregulated transactions, it is very important to disrupt illegal gun markets.[44] Stricter license requirements for dealers in the last few years has decreased their numbers by 19% from the peak of 284,100 in 1992, and the number is expected to drop below 100,000 within 5 years.[13] In terms of commercial transfers, the seller could be made responsible for checking the purchaser's background and recording the transaction, and for any misadventures that occurred following violation of such laws. This would require an adequate and accessible database of people convicted of certain crimes or with dangerous mental diseases, which is not yet in place.

There are other possible areas of control. Many seem so logical it would seem difficult to muster any reasonable arguments against them. Minors should not be permitted to own guns. There should also be a "cooling-off" period to prevent purchase during an emotional crisis which might lead to suicide or homicide. The law could also require a written and practical examination demonstrating competence in using a weapon, such as that required to obtain a driver's license. These requirements should also apply to private transfers, including gifts. In order to insure that liability can be assigned accurately

for failure to insure only appropriate sale or transfer, it would be necessary to require that all guns be registered. In addition, the number of guns that could be purchased in a given time period could be limited to prevent gun running, as has happened recently in Virginia. A limit on the number of guns purchased has been shown to disrupt the illegal interstate transfer of firearms.[62] Possession of stolen guns should be a violation of the law.

Safe storage of guns might also be required. Two problems related to inappropriate storage are accidents and thefts. Nonfatal and fatal accidents occur when children find and play with guns. Since 1989, several state legislatures have passed laws allowing charges against parents or other adults who fail to secure guns from children.[48] Additionally, many criminals obtain guns by theft (250,000/year), and adequate storage could prevent this. However, it can be argued that if guns are required for protection at home, they must be loaded and available. This is only partially true. For example, if a burglar is heard, there is time to unlock a weapon, but if one is surprised, the weapon must be at hand. It is not clear how often each sort of episode arises.

Carrying weapons, particularly concealed weapons, certainly facilitates criminal activity. The argument is that citizens need to be able to carry guns to defend themselves and that carrying protects all citizens, although it has not been shown that this is true. A license to carry a concealed gun can be obtained in well over half the states, either with or without need.[10] Laws allowing the carrying of concealed weapons are opposed by law-enforcement organizations.[59] Indeed, rules to prevent carrying concealed weapons, aggressive enforcement with checks including security gates, and severe penalties for carrying weapons have been shown to decrease gun-related crimes, and could be promulgated. Such an approach has been said to be the reason for the recent dramatic decrease in murders in New York City. Conversely, it appears that the permissive law in Florida may have increased the number of murders.[59] Of course, if nobody was carrying guns, this would obviate the problem.

Lastly, there is the actual use of guns, particularly in crimes. There have been laws mandating add-on penalties when guns are used in crimes. Such laws do need to include some flexibility to allow plea-bargaining, but reasonable middle-ground rules can be developed.

In many states, suicide is a crime. If the person dies, the question is moot. If the person survives, such laws are not enforced. A more humane response than legal action is indicated, and counseling and treatment of psychiatric problems should be pursued.

Thus, there are a number of laws which either theoretically or based on some evidence would seem to have the potential to control the use of guns,[32,44,54,63] although some studies are contradictory regarding the effectiveness of gun control laws.[32] For comparison, Seattle, Washington, and Vancouver, British Columbia are close in proximity and of similar size. However, Vancouver has much more restrictive gun laws and far fewer guns. The firearm homicide rate in Seattle is four times higher than in Vancouver.[50] Other studies of places where restrictive gun laws were enacted indicate that the laws resulted in decreased rates of violence and crime.[32,44] However, until "leakage" from a state with permissive laws to one with stricter laws has been stopped and the pool of accessible guns is decreased, the full impact of such laws will not be known.

Optimal gun control will require federal laws, particularly in such areas as manufacture/import and sale/transfer, or there will continue to be "leakage" of weapons across state lines. But this raises complex issues relative to states' rights as specified in the 10th and 11th Amendments. For example, in *In re United States v. Lopez* (115 SCt 1624 (1995)), the U.S. Congress was found to have exceeded its authority in making it a federal crime to carry a gun within 1,000 feet of a school. Also, the Fifth Circuit Court of Appeals recently struck down the section of the 1994 Brady Handgun Violence Protection Act (Brady Bill) which requires local law enforcement officials to make background checks of handgun purchasers.[14]

Another problem that must be kept in mind is the immense numbers of guns in the country and particularly in the hands of criminals. It is obvious that control of this pool of weapons would take many years and would require considerable expense, but only when gun control laws have succeeded in substantially reducing the pool of available weapons can the full impact of such laws be determined.

RESPONSIBILITY OF THE FEDERAL GOVERNMENT TO REGULATE GUN USE

The major duties of the federal government, as stated in the Preamble of its founding document, the Constitution, are to "insure domestic tranquility" and "promote the general welfare." While state governments have the primary responsibility to protect the health, safety, and welfare of their citizens in the exercise of their "police power," experience has demonstrated the need for federal gun control legislation because not all states are likely to enact such laws and the efforts of those that do would be undermined by the ability of their citizens to acquire guns from adjacent states. The power of the federal government to enact gun control legislation derives from the Commerce Clause of the Constitution, which grants Congress the power to regulate activities that substantially affect interstate commerce.

Interpreting the scope of federal power under the Commerce Clause, Chief Justice John Marshall in *Gibbons v. Ogden* in 1824 emphasized "[t]he power vested in the legislature by the constitution to make ... laws ... for the good and welfare of the commonwealth, and the subjects of the same."[42] Trying to reduce the number of gun-related injuries and deaths would seem to be an appropriate goal of federal regulation, and the courts have upheld the power of Congress under the Commerce Clause to enact federal gun control legislation.

One opposing argument has been that any regulation of guns compromises the fundamental right of a citizen to personal freedom. This concept is embodied in the vision of a self-sufficient American of the frontier and the citizen soldier of the Revolutionary War.[17] However, it is important to remember that no society can survive without some constraints on its people or there would be anarchy. A middle ground must be found where reasonable rights are protected but where citizens relinquish complete freedom in order to insure stability and the safety of others. This tradition of the balance of rights and privileges vs. responsibilities in a democracy began in Greece and was continued in Britain and the United States. An analogy can be drawn with the control of driving. It is accepted that a driver's license is required to ensure that anyone driving a vehicle has the necessary knowledge and skill to do so safely and that motor vehicles must be registered to ensure that their owners are made liable for any misuse of the vehicle.

Some have contended that the right to own guns is made implicit by the Second Amendment: "A well regulated Militia, being necessary to the security of a free State, the right of the people to keep and bear Arms, shall not be infringed"[45] and that this has been explicitly confirmed by Congress in such laws as the Freedmen's Bureau Act (14 Stat. 176-177 (1866)), The Property Requisition Act (55 Stat. 742 (1941)), and the Firearms Owners' Protection Act (18 USC §921 et seq (1986)).[18] Interpretation of the Constitution ranges from the very literal to utilizing its clauses to capture the general intent of the authors as expressed in the Preamble.[34,44] Indeed, many scholars believe that although the Second Amendment is not clear, it was written to enable the states to establish "well regulated" citizen armies (now the National Guard) and that there was no intent to establish an unfettered right to own guns.[16]

The Constitution was meant to be a living document which can be interpreted in terms of changing conditions, and it was designed so that it can be amended when necessary. In addition, rights imply responsibilities and need not be interpreted as absolute. Regulation does not necessarily destroy a right, but may only limit its abuse. For example, the right of free speech does not allow slander or incitement of violence.

Indeed, there are said to be over 20,000 federal, state, and local laws regulating guns. Federal laws include two laws enacted in 1994: 1) the Brady Bill, which requires a waiting period for the purchase of handguns and a background check on the buyer, and 2) a law which limits the importation and manufacture of some assault weapons. The effect of these laws has been impressive. In the first year of enforcement of the Brady Bill, spot checks revealed denials for 15,506 (3.5%) of 441,545 applicants, including denials for 945 fugitives as well as convicted felons, persons under indictment, persons under restraining orders, drug users, and minors. Thus, a significant number of "bad guys" were pre-

vented from buying handguns and criminals were apprehended, while most people were not "unduly inconvenienced."[43] To improve and speed the screening process for purchasers, $200 million has been allocated to the Department of Justice to establish a national computerized felon identification system so that 5 years after the passage of the Brady Bill, screening can be accomplished at the time of purchase. In addition, the number of assault weapons used in crimes fell 18% (vs. 6% for all guns) in the first 8 months of 1994.[12]

Various of these laws have been tested in hundreds of court cases, including over 50 appelate decisions, two dozen federal cases, and three cases heard in the U.S. Supreme Court, all of which have interpreted the Second Amendment not to mean that citizens should have unregulated access to guns.[6,9,16,17] Experts who have occupied the highest judicial and executive legal positions have championed this position.[16] Warren Burger, former Chief Justice of the Supreme Court, reviewed the legal status of the Second Amendment for the Center to Prevent Hand Gun Violence:

> As a matter of law, the meaning of the Second Amendment has been settled since the ruling of the U.S. Supreme Court in *U.S. v. Miller*, 307 U.S. 174 (1939). In that case, the High Court wrote that the "obvious purpose" of the Second Amendment was "to assure the continuation and render possible the effectiveness" of the state militia. The Court added that the Amendment "must be interpreted and applied with that end in view." Since *Miller*, the Supreme Court has addressed the Second Amendment in two cases. In *Burton v. Sills*, 394 US 812 (1969), the Court dismissed the appeal of a state court ruling upholding New Jersey's strict gun control law, finding the appeal failed to present a "substantial federal question." And in *Lewis v. United States*, 445 US 55 (1980), the Court upheld the federal law banning felons from possessing guns. The Court found no "constitutionally protected liberties" infringed by the federal law.
>
> Since *Miller* was decided, lower federal and state courts have addressed the meaning of the Second Amendment in more than thirty cases. In every case, the courts have decided that the Amendment guarantees a right to be armed only in connection with service in a "well regulated Militia."

TABLE 3

PUBLIC SUPPORT FOR GUN POLICY OPTIONS, SELECTED QUESTIONS, 1987-1992*

Gun Policy Option	Approval Range
Ban manufacture of Saturday night specials	68%-73%
Ban manufacture of assault weapons	72%-73%
Stricter regulation of firearm sales	60%-78%
Stricter regulation of handgun sales	60%-65%
Ban sale of all handguns	40%-42%
Ban sale of Saturday night specials	68%-73%
Ban sale of assault weapons	72%-75%
Seven-day handgun waiting period	80%-95%
Ban possession of all firearms	29%
Ban possession of handguns	29%-43%
Ban possession of Saturday night specials	68%-71%
Ban possession of assault weapons	72%-73%
Register possession of all firearms	67%-79%
Register possession of all handguns	72%-84%
License carrying of guns outside the home	81%-88%
Individual right to bear arms protected by Constitution	68%-90%

* Reprinted by permission of Project HOPE, Public opinion polling on gun policy, *Health Affairs*, Vol 12, p 201, Copyright 1993, *The People-to-People Health Foundation.*

It has been suggested that a major problem in the regulation of guns is that the public has not been well informed about the legal principles involved and that they have primarily been exposed to simplistic arguments by interest groups opposing gun control.[16] Indeed, some physicians share this view, as reflected in several letters to the editor in the *New England Journal of Medicine* in reply to an article defending the efforts of the Centers for Disease Control[61] and in a series of articles, editorials, and letters to the editor in the *Journal of the Medical Association of Georgia* in January 1994, March 1994, June 1994, and June 1995, in which the philosophical underpinnings and databases of both sides and their problems are recapitulated. The ongoing debate centers around the failure of the opponents of gun control to accept that gun control does not necessarily mean forbidding gun ownership but can encompass reasonable regulation, and that while information about

the protective usage of guns is problematic, the data about the danger of possessing handguns with regard to homicide, suicide, and accidents cannot be ignored. Arguments against gun control imply that one major aspect of the problem of gun-related violence, namely easy accessibility to firearms, can be tolerated based on a simplistic argument against regulation.

PUBLIC OPINION

Most people believe in the right to have private ownership of guns (Table 3).[57] A detailed review of 14 opinion surveys from 1959 to 1996[3] specifies who owns guns (men, whites, Republicans, those whose parents owned a gun) and why (hunting, target shooting, protection), a trend toward decreased gun ownership (especially long guns in cities), decreased use for game hunting, and increased handgun ownership in cities and rural settings. After stratifying for gun ownership, these surveys reveal that both owners and nonowners support many gun control measures, including the Brady Bill, the ban on semiautomatic weapons, the registration of handguns, and a limit in the number of gun purchases each month. Most also believe stricter laws will eventually lead to confiscation of all guns, yet a majority oppose this. It is reasonable to assume, therefore, given the intensity of feeling by a passionate minority against gun control and the slow progress to date, that increased gun control will likely be incremental and happen over a long period of time.[3]

CONCLUSION

Complete elimination of gun-related violence would require solving societal socioeconomic problems and creating citizens with the desire and skill to resolve all their disputes peaceably. This utopia is certainly a long way from realization, and, in the view of many, may never occur. Consequently, it is important to devise actions that can minimize the current problems, and gun control would seem to be an important component of such an effort. This will require preventing the manufacture and importation of "hyperhazardous" guns, controlling the sale/transfer of guns, requiring gun owners to have an ownership license, registering all guns, expropriating guns that no one should own, and taking guns away from people who should not own them, including those with criminal records of a variety of types and those with certain mental illnesses, minors, and those who cannot meet licensure requirements. Laws must be national and strictly enforced or they will not be effective and their true potential will not be realized.[32,44]

Given the scope of the problem of guns, perhaps a million gun-related crimes, 300,000 injuries, 40,000 deaths, and a cost of probably over $100 billion a year, the institution of such laws as those described here seems reasonable and appropriate, should aid in reducing gun-related violence, and is urgently required. Limited regulation would allow those who qualify to own guns to possess them. For those qualified, such laws would cause no more inconvenience than

the laws required for car ownership and use, and the cost engendered would not be excessive.

Would such laws prevent all gunshot wounds? No! Would they decrease death and injuries significantly over the next few decades, as efforts in automobile safety have done in the last several decades? They logically should!

RESPONSIBILITIES OF THE PHYSICIAN

The main concerns for the physician, besides caring for the patient, include reporting requirements and the need to obtain and preserve evidence, both discussed in other chapters. In addition, gun-related injuries are a major public health problem, and it is the obligation of the physician as a health care professional and as a citizen to take an active part in trying to prevent them. As noted by former Surgeon General C. Everett Koop:

> Throughout our history, Americans have remained committed to a social contract that respects the rule of law, that promotes peaceful intercourse among citizens, and that has as its highest value the protection of human life. . . .
>
> Our citizens want to live in peace, but each year many thousands of them become victims of violence . . . society has somehow failed them. . . .
>
> Identifying violence as a public health issue is a relatively new idea . . . the professions of medicine, nursing, and the health related social services must come forward and recognize violence as their issue and one that profoundly affects the public health.
>
> . . . progress in this area that is of such great significance for the health and well-being of all Americans and of our society as a whole . . . will be a major contribution toward the strengthening of our nation's social contract.[33]

REFERENCES

1. Annest JL, Mercy JA, Gibson DR, et al: National estimates of nonfatal firearm-related injuries. Beyond the tip of the iceberg. JAMA 273:1749-1754, 1995
2. Baker SP, O'Neill B, Ginsburg MJ, et al: **The Injury Fact Book.** 2nd ed. New York, NY: Oxford University Press, 1992, 344 pp
3. Blendon RJ, Young JT, Hemenway D: The American public and the gun control debate. JAMA 275:

1719-1722, 1996

4. Blumstein A, Heinz HJ III: Youth violence, guns and the illicit-drug industry, in Block C, Block R (eds): **Trends, Risks and Interventions in Lethal Violence: Proceedings of the Third Annual Spring Symposium of the Homicide Research Working Group.** Washington, DC: US Department of Justice, National Institute of Justice, 1995, pp 3-25

5. Brent DA, Perper JA, Goldstein CE, et al: Risk factors for adolescent suicide. A comparison of adolescent suicide victims with suicidal inpatients. **Arch Gen Psychiatry 45:**581-588, 1988

6. Bruce-Briggs B: The great American gun war, in Nisbet L (ed): **The Gun Control Debate. You Decide.** Buffalo, NY: Prometheus Books, 1990, pp 63-85

7. Callahan CM, Rivara FP: Urban high school youth and handguns. A school-based survey. **JAMA 267:** 3038-3042, 1992

8. Cook PJ, Cole TB: Strategic thinking about gun markets and violence. **JAMA 275:**1765-1767, 1996

9. Council on Scientific Affairs, American Medical Association: Assault weapons as a public health hazard in the United States. **JAMA 267:**3067-3070, 1992

10. Cramer CE, Kopel DB: "Shall issue:" the new wave of concealed handgun permit laws. **Tenn Law Rev 62:** 679-757, 1995

11. Division of Violence Prevention, National Center for Injury Prevention and Control, CDC: Firearm-related years of potential life lost before age 65 years—United States, 1980–1991. **JAMA 272:**1246, 1994

12. Editorial: Gun law is working: why would Congress repeal it. **USA TODAY.** Dec 19, 1995, p 10A

13. Gage R: Gun dealers: "weeding out the trash." **US News World Report.** Feb 27, 1995, p 10

14. Greenhouse L: Taking states seriously. **New York Times.** Apr 14, 1996, p E3

15. Hemenway D, Solnick SJ, Azrael DR: Firearm training and storage. **JAMA 273:**46-50, 1995

16. Henigan DA, Nicholson EB, Hemenway D: **Guns and the Constitution. The Myth of Second Amendment Protection for Firearms in America.** Northampton, MA: Aletheia Press, 1995

17. Hofstadter R: America as a gun culture, in Nisbet L (ed): **The Gun Control Debate. You Decide.** Buffalo, NY: Prometheus Books, 1990, pp 25-34

18. Holbrook SP: Congress interprets the Second Amendment: Declarations by a co-equal branch on the individual right to keep and bear arms. **Tenn Law Rev 62:**597-641, 1995

19. Johnson K: Arrests for guns among teens double. **USA TODAY.** Nov 13, 1995, p 1A

20. Jones L: Gun advocates try to shoot down Brady Bill. **Am Med News.** May 27, 1991, pp 4-5

21. Kates DB Jr: Defensive gun ownership as a response to crime, in Nisbet L (ed): **The Gun Control Debate. You Decide.** Buffalo, NY: Prometheus Books, 1990, pp 251-269

22. Kates DB Jr: Gun accidents, in Nisbet L (ed): **The Gun Control Debate. You Decide.** Buffalo, NY: Prometheus Books, 1990, pp 300-303

23. Kates DB Jr: The law-abiding gun owner as a domestic and acquaintance murderer, in Nisbet L (ed): **The Gun Control Debate. You Decide.** Buffalo, NY: Prometheus Books, 1990, pp 270-274

24. Kaufman HH: Civilian gunshot wounds to the head. **Neurosurgery 32:**962-964, 1993

25. Kaufman HH, Loyola WP, Makela ME, et al: Civilian gunshot wounds: the limits of salvageability. **Acta Neurochir 67:**115-125, 1983

26. Kellermann AL: Obstacles to firearm and violence research. **Health Affairs 12:**142-153, 1993

27. Kellermann AL: Reply to letters to the editor. **JAMA 275:**281, 1996

28. Kellermann AL, Lee RK, Mercy JA, et al: The epidemiologic basis for the prevention of firearm injuries. **Annu Rev Public Health 12:**17-40, 1991

29. Kellermann AL, Reay DT: Protection or peril? An analysis of firearm-related deaths in the home. **N Engl J Med 314:**1557-1560, 1986

30. Kellermann AL, Rivara FP, Rushforth NB, et al: Gun ownership as a risk factor for homicide in the home. **N Engl J Med 329:**1084-1091, 1993

31. Kellermann AL, Rivara FP, Somes G, et al: Suicide in the home in relation to gun ownership. **N Engl J Med 327:**467-472, 1992

32. Kleck G: **Point Blank. Guns and Violence in America.** New York, NY: A de Gruyter, 1991

33. Koop CE: Foreword, in Rosenberg ML, Fenley MA (eds): **Violence in America. A Public Health Approach.** New York, NY: Oxford University Press, 1991, pp v-vi

34. Levinson S: The embarrassing Second Amendment, in Nisbet L (ed): **The Gun Control Debate. You Decide.** Buffalo, NY: Prometheus Books, 1990, pp 311-332

35. Marzuk PM, Leon AC, Tardiff K, et al: The effect of access to lethal methods of injury on suicide rates. **Arch Gen Psychiatry 49:**451-458, 1992

36. Max W, Rice DP: Shooting in the dark: estimating the cost of firearm injuries. **Health Affairs 12:**171-185, 1993

37. McDowall D, Wiersema B: The incidence of defensive firearm use by U.S. crime victims, 1987 through 1990. **Am J Public Health 84:**1982-1984, 1994

38. McGinnis JM, Lee PR: Healthy People 2000 at mid decade. **JAMA 273:**1123-1129, 1995

39. McGinnis JM, Richmond JB, Brandt EN Jr, et al: Health progress in the United States: results of the 1990 objectives for the nation. **JAMA 268:**2545-2552, 1992

40. Meier B: Guns don't kill, gun makers do? **New York Times.** Apr 16, 1995, p 3

41. Mercy JA, Rosenberg ML, Powell KE, et al: Public health policy for preventing violence. **Health Affairs 12:**7-29, 1993

42. National Committee for Injury Prevention and Control: **Injury Prevention: Meeting The Challenge.** New York, NY: Oxford University Press, 1989

43. **One-Year Progress Report: Brady Handgun Violence Prevention Act.** Washington, DC: Bureau of Alcohol, Tobacco, and Firearms, Department of the Treasury, 13 pp, 1995 (Internal document)

44. Reiss AJ Jr, Roth JA (eds): **Understanding and Preventing Violence.** Washington, DC: National Academy Press, 1993/1994

45. Reynolds GH: A critical guide to the Second Amendment. **Tenn Law Rev 62:**461-512, 1995

46. Rice DP, MacKenzie EJ, and Associates: **Cost of Injury in the United States: A Report to Congress.** San Francisco, Calif: Institute for Health and Aging, University of California and Injury Prevention Center, The Johns Hopkins University, 1989

47. Rosenberg ML, Fenley MA (eds): **Violence in America. A Public Health Approach.** New York, NY: Oxford University Press, 1991

48. Sharp D: Gun laws target parents. Parents whose children injure or kill others with guns are being prosecuted. **USA TODAY.** Aug 29, 1995, p 2A

49. Sinauer N, Annest JL, Mercy JA: Unintentional, nonfatal firearm-related injuries. A preventable public health burden. **JAMA 275:**1740-1743, 1996

50. Sloan JH, Kellerman AL, Reay DT, et al: Handgun regulations, crime, assaults, and homicide. A tale of two cities. **N Engl J Med 319:**1256-1262, 1988

51. Sosin DM, Sniezek JE, Waxweiler RJ: Trends in death associated with traumatic brain injury, 1979 through 1992: success and failure. **JAMA 273:**1778-1780, 1995

52. Stone A: If you're afraid, you're a victim of crime. **USA TODAY.** Dec 9, 1994, p 4A

53. Teret SP: The firearm injury reporting system revisised. **JAMA 275:**70, 1996 (Editorial)

54. Teret SP, Wintemute GJ: Policies to prevent firearm injuries. **Health Affairs 12:**96-108, 1993

55. Teret SP, Wintemute GJ, Beilenson PL: The firearm fatality reporting system. A proposal. **JAMA 267:** 3073-3074, 1992

56. US Department of Health and Human Services, Public Health Service: **Healthy People 2000: National Health Promotion and Disease Prevention Objectives.** Washington, DC: US Government Printing Office, 1990, 154 pp

57. Vernick JS, Teret SP, Howard KA, et al: Public opinion polling on gun policy. **Health Affairs 12:**198-208, 1993

58. Violence Prevention Task Force of the Eastern Association for the Surgery of Trauma: Violence in America: A public health crisis—the role of firearms. **J Trauma 38:**163-168, 1995

59. Voelker R: States debate: "carrying concealed weapons" laws. **JAMA 273:**1741, 1995

60. Waxweiler RJ, Rosenberg ML, Fenley MA: **Injury Control in the 1990s: A National Plan for Action.** Des Plaines, Ill: Association for the Advancement of Automotive Medicine, 1993

61. Weddle RD: The attack on the National Center for Injury Prevention and Control. **N Engl J Med 334:** 191-194, 1996 (Letter to the editor and comments)

62. Weil DS, Knox RC: Effects of limiting handgun purchases on interstate transfer of firearms. **JAMA 275:** 1759-1761, 1996

63. Wintemute GJ: **Defensive Uses of Firearms.** Subcommittee on Crime, Committee on the Judiciary, United States House of Representatives, Hearing, March 31, 1995

64. Wintemute GJ: The relationship between firearm design and firearm violence. Handguns in the 1990s. **JAMA 275:**1749-1753, 1996

65. Wright JD, Rossi PH: The great American gun war: some policy implications of the felon study, in Nisbet L (ed): **The Gun Control Debate. You Decide.** Buffalo, NY: Prometheus Books, 1990, pp 108-122

66. Zawitz MW: Guns used in crime. **Bureau of Justice Statistics, Selected Findings.** Washington, DC: US Department of Justice, 1995, pp 1-7

67. Zimring FE: Policy research on firearms and violence. **Health Affairs 12:**109-122, 1993

CHAPTER 14

Alcohol Use and the Physician's Role in Treatment

Howard H. Kaufman, MD

Alcohol is a drug that produces pleasurable and anxiety-reducing sensations, and its use is associated with reinforcement.[25] Until the later 19th century, alcohol was believed to have both nutritional and therapeutic value.[16] In fact, it does appear to prevent cardiovascular problems when used in moderation,[9,22,28] and the National Institutes of Health is interested in studying the benefits of the use of alcohol. Federal guidelines suggest that men may benefit from up to two drinks a day and women one.

However, the consumption of too much alcohol can be problematic. Alcohol abuse is defined as excessive drinking of alcohol (called binge drinking when it is episodic) sufficient to impair health or social functioning. Alcoholic dependence or alcoholism is an addiction to alcohol, with dependence and tolerance.

Alcohol abuse is based on a craving due to experience superimposed on a genetic vulnerability.[12] There appear to be two kinds of alcoholism, a severe early type which is associated with antisocial behavior and a milder type with later onset.[2,6,25] Social (e.g., parental and peer influences) and psychological (e.g., personality patterns, expectations, and effects such as decrease of internal conflicts or release of inhibitions) elements also play a role.[18,25] Alcohol abuse is associated with psychiatric problems, in particular the antisocial personality disorder, which affect the patient's subsequent course and treatment.[25] For a variety of reasons, women and the elderly are more susceptible to the acute and chronic effects of alcohol.

Several definitions can be used when diagnosing patients with alcohol problems, including the "International Classification of Diseases, 10th Revision" (ICD-10), and the "Diagnostic and Statistical Manual of Mental Disorders, Revised Fourth Edition" (DSM-IV-R) of the American Psychiatric Association. In the ICD-10 classification, there are two categories, harmful use and dependence, while in the DSM-IV-R there are also two categories, abuse and dependence. The advantage of the DSM-IV-R system, which is used more widely, is that it explicitly considers the social and legal consequences of problems with alcohol.[20] Another definition is that of the National Council on Alcoholism and Drug Dependence (NCADD) and the American Society of Addiction Medicine (ASAM):

> ... a primary, chronic disease with genetic, psychosocial and environmental factors influencing its development and manifestations. The

disease is often progressive and fatal. It is characterized by impaired control over drinking, preoccupation with the drug alcohol, use of alcohol despite adverse consequences, and distortions in thinking, most notably denial.[19]

Men tend to consume more alcohol than women; a known exception is for persons aged in their twenties. Alcohol consumption by adolescents is a concern to adults, although some believe that its use is declining. Excessive drinking is also a problem among the elderly. Indeed, 7% of all Americans are said to drink in excess.

It is encouraging that alcohol abstinence is increasing and heavy drinking is decreasing. This decrease has been associated with a decreased incidence of cirrhosis as well as of alcohol-related traffic fatalities. However, certain problems are particularly troublesome, such as binge drinking in college. It is said that 44% of students are binge drinkers and suffer adverse effects and 80% of students have problems due to the binge drinking of others.[29]

Drinking among the elderly is complex and related to past patterns and changes in activities/situations, mental diseases (especially depression), and interaction with about 100 of the drugs most commonly prescribed for the elderly. Alcohol consumption may promote mental deterioration. The elderly are more sensitive to excess alcohol use because of decreased body water. But treatment of alcohol abuse among the elderly can be very helpful, especially in those who begin drinking later in life.[1,5,25]

Inappropriate acute or chronic consumption of alcohol contributes to 100,000 deaths or 5% of all deaths each year in the United States. When used in excess, alcohol is associated with interpersonal violence, accidents, and suicide as well as other high-risk behavior, including high-risk sexual practices,[25] and is thus associated with injuries as well as with many medical problems and increased mortality rates.[22] Injuries and cirrhosis are the two greatest health problems associated with excessive alcohol consumption.[25]

One-half of emergency room trauma patients arrive intoxicated and three-fourths of these are alcoholics. Of all hospitalized patients, 20% to 40% have alcohol-related problems. Alcohol abuse and alcoholism led to $136 billion in medical and socioeconomic costs in 1990. These costs include medical care, lost opportunities due to impaired education and work, and criminal activities related to alcohol use. This is far more than the revenues of $70.3 billion generated by the alcohol industry.[3,6,19,23,25]

TRAUMA

Information about the relationship of alcohol consumption to traumatic deaths is more detailed than information about nonfatal injuries and reveals that blood alcohol levels are elevated in homicide victims, unintentional injury victims, and suicide victims.

Alcohol is associated with 50% to 70% of assaults and robberies. Domestic violence (e.g., that directed toward a spouse or child) and criminal violence are linked with the consumption of alcohol by both perpetrator and victim. The perpetrator has impaired moral judgment, decreased inhibition, and increased aggression. The victim, who tends to associate with other drinkers, is less aware of the developing conflict and is less able to resist. But many people who use alcohol do not become violent. The nature of the relationship between alcohol and violence is complex and relates to biological and social factors. More studies are required to understand these issues fully[8,23,24] and so to be able to develop prevention strategies.

Risks from unintentional injuries are several times higher in those abusing alcohol. About one-half of all automobile crashes involving a fatality are associated with alcohol use (the higher the level, the higher the risk) (Figure 1), as are general aviation accidents, bicycle accidents, drownings, and fires involving a fatality.

It is encouraging that the numbers and percentages of accidents involving drunk drivers have decreased over the last several years. This appears to be due to changing laws (e.g., increased legal drinking age and prompt motor-vehicle license suspension), stricter enforcement of laws, education, and altered attitudes toward drinking promoted by the work of voluntary groups. The largest of these groups, Mothers Against Drunk Driving (MADD), with three million members, has helped with such efforts. Indeed, alcohol-related traffic fatalities decreased from 23,646 in 1984 to 16,589 in 1994. The percentage of fatalities that were alcohol-

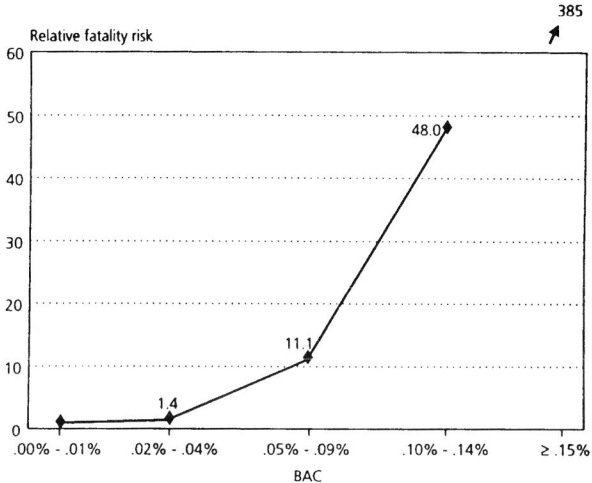

Figure 1: Estimated increased fatality risk for drivers in single-vehicle crashes at different blood alcohol concentrations (BACs). (Reprinted with permission from Zador PL: Alcohol-related relative risk of fatal driver injuries in relation to driver age and sex. *J Studies Alcohol 52:*302-310, 1991)

related decreased from 53% to 41%, particularly for those aged 15 to 20 years (44%).[4,7] To further decrease these numbers, it has been proposed that limits for blood alcohol concentration be decreased from 0.10 gm/dl to 0.08 gm/dl for drivers over 21 years of age and decreased even more for those younger than 21 years.[4]

Alcoholism and alcohol intoxication are also associated with suicide. Suicide victims are often alcoholics and they are frequently inebriated at the time they commit suicide.

MEDICAL COMPLICATIONS

Affective processes are influenced by the consumption of alcohol, and the changes range from euphoria to combativeness to drowsiness. Cognitive processes are also influenced.[20,24] Physical skills begin to deteriorate at a blood alcohol concentration of 0.025%, which may be achieved by consuming fewer than two drinks in an hour. Blood alcohol concentration (threshold 100 mg/dl or 0.10 gm/dl) or a breath analyzer can be used to confirm intoxication.[10] For a variety of reasons (including gender, age, body weight, fatigue, illness, tolerance, spacing of drinks, metabolic rate, recent food consump-

tion, and drinker's expectations), some people are more sensitive than others.

Some of the acute medical syndromes related to alcohol include acute alcohol intoxication/poisoning and alcohol withdrawal syndrome. About 300 people die each year of acute alcohol poisoning. Withdrawal from alcohol consumption may cause adverse mental and physiological changes and may also prove fatal.

Chronic alcohol-related medical disorders affect many systems and organs, including the liver, nervous and cardiovascular systems, pancreas, gut, muscle, and bone, as well as endocrine and reproductive functions (Table 1). Alcohol use can also adversely affect levels of metabolites, nutrition, electrolytes, and the immune system, and it is related to some cancers (e.g., mouth, upper airway, and liver).[6,12,14,25]

Alcohol use by pregnant women has adverse effects on the developing fetus, causing the well-known fetal alcohol syndrome and other fetal alcohol effects (Table 2), and being associated with babies born with Down's syndrome and spina bifida.[25,26] Although any use of alcohol by pregnant women is generally proscribed, the lower tolerable limits have not been defined, and it is not certain that occasional social use is harmful to the fetus.

TABLE 1

BODY ORGANS AFFECTED BY ALCOHOL INGESTION*

Liver
  Fatty liver, alcoholic hepatitis and fibrosis, and
    cirrhosis
Nervous system
  Acute intoxication
  Abstinence withdrawal syndrome
  Nutritional disease
    Wernicke-Korsakoff syndrome and subtle
      deficits
  Fetal alcohol syndrome
  Disease of unknown etiology
    Alcoholic dementia
  Secondary disorders
    Hepatic encephalopathy
Cardiovascular system
  Hypertension, weakened heart muscle, and
    arhythmias
  Hemorrhagic stroke
Pancreas
Gut
Muscle
Bone
Endocrine and reproductive functions
Metabolytes
Nutrition and electrolytes
Immune system
  Infections (? human immunodeficiency virus)
  Cancers (mouth, upper airway, and liver)

* Reproduced from the *Eighth Special Report to the U.S. Congress on Alcohol and Health.*[25]

TABLE 2

EFFECTS OF ALCOHOL USE ON THE DEVELOPING FETUS*

Fetal alcohol syndrome
- Growth retardation
- Abnormalities of brain structure and function
- Characteristic face
- Many other problems

Fetal alcohol effects, alcohol-related birth defects
- Only some attributes
- Genetic and maternal variables

* Reproduced from the *Eighth Special Report to the U.S. Congress on Alcohol and Health.*[25]

PREVENTION

Even occasional heavy alcohol use, particularly in the wrong setting, can be problematic. Prevention of alcohol abuse and alcoholism is therefore of paramount importance and was targeted in the national health care plan, *Healthy People 2000,*[27] as a major priority[23] (Table 3). The development of effective strategies for prevention was considered paramount by the Panel on Alternative Policies Affecting the Prevention of Alcohol Abuse and Alcoholism of the National Research Council, sponsored by the National Institute of Alcohol Abuse and Alcoholism (NIAAA). In 1981, they published their proposed strategies.[11,17] Reviewing historical, current, and proposed policies, this panel organized its proposals into three areas: 1) control availability through taxes, minimum age requirements, and regulation of outlets and availability and times of sale; 2) shaping drinking practices regarding appropriate and safe behavior; and 3) making the surrounding environment safer by such procedures as redesigning vehicles and other consumer products and arranging "designated drivers."

Such efforts have been tried for a number of years. Raising the cost of alcohol reduces the consumption, as does limiting the number of stores where it is available and the hours of operation of the stores. In terms of the law, strict enforcement of the legal drinking age is effective in limiting use of alcohol in underage persons, as is use of swift and certain penalties for drunk driving, such as administrative license suspension and the imposition of liability on servers for drinking-related problems.[20] Social standards can be changed, and this approach has been used for youths, male blue-collar workers, the military personnel, and executives—all of whom are at increased risk. "Designated drivers" are an example of such strategies. The media can de-emphasize the glamour of heavy drinking and provide education. Educational efforts have been targeted at the whole of society as well as specific groups at risk, particu-

TABLE 3
LIST OF OBJECTIVES CONCERNING USE OF ALCOHOL AND OTHER DRUGS*

Health Status Objectives
  · Reduce deaths from alcohol-related motor-vehicle crashes
  · Reduce cirrhosis

Risk Reduction Objectives
  · Increase the average age of first use of alcohol
  · Reduce the proportion of young people using alcohol
  · Reduce the proportion of high school students and college students engaging in heavy drinking
  · Reduce alcohol consumption by people aged 14 years and older
  · Increase the proportion of high school students who perceive social disapproval associated with the heavy use of alcohol
  · Increase the proportion of high school students who associate risk of physical or psychological harm with the heavy use of alcohol

Services and Protection Objectives
  · Establish and monitor in 50 states comprehensive plans to ensure access to alcohol treatment programs
  · Provide education programs on alcohol in all schools
  · Extend adoption of alcohol policies for the work environment
  · Extend to all states administrative driver's license suspension/revocation laws or programs of equal effectiveness for drivers under the influence of alcohol
  · Increase to 50 the number of states that have enacted and enforced policies, beyond those in existence in 1989, to reduce access to alcoholic beverages
  · Increase to at least 20 the number of states that have enacted statutes to restrict promotion of alcoholic beverages that is focused principally on young audiences
  · Extend to all states legal blood alcohol concentration tolerance levels of .04% for motor vehicle drivers aged 21 years and older and .00% for those younger than age 21.
  · Increase to at least 75% the proportion of primary care providers who screen for alcohol and other drug use problems and provide counseling and referral as needed.

* Reproduced from *Healthy People 2000.*[27]

larly high school and college students, but the effectiveness has been questioned. On the other hand, the environment can be altered in many ways which have been shown to be helpful. Breath analysis machines can be installed to prevent people who have a high blood alcohol concentration from starting cars. Passive protection such as seat belts and airbags, as well as stronger cars and safer roads can help. Given evidence such as the decline in the number and percent of alcohol-related traffic fatalities, these proposals and efforts seem to have had considerable effect already.

SCREENING

Because drinking is a common and costly problem, because proven screening instruments are available, and because brief treatment is helpful for nondependent problem drinkers (of whom there are 15-20 million in the U.S.), screening and brief intervention for patients with apparent alcohol-related problems is recommended. This approach even has the potential to detect people who are apparently asymptomatic, and this issue is now being considered.[9,16,21,25]

TABLE 4

SHORT MICHIGAN ALCOHOL SCREENING TEST QUESTIONS CONCERNING ALCOHOL USE

1. Do you feel you are a normal drinker? (By normal, we mean you drink less or the same as most other people.)

2. Does your wife, husband, a parent, or other near relative ever worry or complain about your drinking?

3. Do you ever feel guilty about your drinking?

4. Do friends or relatives think you are a normal drinker?

5. Are you able to stop drinking when you want to?

6. Have you ever attended a meeting of Alcoholics Anonymous?

7. Has your drinking ever created problems between you and your wife, husband, a parent or other near relative?

8. Have you ever gotten in trouble at work because of drinking?

9. Have you ever neglected your obligations, your family, or your work for two or more days in a row because you were drinking?

10. Have you ever gone to anyone for help about your drinking?

11. Have you ever been in a drinking hospital because of drinking?

12. Have you ever been arrested for drunken driving, driving while intoxicated, or driving under the influence of alcoholic beverages?

13. Have you ever been arrested, even for a few hours, because of other drunken behavior?

Concerns with alcohol involve three domains: 1) pattern or quantity/frequency of ingestion, 2) symptoms of dependence upon alcohol, and 3) associated problems caused by alcohol. These can be detected by using any of a number of well-tested questionnaires, including: 1) the short Michigan Alcohol Screening Test (sMAST) (13 questions) (Table 4); 2) "CAGE" test (Table 5); 3) the Alcohol Use Disorders Identification Test (AUDIT) from the World Health Organization (10 questions); 4) the National Institute of Mental Health Diagnostic Interview Schedule form III-R (DIS) (22 items); and 5) the Short Alcohol Dependence Data (SADD) questionnaire (15 items). One strategy is to administer the sMAST to determine if there is a problem and, if positive, the SADD, which concentrates on the issue of dependence, although the CAGE is faster and the AUDIT may be more sensitive.[10,13] Other instruments, such as the Addiction Severity Index and the Clinical Institute Alcohol Withdrawal Scale, can be used to determine the severity and nature of specific aspects of alcoholism.

Persons who are admitted for alcohol-related trauma should be screened, referred, and treated appropriately.[10] Admission provides the opportunity to address the underlying problem and the motivation to do so. Brief interventions in these circumstances have been shown to decrease drinking and recurrent admissions.

TREATMENT FOR ALCOHOLISM

Treatment for alcohol abuse is widespread but its effectiveness remains problematic. In 1991, 500,000 people underwent treatment, including 11% in inpatient settings and 87% in outpatient settings. Most were between 25 and 44 years old.

Modes of treatment have improved (Table 6) and are being further refined, with attempts made to target particular groups (i.e., youth,

TABLE 5
"CAGE" QUESTIONS CONCERNING ALCOHOL USE

Have you ever tried to cut down on your drinking?

Are you annoyed when people complain about your drinking?

Do you ever feel guilty about your drinking?

Do you ever drink eye openers?

TABLE 6
TREATMENT FOR PERSONS WHO ABUSE ALCOHOL*

Minnesota Model of Treatment (multimodality)
 Education
 Individual and group therapy
 Participation in Alcoholics Anonymous

Pharmacological Agents
 Withdrawal management
 Adversive reactions (disulfiram)
 Decreased desire/consumption (reverse intoxication, depression—in development)
 Treat coexisting psychiatric disorders

Marital and family therapy

Relapse prevention/aftercare based on conditioning

* Reproduced from the *Eighth Special Report to the U.S. Congress on Alcohol and Health.*[25]

older adults, women, and ethnic minorities). Depending on the severity of the problem, treatment may involve brief intervention, outpatient treatment, or a more intensive inpatient program.[10] Abstinence is thought by most to be the only permanent way of controlling alcoholism. An alternative approach views alcohol abuse as a continuum and posits that people who have relatively good control can cut back on consumption. Two programs, DrinkWise and Moderation Management, use this philosophy.[15] Alcoholics "on the wagon" need understanding, support, and reintegration into society.[21,25] Various support groups address this need, with Alcoholics Anonymous being the most well known.

It must be remembered that it is a part of routine care to offer treatment to any patient suspected of abusing alcohol. If it appears a patient is a danger to self or others, a physician or indeed any adult can petition for a formal hearing by a magistrate, circuit court judge, or mental hygiene commissioner (depending on the jurisdiction) to decide if a psychiatric evaluation is indicated. If a hearing reviewing such an evaluation determines that it is necessary, an involuntary committment for treatment can be mandated.

When a patient who has been drinking leaves a physician's office or hospital, it is advisable that they not drive and that they be in the care of a responsible individual.

RECORDING AND REPORTING

To encourage persons with alcohol-related problems to seek care, federal regulations protect the privacy of information about these problems, requiring separate records from the routine hospital chart. An exception occurs for emergency treatment, when a patient grants informed consent which allows screening and diagnostic testing for conditions that must be understood to manage the presenting problem; such information can be recorded in the medical record. The issue is how to legally determine when a driver is inebriated while preserving the right to due process. The regulations about police access to a blood alcohol concentration level in someone who is seen in a hospital after an accident vary from state to state. The blood alcohol concentration level may be inadmissable in court if the rules are not followed or there is no chain of custody.[10] This subject is discussed elsewhere. There is no stipulation that physicians must report alcohol abuse or use to the local police, and in many circumstances there may be a duty to actually conceal evidence of alcohol use by keeping separate records. This subject is also discussed elsewhere.

One particular observation which a physician should record is when one detects the odor of alcohol on a patient, since this is the type of observation a reasonable physician would be expected to make. It probably is not appropriate to specify that there is alcohol on the breath. Although smelling alcohol does not require a physician to obtain a blood alcohol concentration level, it does make it obligatory to determine if the patient is competent to make decisions.

Some states have laws against public drunkenness which are intended to keep people who are drunk from harming and offending others and to prevent themselves from becoming victims of crime, exposure, or illness. More recent laws have been associated with decriminalization of drunkenness and with provision of appropriate social and medical services, hopefully promoting prompt referral. The effect of these combined efforts is not yet known.[21] These laws may permit or even require the physician to alert the police about someone who is inebriated and who may have been involved in an accident.

The physician must consider the medical needs of the patients and must be aggressive in detecting and providing treatment for alcohol abuse. Patient confidentiality must be protected, however. As an informed citizen, the physician also should promote and support public health efforts aimed at developing laws and encouraging strict enforcement in order to combat problems caused by those who abuse alcohol.

REFERENCES

1. American Medical Association, Department of Geriatric Health: **Alcoholism in the Elderly. Diagnosis, Treatment, Prevention.** Chicago, Ill: American Medical Association, 1995
2. Babor TF, Hesselbrock V, Meyer RE, et al (eds): Types of alcoholics. Evidence from clinical, experimental, and genetic research. **Ann NY Acad Sci 708:**1-258, 1994
3. Baker SP, O'Neill B, Ginsburg MJ, et al: **The Injury Fact Book.** 2nd ed. New York, NY: Oxford University Press, 1992
4. Centers for Disease Control and Prevention: Update: Alcohol-related traffic crashes and fatalities among youth—United States, 1982–1994. **JAMA 274:** 1904-1905, 1995
5. Council on Scientific Affairs, American Medical Association: Alcoholism in the elderly. **JAMA 275:** 797-801, 1996
6. Diamond I: Alcoholism and alcohol abuse, in Wyngaarden JM, Smith LH Jr, Bennett JC (eds): **Cecil Textbook of Medicine.** 19th ed. Philadelphia, Pa: WB Saunders, 1992, pp 44-47
7. Editorial: Tough new drinking laws cut road deaths sharply. **USA TODAY.** Dec 27, 1995, p 10A
8. Fagan J: Interactions among drugs, alcohol, and violence. **Health Affairs 12:**65-79, 1993
9. Fuchs CS, Stampfer MJ, Colditz GA, et al: Alcohol consumption and mortality among women. **N Engl J Med 332:**1245-1250, 1995
10. Gentilello LM, Donovan DM, Dunn CW, et al: Alcohol interventions in trauma centers. Current practice and future directions. **JAMA 274:**1043-1048, 1995
11. Gerstein DR (ed): **Toward the Prevention of Alcohol Problems. Government, Business, and Community Action.** Washington, DC: National Academy Press, 1984
12. Gordis E: Unraveling the brain chemistry behind alcohol abuse. **JAMA 272:**1733, 1994
13. Kitchens JM: Does this patient have an alcohol problem? **JAMA 272:**1782-1787, 1994
14. Lieber CS: Medical disorders of alcoholism. **N Engl J Med 333:**1058-1065, 1995
15. Manning A: New alcohol programs turn focus to moderation. **USA TODAY.** Jan 16, 1996, p 6D
16. Martensen RL: Alcoholism. **JAMA 272:**1895, 1994
17. Moore MH, Gerstein DR (eds): **Alcohol and Public Policy: Beyond the Shadow of Prohibition.** Washington, DC: National Academy Press, 1981
18. **Morbidity and Mortality Weekly Report.** Waltham, Mass: Massachusetts Medical Society, Dec 1994, Vol 43, pp 861-880
19. Morse RM, Flavin DK, for the Joint Committee of the National Council on Alcoholism and Drug Dependence and the American Society of Addiction Medicine to Study the Definiton and Criteria for the Diagnosis of Alcoholism: The definition of alchoholism. **JAMA 268:**1012-1014, 1992
20. National Committee for Injury Prevention and Control: **Injury Prevention: Meeting the Challenge.** New York, NY: Oxford University Press, 1989
21. Olson S, Gerstein DR: **Alcohol in America. Taking Action to Prevent Abuse.** Washington, DC: National Academy Press, 1985
22. Poikolainen K: Alcohol and mortality: a review. **J Clin Epidemiol 48:**455-465, 1995
23. Reiss AJ, Roth JA: **Understanding and Preventing Violence.** Washington, DC: National Academy Press, 1993
24. Rosenberg ML, Fenley MA (eds): **Violence in America. A Public Health Approach.** New York, NY: Oxford University Press, 1991
25. Secretary of Health and Human Services: **Eighth Special Report to the U.S. Congress on Alcohol and Health.** Washington, DC: US Department of Health and Human Services, 1993
26. Shephard BD: Say no to drugs (in pregnancy). **1995 Medical and Health Annual. Encyclopedia Brittanica.** Chicago, Ill: Encyclopedia Brittanica, 1994, pp 419-423
27. US Department of Health and Human Services: **Healthy People 2000. National Health Promotion and Disease Prevention Objectives.** Washington, DC: US Department of Health and Human Services, 1990
28. Victor RG, Hansen J: Alcohol and blood pressure—a drink a day. **N Engl J Med 332:**1782-1783, 1995
29. Wechsler H, Davenport A, Dowdall G, et al: Health and behavioral consequences of binge drinking in college. A national survey of students at 140 campuses. **JAMA 272:**1672-1677, 1994

CHAPTER 15

EFFECTS OF TOBACCO AND CONTROL OF USE

HOWARD H. KAUFMAN, MD

> *. . . Is it not both great vanity and uncleanliness, that at the table . . . men should . . . sit . . . making the filthy smoke and stink thereof . . . when very often men that abhor it are at their repast?*
>
> *Surely smoke becomes a kitchen far better than a dining chamber, and yet it makes a kitchen also oftentimes in the inward parts of men, soiling and infecting them with an unctuous and oily kind of soot, as hath been found in some great tobacco takers that after their death were opened. . . . It is a custom loathsome to the eye, hateful to the nose, harmful to the brain, dangerous to the lungs, and in the black, stinking fume thereof, nearest resembling the horrible Stygian smoke of the pit that is bottomless.[6]*
>
> King James I
> A Counterblast to Tobacco, early 1660s

The smoking of tobacco originated with the American Indians, who considered tobacco a gift of their spirits and their most sacred plant. Smoked in sacred pipes, tobacco was used as an offering to "renew the relationship between men and spirits" and to carry words and thoughts to the spirits. Varieties more potent than those used commercially today were cultivated, traded, and used everywhere in North America except along the Northwest Coast.[46] Tobacco's addictive properties were noted soon after it was introduced in Europe.

> Those who have once become accustomed thereto [to smoking] can hardly be restrained therefrom.[6]
>
> Francis Bacon, 1622

Widespread smoking in the United States began in the early 20th century (Figure 1). The factors that led to this included the development of machines to make cigarettes in the late 1800s as well as the development of the safety match at the turn of the century. Use of milder, blended tobacco, which was easier to inhale, began about 1913 in Camel cigarettes. This was accompanied by a change in pH that prevented absorption of nicotine in the oral mucosa and so required deep inhalation, exposing the lungs to toxic substances. Mass marketing began, and World War I saw the beginning of the tradition of smoking as an initiation rite of manhood.[41-43]

In the last few years, there has been a marked decline in the prevalance of smoking related to the realization of the dangers of smoking and a variety of educational and legal actions to decrease it (Figure 2). Data produced by the U.S. Department of Agriculture indicate that the total consumption of cigarettes declined from 640 billion in 1981 to 480 billion in 1994. Per capita consumption declined from 4,287 cigarettes in 1966 to 2,470 cigarettes in 1994.

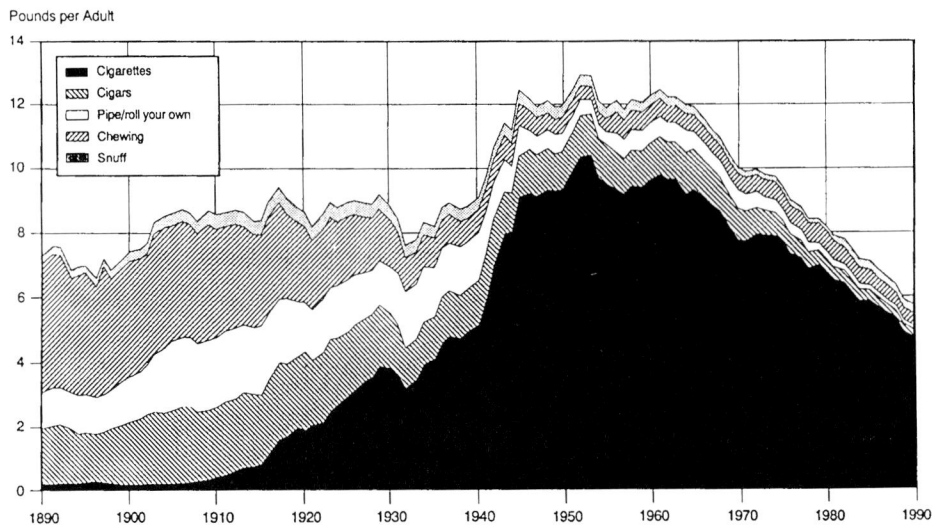

Figure 1: Trends in per capita tobacco consumption by major product category in the U.S., 1890 to 1990.

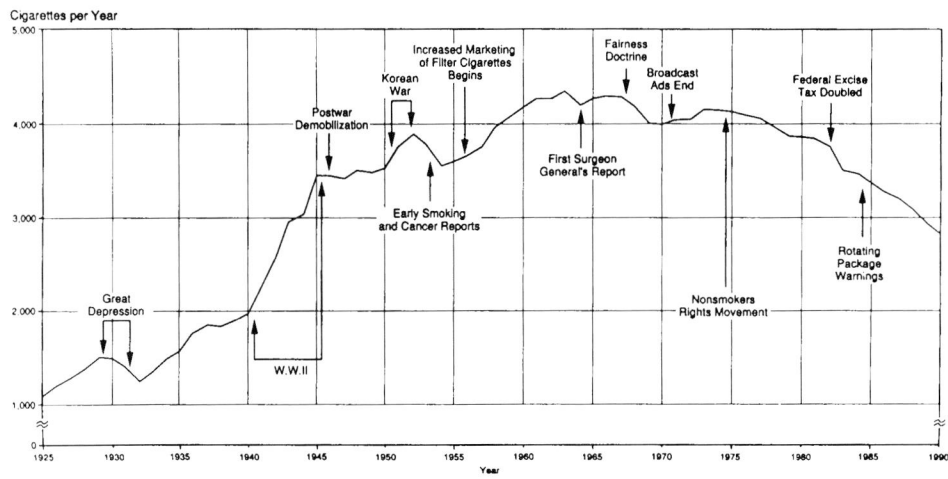

Figure 2: Per capita cigarette consumption for adults aged 18 years and older in the U.S., 1925 to 1990.

Approximately 45 million people who once smoked have stopped, although about 48 million people continue to smoke. Smoking is related inversely to educational level and income, as well as to cultural factors. Prevalence level may have reached a plateau, decreasing among adults but increasing among teenagers, possibly related to increased advertising by the tobacco companies and decreased prices of cigarettes.[29]

EFFECTS OF TOBACCO

Smoking (and smokeless tobacco) has many attractive effects. Nicotine from tobacco activates cholinergic receptors, which leads to the release of other neurotransmitters. The result is pleasure, reduced anxiety and tension, arousal, enhanced cognitive performance, and appetite suppression.

The nicotine in tobacco is highly addicting. In addition, tobacco smoke, an aerosol, contains about 4,000 chemicals, many of which are harmful. Smoke also causes damage through particulate matter, including tar which is carcinogenic, as well as gases which are ciliotoxic. The impact of smoking depends upon the age that smoking is started, the number of cigarettes consumed over time, and the depth of inhalation.[3,23,26] Environmental factors, such as asbestos, also affect the impact of cigarettes.

The adverse effects of smoking began to be considered as lung cancer in men rose during the 1930s and 1940s. The scientific community became convinced of its adverse effects in the 1950s. The federal effort in smoking control and prevention began with the landmark 1964 publication, *Smoking and Health, Report of the Advisory Committee to the Surgeon General of the Public Health Service.*[41,43] This was the first of many government reports which now are published annually, as mandated by a federal law passed in 1969. The 25th such report was published in 1996. These comprehensive reports cover a multiplicity of subjects (Table 1). The primary literature on tobacco products is immense. Between 1960 and 1990, over 60,000 scientific publications worldwide linked tobacco to health problems.[39]

The diseases caused by cigarette smoking and other tobacco use constitute the largest preventable public health problem in the U.S. Of the two million deaths each year in the U.S., 400,000 (20%) are attributable to smoking-related diseases. Tobacco smoking causes more deaths than alcohol, motor crashes, acquired immune deficiency syndrome, suicide, homicide, illegal drugs, and fires together. The costs of smoking are estimated to total $68 billion each year and include $20.8 billion in direct health costs, $6.9 billion from lost productivity due to disability (particularly lung disease) costs, and $40.3 billion from lost productivity due to death. (Other estimates have been as high as $50 billion in direct costs and $100 billion in total costs each year.) Male smokers' medical costs increase 28%, while female smokers' medical costs increase 21%. A smoker's life expectancy is decreased 15 years, and one-third die prematurely. Smoking causes a loss of 6 million years of productive life each year.[23]

Smoking affects many tissues and organs in the human body. Cardiovascular disease is caused by damage to vessel walls and increased thrombosis and embolism as well as increased heart rate and blood pressure, decreased oxygen-carrying capacity of the blood, and increases in the threshhold for ventricular fibrillation. Atherosclerosis, which results from smoking, leads to coronary artery disease (and is its largest avoidable cause, thought to be a contributing factor in 21% of victims), peripheral vascular disease (smokers constitute 90% of the cases), and stroke.[44] In terms of atherosclerotic disease, smoking has a synergistic effect with hypertension and hypercholesterolemia. In women, smoking increases the risk for myocardial infarction and subarachnoid hemorrhage. In women taking oral contraceptives, the risk for cardiovascular disease is increased.[3,23,26] In pregnant women, the birth process is compromised by an increased incidence of placenta previa and abruptio placentae. Children born of mothers who smoke have smaller birth weights and a higher incidence of perinatal mortality.[3,23,26]

Smoke impedes lung growth and development in children. Smoking causes chronic obstructive pulmonary disease, producing cough and mucus hypersecretion, bronchitis with airflow obstruction, and emphysema.[3,23,26]

Smoking also affects the gastrointestinal tract, causing gastric and duodenal ulcers as well as gastric reflux. It impairs liver function, altering hepatic metabolism of drugs and vitamins.

Cancer is another major result of smoking. Thirty percent of all cancers occur because of smoking. Smoking causes lung cancer of all types and accounts for over 85% of the mortality due to lung cancer. Cancers of the aerodigestive tract, pancreas, kidney, bladder, and cervix are also attributable to smoking.[3,23,26] Smoking-related diseases can interact synergistically (i.e., chronic obstructive pulmonary disease and lung cancer).[3,26]

For those who already smoke, cessation is very worthwhile. The effects of smoking are not necessarily permanent. A 1990 federal report, *The Health Benefits of Smoking Cessation,*[38] concludes that cessation has "major and immediate benefits for men and women of all ages, even if they already have smoking-related diseases. If one quits before 50 years of age, the risk of

TABLE 1

REPORTS BY THE SURGEON GENERAL, PUBLISHED BETWEEN 1964 AND 1996

Smoking and Health: Report of the Advisory Committee to the Surgeon General of the Public Health Service. 1964

The Health Consequences of Smoking: A Public Health Service Review. 1967

The Health Consequences of Smoking: 1968 Supplement to the 1967 Public Health Service Review. 1968

The Health Consequences of Smoking: 1969 Supplement to the 1967 Public Health Service Review. 1969

The Health Consequences of Smoking: A Report of the Surgeon General. 1971

The Health Consequences of Smoking: A Report of the Surgeon General. 1972

The Health Consequences of Smoking, 1973.

The Health Consequences of Smoking, 1974.

The Health Consequences of Smoking, 1975.

The Health Consequences of Smoking: Selected Chapters from 1971 through 1975 Reports. 1976

The Health Consequences of Smoking, 1977-1978. 1978

Smoking and Health: A Report of the Surgeon General. 1979

The Health Consequences of Smoking for Women: A Report of the Surgeon General. 1980

The Health Consequences of Smoking—The Changing Cigarette: A Report of the Surgeon General. 1981

The Health Consequences of Smoking—Cancer: A Report of the Surgeon General. 1982

The Health Consequences of Smoking—Cardiovascular Disease: A Report of the Surgeon General. 1983

The Health Consequences of Smoking—Chronic Obstructive Lung Disease: A Report of the Surgeon General. 1984

The Health Consequences of Smoking—Cancer and Chronic Lung Disease in the Workplace: A Report of the Surgeon General. 1985

The Health Consequences of Involuntary Smoking: A Report of the Surgeon General. 1986

The Health Consequences of Smoking—Nicotine Addiction: A Report of the Surgeon General. 1988

Reducing the Health Consequences of Smoking—25 Years of Progress: A Report of the Surgeon General. 1989

The Health Benefits of Smoking Cessation: A Report of the Surgeon General. 1990

Smoking in the Americas: A Report of the Surgeon General. 1992

Preventing Tobacco Use Among Young People: A Report of the Surgeon General. 1994

Surgeon General's Report on Physical Activity and Health. 1996

---

dying is halved for the next 15 years. If a healthy male smoker aged 60-64 years quits, he decreases his risk of dying by 10% over the next 15 years. (It should be remembered that smoking is a major risk factor for six of the 14 leading causes of death and is a risk factor for three other causes for those 60 years and older.) The effects of cessation include decreases in the incidence of lung cancer and other cancers, heart attack, stroke, and chronic lung disease. After 10-15 years of abstinence, the smoker's risks return to baseline. The benefits are believed to far exceed the expected 5-pound weight gain and any adverse psychological effects, which are generally early and brief.[4]

In addition, women who stop smoking within the first three or four months of pregnancy reduce the risk of having a low-birth-weight baby to that of nonsmoking women. Smoking cessation could prevent 5% of perinatal deaths, 20% of low-birth-weight births, and 8% of preterm deliveries. Of course, if parents did not smoke, many children would not be susceptible to respiratory infections and middle ear effusions.

Since the 1970s, it has been shown that passive or second-hand smoke (environmental tobacco smoke) is a major health problem, especially for those with allergies and pre-existing lung or heart disease. Environmental tobacco smoke is the only agent classified by the Environmental Protection Agency (1992) as a carcinogen at environmental levels[41] (although the tobacco companies have protested this in a lawsuit). It has been estimated that 3,000 lung cancers each year are caused by second-hand smoke, and as many as 53,000 deaths from all diseases. Between 150,000 and 300,000 cases of lung infections (such as bronchitis and pneumonia) in children up to 18 months of age have been attributed to passive smoke, as well as many middle ear effusions. Between 200,000 and one million asthmatic children are harmed by environmental tobacco smoke, and new cases may be precipitated. Lung function is decreased in children. It is believed that more than 700 cases of sudden infant death syndrome have been attributable to maternal smoking.[3,23,26,39,41]

A disturbing new development is the increase in the use of smokeless tobacco, which can cause cheek and gum recession and leukoplakia as well as oral cancer and, of course, nicotine addiction. The use of smokeless tobacco is a growing problem. Smokeless tobacco is addicting and harmful and its use should be prevented or stopped, as the user encounters issues similar to smoking; similar strategies are being evolved to combat its use.[3,23,26]

Allegedly to obviate the adverse health effects of smoking, tobacco companies are marketing cigarettes that supposedly result in less tar and nicotine consumption. However, analysis by smoking machines of such products does not correlate with the actual effect on smokers because smokers may occlude vents on the filters as they smoke, may inhale more deeply, and may compensate by using more cigarettes.

CONTROL OF TOBACCO USE

Overview

One of the most important of the federal reports was published in 1991, entitled *Strategies to Control Tobacco Use in the United States,*[43] which stated that a persistent, inescapable message must be put out that it is important to quit or never start smoking, that this requires continuous reinforcement, and that environmental changes are required to help the effort. The steps that lead to smoking and the factors that contribute to developing and maintaining the addiction and to controlling it are indicated in Figure 3, and understanding them forms the basis of controlling this public health problem. Information about what works can be gleaned from numerous prior studies. The state of the art:

> . . . recognizes that no single approach is best for all smokers and that different smokers are most attracted to and most affected by different programs. Perhaps more importantly, it recognizes that no single channel reaches all smokers and that no single time is best for all smokers to make an attempt to quit. Comprehensive strategies are characterized by the delivery of persistent and inescapable messages to quit, or not to start, smoking, coupled with continuously available support for individual cessation efforts provided through multiple channels, and reinforced by environmetal incentives for nonsmokers.[43]

The optimal strategy involves political, economic, educational, media, health care professionals, and voluntary health organization activities. Approaches directed to individuals include public education campaigns, school-based education campaigns, and programs and clinics for people who want to quit. Information about the harmfulness of smoking, although shown to decrease cigarette consumption, is not enough to eliminate tobacco use. Environmental influences include adverse public opinion, limiting access of adolescents to tobacco, restricting where smoking is allowed, and increasing the direct and indirect costs of tobacco. Economic pressures include awarding nonsmokers preference in hiring and promotion, differential health and other insurance rates for smokers and nonsmokers, and eliminating governmental price supports to tobacco farmers. Groups that are particularly susceptible to smoking, such as adolescents, women, blacks, and Hispanics, need to be targeted. The optimal strategy encompasses cooperation and coordination between various sectors of society, including health care professionals and grass roots organizations.[43]

An editorial signed by the officers of the American Medical Association (AMA) and the editor of the *Journal of the American Medical Association* (*JAMA*) in 1995 suggested the justification and need for a regulatory approach.[37]

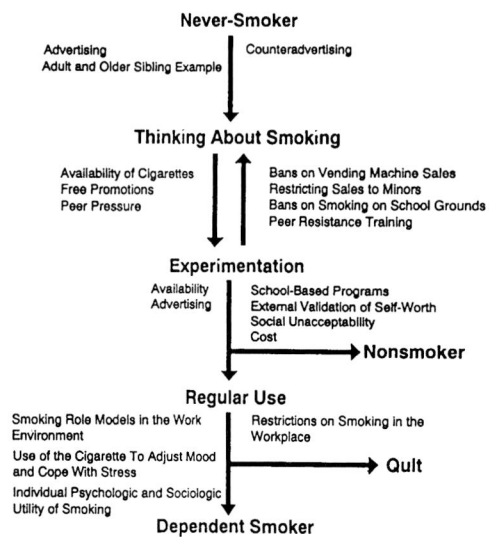

Figure 3: Forces that influence adolescent progression into adult smoking.

There are three subjects to consider when discussing elimination of tobacco use: 1) how to prevent people from starting, 2) how to stop those that already use tobacco, and 3) how to protect people from environmental tobacco smoke. Some of the strategies for each will affect one or both of the others.

Prevention

The easiest way to control the problem is to prevent it from beginning, which requires an understanding of who begins to use tobacco, why, and what are the most effective ways to prevent this. A 1994 book in the federal series, *Preventing Tobacco Use Among Young People*,[40] and a monograph from the Institute of Medicine, *Growing Up Tobacco Free*,[23] emphasize that most people who smoke begin before age 18 years (70%) or at least by age 21 years (90%), that because of a variety of factors they are most susceptible at this age to outside influences, particularly advertising linking smoking to glamorous, successful lifestyles, and family/friends.[31] New studies trace the impact of tobacco advertising, and because preventing smoking is much more successful than trying to stop someone who already smokes (70% of adolescent smokers wish they could stop), a primary public health effort must be expended to encourage adolescents and young adults to never begin smoking.

Young people smoke for a variety of reasons. As part of becoming adults, they act in ways to assert their independence and achieve their image of adult status as well as identifying with and establishing bonds with their peers, and they associate smoking with all of these. By nature, young people are more concerned with short-term goals than long-term ones. In addition, they overestimate the number of people who smoke and think it is more acceptable to other people than it is. Another problem is lack of appreciation of the strength of the addiction to tobacco. Adolescents believe, although wrongly so, that they will be able to stop smoking within a few years when they choose to do so.[23] Indeed, one-third to one-half of adolescents who try smoking become regular smokers. And although seven of 10 young smokers regret starting, three of four try to quit but fail.[20]

Several specific risk factors have been identified, including low school achievement, lack of skills to resist pressure to smoke, a low self image, and friends (and parents) who smoke. Low socioeconomic status is a factor. Smoking is also facilitated by the ease of purchase and the low cost of cigarettes. In addition, use of tobacco by youths is promoted by aggressive advertising, much of which is targeted at adolescents/young adults who have been shown to be particularly vulnerable. Indeed, in 1992 tobacco was the second most advertised product, and expenditures for advertising were more than $5.2 billion for a product with revenues of over $40 billion per year.[23,40]

Smoking is also associated with other problems. Youths who smoke often go on to use other drugs, are violent, engage in high-risk sex, and commit suicide. Of course, these behaviors may all be related to the same underlying personality patterns,[40] but this is another reason to attend to this group.

Attempts so far to convince young people to not start smoking have not been particularly successful. Although the proportion of Americans who smoked dropped from 40.4% in 1965 to 25.7% in 1991, and although 43 million Americans have quit, 28% of high school seniors smoke, and the proportion is increasing.

The effects of various antismoking policies have been analyzed. Informing the students about the health problems caused by smoking has not been very successful, but can be made more effective by general health education and programs in the community. Even more important is to promote a cultural change so that nonsmoking is the norm and smoking is not acceptable. In addition, young people can be denied access to cigarettes.

One attempt to enforce national standards to prevent youth from smoking involves the Synar rules, first published in 1992 and made final January 19, 1996. These required all states to have laws preventing the sale of tobacco products to individuals younger than 18 years, reasonable enforcement, unauthorized annual random inspections of at least 20% of outlets in the state a year, and mandated designation of a state office or agency to ensure compliance.[18] Compliance is to be supervised by the U.S. Department of Health and Human Services and failure can result in loss of up to 40% of Substance Abuse and Prevention and Treatment block grants, which can amount to millions of dollars in each state. However, state laws have varied in strength and enforcement has been a problem. It has been suggested that the age be raised to 21 years, which would parallel alcohol restrictions and thus be more convenient to enforce. One difficulty is controlling vending machines, although these could be eliminated completely.

One of the most effective ways of preventing young people from starting to smoke is to increase the price of tobacco products by increasing taxes, and this has been done at the federal, state, and local levels. (This approach is not as helpful in decreasing consumption or leading to complete cessation.) Every price increase of several cents to purchase a pack of cigarettes prevents a few percent of people from starting, and men are more susceptible to price hikes. It has been suggested that several hundred thousand lives have been saved by the increases in taxes of the last several years.

Warning labels have been studied. Although not especially effective in their present forms, there are ways to increase their effectiveness. Of course, promotion and advertising by tobacco manufacturers, particularly that aimed at youth, could be completely forbidden.[23,40]

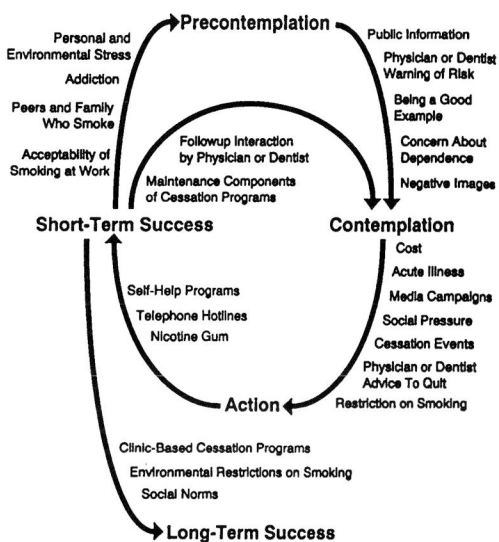

Figure 4: Process of cessation of tobacco usage.

Quitting

Once started, it is difficult to stop smoking. About one-third of smokers attempt to quit each year, but it is estimated that at least 90% ultimately fail. In fact, only 20% to 40% of those who attempt to quit smoking are abstinent after 1 year. People can be helped with encouragement from health care practitioners and by pharmacological aids such as nicotine supplementation, which can increase success rates two- to threefold.[15] It is said that unassisted, perhaps 8% to 20% are successful, while those who undergo smoking cessation programs are successful 20% to 40% of the time.[38,43] The various programs available have been reviewed in detail.[43] The dynamics of quitting are indicated in Figure 4. The best method appears to be stopping "cold turkey." Current knowledge is summarized in the "Smoking Cessation Clinical Practice Guidelines" published in 1996 by the U.S. Agency for Health Care Policy and Research, which suggest multiple counseling sessions and nicotine replacement therapy, specifically with the easily used patch, in an infrastructure with identification of users, dedicated and trained personnel, and funding for such efforts.[35] Recently, nicotine gum and nicotine patches have been released by the Food and Drug Administration (FDA) for over-the-counter sale. They are being intensely promoted, and their sales may exceed $1 billion a year.[9] However, it is not clear whether using nicotine without a physician's advice will be particularly successful.[11]

In addition, people can be helped by changes in the environment such as: 1) making smoking socially unacceptable; 2) increasing the cost of cigarettes; 3) preventing smoking in locations such as government buildings, including schools, private establishments such as health care facilities, religious facilities, restaurants, and workplaces (which would also eliminate the exposure of nonsmokers to environmental tobacco smoke); 4) controlling access to or eliminating vending machines; 5) preventing distribution of samples to youths; and 6) requiring licenses to sell tobacco. Strict enforcement is required.[3,26,39]

There are several voluntary efforts to help people stop smoking. One is American Stop Smoking Intervention Strategy for Cancer Prevention (ASSIST), which provides direct funding for smoking interventions at the community level in 17 states where it is intended to decrease smoking prevalence to 15% or less. It is estimated that by the year 2000, this media-aided grass roots effort will have prevented two million people from beginning smoking, led 4.5 million people to stop smoking, and saved 1.2 million lives including prevention of 400,000 deaths from lung cancer—at a cost of $130 per life. Another voluntary effort includes such organizations as the American Cancer Society, the American Lung Association, and the American Heart Association, the three of which have currently joined together in a coalition, the Coalition on Smoking and Health.[26] The AMA has also begun an effort entitled Physicians for a Tobacco-Free America. Voluntary activities are also summarized in *State Tobacco Control Highlights—1996*, a book prepared by the Centers for Disease Control and Prevention (CDC).[5]

Regulation

Federal laws enacted have resulted in the following: requiring printed health warnings on cigarettes (1965); requiring one educational announcement for every three to four cigarette ads (1969); banning broadcast advertising (1970); prohibiting smoking on domestic flights (1989), increasing the excise tax on cigarette packages from 16 cents to 24 cents (1990); and banning smoking on buses while on bus routes (1990). Also, U.S. airlines are beginning to voluntarily ban smoking on international flights. On October 4, 1994, the Occupational Safety and Health Administration (OSHA) published a proposed rule for a workplace smoking ban to prevent smoking in restaurants, bars, and nightclubs; taxis; offices; and stores, malls, building lobbies, and airline terminals. This was folded into a Clean Air bill in 1995, but early in 1996, the Action on Smoking and Health (ASH) filed a federal suit in Washington, D.C. for finalization of the rules.

Since the 1970s, many tobacco control ordinances have been passed at state and local levels and include prohibiting smoking in public places and increasing local taxes. Sites where smoking is forbidden include health care facilities, day care centers, schools, malls, restaurants, sports facilities, religious facilities, and workplaces. Recently, smoking has even been banned in some public parks and beaches. By 1990, 45 states and the District of Columbia, as well as 51% of cities with over 25,000 inhabitants, had laws to this effect. A recent summary of state laws had been prepared by the CDC.[5] Recently, most ordinances are more strongly worded. These have been upheld in the courts. Model laws are available.[39]

One admirable quasi-official effort was that of the Joint Commission on Accreditation of Healthcare Organizations (JCAHO), which established the first industry-wide ban on workplace smoking. Because of its leadership position, the commission developed rules to protect both workers and patients which were announced in November 1991, and required plans to be developed by February 1992 and to be in place by December 1993, at which time 96% of hospitals were in compliance.[21]

Recent Developments

An interesting series of events that started in April 1995 may eventually lead to a national approach to prevent young people from becoming addicted. On April 4, 1995, executives from the seven leading tobacco companies testified at Congressional hearings that nicotine was not addictive, that cigarettes did not cause disease, and that the companies did not manipulate nicotine levels in cigarettes. However, in July 1995 confidential records that indicated the opposite were revealed on the U.S. House floor, obtained from Phillip Morris Co. as well as from Brown and Williamson; these records were published extensively in publications including the *JAMA*.[22] The revelation led to convening of U.S. grand juries to determine if there had been fraud and perjury and whether criminal charges should be entered against these executives.[22,24,27] Three books published in 1996 detail information about the tobacco companies understanding of the dangers of cigarette smoking and their efforts to promote smoking.*[16,33,36]

Other lawsuits are in progress. It should be noted that since 1954 over 820 lawsuits have been entered against tobacco companies, although only a handful have gone to trial. In a potentially successful 1988 suit, a retrial was ordered by the U.S. Supreme Court, but the family could not afford to pursue it.

However, the legal situation may be changing. On August 9, 1996, a Florida jury awarded $750,000 to a smoker of 44 years who lost part of a lung to cancer. The case was based on the failure to warn about known adverse effects, using for the first time internal documents of a tobacco company.[19] In addition, several states, beginning with Florida, Louisiana, Massachusetts, Minnesota, Mississippi, Texas, and West Virginia, have sued the tobacco companies to recover their costs for medical care for indigents with tobacco-related illnesses.[1] By October 1996, the number of states had grown to 17. A remarkable development has been the decision of the Liggett Group, the fifth largest tobacco company, to pay millions of dollars (mostly for cessation programs) to end its involvement in a class action suit in New Orleans[34] (although the suit was eventually rejected) and to partially reimburse the seven state governments for the cost of treating Medicaid patients for tobacco-related diseases. The terms arrange for immediate payments plus percentages of profits. In addition, the company agreed to comply with some of the proposed FDA requirements (vide infra). This may also be a maneuver to allow Reynolds Tobacco, the second largest tobacco company, to share in the terms of the settlement if they merge with the Liggett Group, Inc., as planned. Although this would result in hundreds of millions of dollars in settlements, it would probably save them far more in legal fees and settlements for costly suits in the future.[13] A suit by Blue Cross/Blue Shield of Minnesota asking for payment from the tobacco companies for tobacco-related diseases was filed in August 1994 and is being considered by the Minnesota Supreme Court.[28] A successful suit in 1995 based on the Americans with Disabilities Act established the right of smoke-sensitive patients to a smoke-free environment in workplaces and public spaces.[32]

Perhaps the most important reaction to the revelation of the tobacco companies' apparent disregard for the public welfare has been that of the FDA to prevent young people from becoming addicted to tobacco. Arguing that the nicotine in tobacco is a drug, defined as a substance meant to alter the function of the body, and that tobacco products are delivery devices, the FDA claimed jurisdiction over tobacco products because nicotine meets the definition of a drug and it is not safe, as is required. On August 11, 1995, the FDA published a proposed rule aimed at meeting the goal of *Healthy People 2000* of decreasing smoking by 50% in 7 years, and particularly at decreasing the number of minors who start smoking from 3,000 to 1,500 a day:[10,17]

> The proposed rule would reduce children's and adolescents' easy access to cigarettes and smokeless tobacco as well as significantly decrease the amount of positive imagery that makes these products so appealing to them. The proposed rule would not restrict the use of tobacco products by adults.[10]

Since it would not be advisable to ban to-

---

* Books detailing knowledge and activities of the tobacco companies include: Glantz S, Slade J, Bero LA, et al: **The Cigarette Papers.** Berkeley, Calif: University of California Press, 1996, 539 pp; Hilts PJ: **Smokescreen. The Truth Behind the Tobacco Industry Cover-Up.** Reading, Mass: Addison-Wesley, 1996, 253 pp; and Kluger R: **Ashes to Ashes. America's Hundred-Year Cigarette War, the Public Health, and the Unabashed Triumph of Philip Morris.** New York, NY: Knopf, 1996, 809 pp.

TABLE 2

FINAL REGULATIONS TO REDUCE CHILDREN'S USE OF TOBACCO

Reduce easy access by children
- Require age verification and face-to-face sale (except for mail orders), and eliminate free samples and the sale of single cigarettes and packages with fewer than 20 cigarettes.
- Ban vending machines and self-service displays except in facilities where only adults are permitted.

Reduce appeal to children
- Ban outdoor advertising within 1,000 feet of schools and publicly owned playgrounds. Permit black-and-white text-only advertising for all other outdoor advertising.
- Permit black-and-white text-only advertising in publications with significant (>15% or two million) youth readership (<18 years).
- Prohibit the sale or giveaway of products such as baseball caps or gym bags that carry cigarette or smoke-less tobacco product brand names or logos.
- Prohibit brand-name sponsorship of sporting or entertainment events, but permit it in the corporate name.

Educate children about real dangers of use of tobacco products
- The FDA will also propose to require each of the six major tobacco companies with significant sales to children to educate young people about the real health dangers associated with the use of tobacco products. This national multimedia campaign, including television spots, would be monitored for its effectiveness.

---

bacco because of the adverse effects to be expected on addicted smokers in the U.S., the rule was not meant to eliminate tobacco products. The discussion of the rule also details the legal analysis relative to FDA jurisdiction over tobacco products, the evidence that nicotine has drug effects on the body, and the "statements, research, and actions by tobacco companies."

Initially, the time for comments was to end November 9, 1995; however, the deadline was extended to January 6, 1996. The FDA received over 60,000 comments, including a 2,000-page document from the tobacco companies, which must be considered. The comment period was reopened in March 1996 when more information about the alleged manipulation of nicotine levels became known.[13] The final amended rule was issued August 28, 1996[30] (Table 2) and enforcement will be phased in beginning 6 months from that time, to be complete in two years.

The FDA rule has received extensive support. An important new entity is the Campaign for Tobacco-Free Kids, a group of over 125 organizations including the AMA.[18] The efforts of the Campaign are being facilitated by grants of $20 million from the Robert Wood Johnson Foundation and $10 million from the American Cancer Society, which has permitted opening of the National Center for Tobacco Free Kids in Washington, D.C., in June 1996.[14]

On the other hand, a significant campaign has been mounted against the rules by the tobacco companies, advertisers, and sports events sponsors, as well as by civil libertarians, who have instituted suits in North Carolina based on freedom of speech and lack of FDA jurisdiction. In addition, a number of bills have been introduced in the U.S. Congress to deny the FDA jurisdiction over tobacco products and Congress has 60 days to review the FDA regulations. Indeed, it must be noted that the tobacco companies contributed $16 million to Congressional candidates between 1984 and 1995 and over $700,000 in the first 6 months of 1995, 80% to Republicans.[18] The amount spent in 1995 was twice that spent in 1993.[13] To put this issue of promotion of cigarette use by tobacco companies in perspective, it should be noted that in 1990 for each dollar the National Cancer Institute spent on research to combat smoking, the tobacco industry spent $80 to promote smoking.

Tobacco was also an issue in the 1996 presidential campaign. Senator Robert Dole, the Republican presidential candidate, stated in a television interview that he was not certain whether tobacco is addictive, although he did speak against its use and mentioned that it contributed to the death of his brother. Vice-President Al Gore, the Democratic vice-presidential candidate, gave an impassioned speech at the Democratic convention about how tobacco contributed to the death of his sister.

The April 24, 1996 issue of *JAMA* (Volume 275, pp 1215-1290) was devoted to the scientific knowledge and legal situation with regard to tobacco use as of that date. It included articles about the biochemistry of addiction, prevalence and changes in smoking rates among various groups, pre-emptive efforts of the tobacco industry using its great resources to recruit users and to impede tobacco controls, efforts to prevent tobacco use, strategies to help people stop smoking, exposure to second-hand smoke, and the economic implications if tobacco sales decreased. A detailed article recounts the tobacco industries' efforts to neutralize governmental controls, which include litigation to prevent FDA regulation, threats to the media, advertising campaigns against governmental controls, contributions to politicians and lobbying, and blocking regulations by submitting huge amounts of materials during mandatory public comment periods for proposed federal regulations.[2,8] In this context, it is important to remember that tobacco companies are part of a $45 billion industry, employ over 700,000 workers, spend $6 million on advertising, and have over 56 million customers. Economic implications of declining tobacco sales are fascinating. Although jobs would be lost in the tobacco industry, redistribution of expenditures to other consumer products actually would create a net increase in jobs.[45] In a discussion about this article, it was noted that costs for care of tobacco-related diseases would drop, but so would income from taxes on tobacco products, whereas total health care costs would be higher because of later and possibly more costly deaths, and longer retirement benefits would be more costly. Thus, looking at the economics alone, ironically it may be financially disadvantageous to stop tobacco use.[25,45]

Two other economic subjects are of interest. One is that medical researchers are accepting funding from tobacco companies which implicitly legitimizes the companies' activities and is used explicitly by the companies to challenge the certainty of scientific evidence of the adverse effects of tobacco. To avoid this legitimization, some organizations have decided not to accept such funding and some professional journals refuse manuscripts developed with such grants. There has even been a proposal that federal granting agencies should deny funds to recipients of such monies.[7] Second, many individuals and groups who are opposed to tobacco use (including medical school pension funds and insurance companies) purchase and hold the stocks of tobacco companies in their parent organizations or mutual funds which include such stocks. Such stocks and funds are being publicly identified by groups such as Co-op America in Washington and investors are being urged to stop investing in these companies.[12]

The major problem is still that large numbers of young people start smoking, particularly the less educated. Unfortunately, trying to help the addicted stop is still problematic. There has been some progress in protecting people from second-hand smoke. However, an increased commitment is required.

> The disgraceful tradeoff in America between profits and good health must stop! But it will stop only when our citizens rise up and say "Enough—no more!"[42]
>
> Louis W. Sullivan, M.D.
> Secretary, U.S. Department of
> Health and Human Services

REFERENCES

1. Anti-tobacco suits building, but impact still uncertain. **Am Med News.** Mar 4, 1996, p 8
2. Arno PS, Brandt AM, Gostin LO, et al: Tobacco industry strategies to oppose federal regulation. **JAMA** 275:1258-1262, 1996
3. Burns DM: Tobacco and health, in Wyngaarden JB, Smith LH Jr, Bennett JC (eds): **Cecil Textbook of Medicine.** 19th ed. Philadelphia, Pa: WB Saunders, 1992, pp 34-37
4. Califano JA Jr: The wrong way to stay slim. **N Engl J Med** 333:1214-1216, 1995 (Editorial)
5. Centers for Disease Control and Prevention: **State Tobacco Control Highlights—1996.** Atlanta, Ga: Centers for Disease Control and Prevention, 1996
6. Cheyney EP: **Readings in English History Drawn From the Original Sources.** Boston, Mass: Ginn, 1935, pp 420-421
7. Cohen J: Tobacco money lights up a debate. **Science**

272:488-494, 1996

8. Davis RM: The ledger of tobacco control. Is the cup half empty or half full. **JAMA** 275:1281-1284, 1996

9. Enrico D: Cashing in on kicking a habit. **USA TODAY.** Sept 13, 1996, pp B1, B2

10. **Federal Register.** Vol 60 (No. 155), 41314-41787 (August 11, 1995)

11. Fiscella K, Franks P: Use of over-the-counter nicotine patch for smoking cessation: prudent or premature? **JAMA** 276:371-372, 1996 (Letter)

12. Goldsmith MF: Mutual fund investors advised to sniff out tobacco. **JAMA** 275:1222, 1996

13. Hearn W: Breach in tobacco ranks. Liggett settlement seen to strengthen anti-tobacco efforts. **Am Med News.** Apr 1, 1996, pp 3, 22

14. Hearn W: Tobacco-Free Kids' Center gears up lobbying effort. **Am Med News.** Apr 15, 1996, p 16

15. Henningfield JE: Nicotine medications for smoking cessation. **N Engl J Med** 333:1196-1203, 1995

16. Houston T: Tobacco. The cigarette papers. **JAMA** 276:997-998, 1996 (Book review)

17. Kent C: Battle over FDA regulation. **Am Med News.** Nov 6, 1995, pp 3, 26

18. Kent C: Long-awaited tobacco control rules get tepid praise. **Am Med News.** Feb 5, 1996, p 4

19. Kent C: Tobacco firm pays for failure to warn. **Am Med News.** Aug 26, 1996, pp 1, 20, 22

20. Kessler DA: Nicotine addiction in young people. **N Engl J Med** 333:186-189, 1995

21. Longo DR, Brownson RC, Kruse RL: Smoking bans in U.S. hospitals. Results of a national survey. **JAMA** 274:488-491, 1995

22. Lundberg GD: Tobacco/Medicare. **JAMA** 274: 189-282, 1995

23. Lynch BS, Bonnie RJ (eds): **Growing Up Tobacco Free. Preventing Nicotine Addiction in Children and Youths.** Washington, DC: National Academy Press, 1994

24. Manning A: Tobacco executives' testimony investigated. **USA TODAY.** July 26, 1995

25. Mansnerus L: Making a case for death. **New York Times.** May 5, 1996, pp 4-1, 4-6

26. Marshall R Jr, Shopland DR: Smoking. **Medical and Health Annual. Encyclopedia Brittanica.** Chicago, Ill: Encyclopedia Brittanica, 1995

27. McCormick B: Criminal investigations add to legal woes for tobacco firms. **Am Med News.** Aug 21, 1995, p 3

28. Minnesota insurer asks to sue tobacco firms. **Am Med News.** Feb 19, 1996, p 21

29. National Center for Chronic Disease Prevention and Health Promotion: Cigarette smoking among adults —United States, 1994. **JAMA** 276:595-596, 1996

30. Nightingale SL: Final regulations to reduce children's use of tobacco issued. **JAMA** 276:1128, 1996

31. Nowak R: New studies trace the impact of tobacco advertising. **Science** 270:573-574, 1995

32. Parmet WE, Daynard RA, Gottlieb MA: The physician's role in helping smoke-sensitive patients to use the Americans with Disabilities Act to secure smoke-free workplaces and public spaces. **JAMA** 276:

909-913, 1996

33. Proctor RN: Tobacco. Smokescreen: The truth behind the tobacco industry cover-up. **JAMA** 276: 998, 1996 (Book review)

34. Public release sought for Philip Morris nicotine papers. **Am Med News.** Sept 18, 1995, p 18

35. Smoking Cessation Clinical Practice Guidelines Panel and Staff, US Agency for Health Care Policy and Research: Smoking cessation clinical practice guidelines. **JAMA** 275:1270-1280, 1996

36. Sugarman SD: Smoking guns. **Science** 273:744-745, 1996 (Book review)

37. Todd JS, Rennie D, McAfee RE, et al: The Brown and Williamson documents. Where do we go from here? **JAMA** 274:256-258, 1995

38. US Department of Health and Human Services, Public Health Service: **The Health Benefits of Smoking Cessation: A Report of the Surgeon General.** Atlanta, Ga: Centers for Disease Control, National Center for Chronic Disease Prevention and Health Promotion, Office on Smoking and Health, 1990, 628 pp (DHHS Publication No. (CDC) 90-8416)

39. US Department of Health and Human Services, Public Health Service: **Major Local Tobacco Control Ordinances in the United States.** Washington, DC: US Government Printing Office, 1993, 139 pp (NIH Publication No. 93-3532)

40. US Department of Health and Human Services, Public Health Service: **Preventing Tobacco Use Among Young People: A Report of the Surgeon General.** Atlanta, Ga: Centers for Disease Control and Prevention, National Center for Chronic Disease Prevention and Health Promotion, Office on Smoking and Health, 1994, 314 pp

41. US Department of Health and Human Services, Public Health Service: **Respiratory Health Effects of Passive Smoking: Lung Cancer and Other Disorders. The Report of the Environmental Protection Agency.** Washington, DC: US Government Printing Office, 1993, 364 pp (NIH Publication No. 93-3605)

42. US Department of Health and Human Services, Public Health Service: **Smokeless Tobacco or Health. An International Perspective.** Washington, DC: US Government Printing Office, 1992 (NIH Publication No. 93-3461)

43. US Department of Health and Human Services, Public Health Service: **Strategies To Control Tobacco Use in the United States: A Blueprint for Public Health Action in the 1990's.** Washington, DC: US Government Printing Office, 1991 (NIH Publication No. 92-3316, 307 pp)

44. Wannamethee SG, Shaper AG, Whincup PH, et al: Smoking cessation and the risk of stroke in middle-aged men. **JAMA** 274:155-160, 1995

45. Warner KE, Fulton GA, Nicolas P, et al: Employment implications of declining tobacco product sales for the regional economies of the United States. **JAMA** 275:1241-1246, 1996

46. Woodhead H (ed): The power in the green stalk, in: **The Spirit World.** Alexandria, Va: Time-Life Books, 1992, pp 85-112

CHAPTER 16

INFECTIOUS DISEASES, PUBLIC HEALTH, AND THE LAW

RAYMOND A. SMEGO, JR., MD, MPH, FACP, DTM&H

Proper maintenance of the public's health and that of individuals within society at times requires some form of legal or legislative action or protection. In the field of infectious diseases, uninfected persons may need to be protected from certain individuals infected with contagious illnesses. Disease surveillance, contact tracing, isolation and/or quarantine when necessary, immunization, and obligatory reporting of a variety of notifiable diseases from anthrax to yellow fever are all crucial elements in the control of major communicable diseases. Such measures may be required at federal, state, or local levels or mandated under international health regulations.[12]

In health care settings, occupational exposure to infectious agents such as hepatitis viruses, cytomegalovirus, and human immunodeficiency virus (HIV) has prompted the promulgation of federal guidelines and requirements in infection control and prevention for health care providers, facilities, and institutions.[18,82] The unprecedented rise in tuberculosis and the emergence of multidrug-resistant tuberculosis as a major public health problem in the United States has changed our approach to tuberculosis management. This new epidemic is due in large part to drug non-compliance among high-risk infected persons such as illicit drug users, patients infected with the HIV, and the homeless.[16,48] Directly-observed anti-tuberculous therapy has become the mainstay of management in many locales, and failure to comply with such treatment legally justifies home quarantine, involuntary commitment, or incarceration of recurrently noncompliant tuberculous-infected patients in most states.[7,18,37]

In recent years, legal reform has offered protection to pharmaceutical manufacturers who provide the nation's immunobiologicals against excessive litigation and claims of vaccine-related injury. The National Childhood Vaccine Injury Act of 1986 reduced the fear of liability for physicians and vaccine manufacturers by creating a federal vaccine injury compensation fund for persons found to have adverse effects from required immunizations.[57]

During the past decade, the evolution of the HIV and acquired immunodeficiency syndrome (AIDS) epidemic, the complex interplay of medical, psychological, sociological, and economic features have impacted notably on the public health of America. HIV/AIDS has become the nation's number one public health priority. Since 1993, the HIV infection has been the most common cause of death among persons aged 25 to 44 years and is the fourth leading cause of years of potential life lost before age 65.[20,22] In addition to its own impact, AIDS has contributed to a resurgence of other infectious diseases such as tuberculosis and syphilis, both in the U.S. and worldwide.

The need to control this deadly disease has demanded a multifaceted approach emphasizing both preventive and therapeutic measures. The highest priority has been given toward education of individuals at highest risk for HIV infection, aimed at avoidance of dangerous sexual and drug-associated needle-sharing behavior most likely to transmit disease. In the health care arena, institution of and adherence to universal precautions have revolutionized the principles and practice of infection control, leading to greater protection of both health care providers and patients against HIV and other blood-borne pathogens.

Coincident with the social phenomena of the AIDS epidemic have come several landmark legal controversies and milestones. Issues involving patient confidentiality, mandatory blood testing, discrimination, forced confinement, and segregation have evoked often conflicting public health and civil libertarian responses, as national organizations and legal systems struggle to influence public policy that is both fair and protective for individuals, institutions, and government.

The presence of HIV/AIDS in the health care workplace poses many intriguing and complicated questions that can be examined from a legal as well as medical perspective:[13,38] Do HIV-infected health care workers endanger their patients? Is there a reasonable risk that the virus will be transmitted accidentally? What constitutes reasonable risk? Should physicians and other health care workers be screened for HIV? Does the patients' right to know if their doctor is HIV seropositive outweigh the physician's right to confidentiality? What aspects of an HIV-infected physician's medical practice poses a risk to patients? Does the risk of transmission warrant restricting infected clinicians from certain procedures, or should a high standard of infection control be emphasized and compliance monitored? Do professional rules limiting the right to practice invasive procedures violate anti-discrimination statutes?

In this chapter we address the above questions and explore the following important topics: voluntary vs. mandatory HIV serological blood testing of patients and health care workers; mandatory HIV reporting; the doctor/patient relationship and the legal issues of confidentiality, right to know, and duty to warn third parties; epidemiological look-back investigations of HIV-infected workplace exposures; lawsuits for emotional distress from fear of contracting AIDS; and the interaction of HIV/AIDS and the Americans with Disabilities Act.

Voluntary vs. Mandatory Blood Testing

The transmission of HIV from infected patients to health care workers has been well documented, and the risks of nosocomial percutaneous and permucosal exposures have been quantified by epidemiological investigation.[17] However, to date only one case of converse transmission (i.e., from an infected health care worker to a patient) has been recorded. The case involved six patients who became infected after receiving care from David Acer, an HIV-infected dentist in Florida, through still undetermined mechanisms.[23,24] Current data indicate that the risk of HIV transmission from health care workers to patients is so low that it cannot be measured accurately. Nevertheless, the potential for transmission to patients raises complex medical, ethical, psychological, and social issues that have major public health implications. One of these issues is that of voluntary vs. mandatory serological blood testing.

The current approach to HIV testing, with its demand for extreme privacy, was evolved out of the concern by homosexual men about confidentiality of their health data and the discrimination encountered by them in all levels of society. Early in the epidemic, HIV infection and AIDS were perceived initially more as civil rights issues rather than as public health issues. Over the course of the last decade, the pendulum has shifted in the direction of treating HIV/AIDS as the premier public health issue that it is.

Currently, most HIV testing in the U.S. is voluntary in nature, performed only after the person to be tested has given informed consent. This is in contrast to most other diagnostic tests, which generally do not require individual informed consent unless an invasive surgical procedure is involved. Our democratic society has widely accepted the public health argument that favors voluntary rather than mandatory public health programs for disease control. While there seems to be a consensus among scholars and public officials that screening high-risk patients is valuable, making screening mandatory has been rejected by most institutions and in most jurisdictions.[3,40,52,53,64,70] Mandatory testing is currently performed only on select patient populations such as prison inmates, members of the military, blood donors, persons seeking immigration to the U.S., and life insurance applicants.

Testing without consent may be appropriate in certain circumstances, such as after accidental exposure of a health care provider to a patient's blood or testing of an unconscious or incompetent patient in the absence of a responsible decision-maker. Some states have enacted legislation that permits testing without individual informed consent in such circumstances. In states where informed consent is mandated by law, some hospitals have incorporated into their admission consent forms a provision indicating that, in case of accidental exposure of a health care worker, the patient's blood may be tested for both hepatitis B virus and HIV infections.

Some surgeons have argued that there exists a "need to know" the HIV status of patients on whom they plan to operate, claiming that the risk of accidental exposure justifies mandatory screening. Most institutions, however, have countered that strict observance of universal precautions, as recommended by the Centers for Disease Control and Prevention (CDC) and required by the Occupational Safety and Health Administration (OSHA) bloodborne pathogens standard,[18,82] obviates the need to know HIV status in the absence of informed consent. Studies have indicated that surgeons and dentists will cut a glove in approximately one in every four cases and sustain a significant skin cut in one of every 40 cases. In a study of risk of exposure of surgical personnel to patients' blood during surgery at San Francisco General Hospi-

tal, Gerberding et al[35] found that accidental exposure to blood (parenteral or cutaneous) occurred in 6.4% of all procedures and parenteral exposure occurred in 1.7% of cases. Neither knowledge of diagnosed HIV infection nor awareness of a patient's high-risk status for such infection influenced the rate of exposure. Double-gloving prevented perforations of the inner glove and cutaneous exposures of the hand.

It is estimated that more than 5,000 physicians are infected with the HIV virus in the U.S.[41] Regarding mandatory testing as an attempt to identify HIV-positive doctors and other health care workers, the elimination of all risk is not possible. HIV infection can occur at any time and thus testing would have to be conducted on a daily basis to identify all infected physicians, and even daily testing would not eliminate all risk. The time line between infection and seroconversion precludes mandatory testing from identifying infected physicians until they have been infected for weeks to months. Furthermore, principles of individual liberty preclude widespread invasion of privacy, and most agree that mandatory HIV testing of surgeons would result in unjustified violations of individual privacy.

Mandatory HIV Reporting

Proposals to require "names reporting" of people who test HIV-positive have been hotly debated over the years. About one-half of all states currently require physicians to report patients who test positive for HIV by name, with a handful of others requiring it in specific situations.[13,74] At issue in the practice of mandatory names reporting is how to control the epidemic without exposing its victims to social and economic risks.

Proponents of names reporting cite that it is a critical part of disease surveillance and prevention efforts. For example, information gleaned from reporting is used to initiate partner notification and referral to counseling and other services.[6,10] In some states, in cases involving infected children, a pediatric AIDS care system ensures that they are referred for follow-up testing and care. Data are also used to plan prevention and treatment programs and to allocate federal Ryan White funding and other resources.[74]

Critics of names reporting, however, credit anonymous testing and public education, rather than mandatory testing and names reporting, for the sharp decline in the rate of persons newly infected with HIV and other sexually transmitted diseases in certain hyperendemic areas such as San Francisco. They believe that names reporting and the coincident fear of loss of privacy is a disincentive to serological testing and impedes earlier diagnosis and treatment. The CDC is currently completing a 3-year project in eight states to evaluate the role of names reporting in an individual's decision to obtain testing for HIV.

PATIENT CONFIDENTIALITY AND RIGHT TO KNOW

The legal and public health environment is performing a delicate balancing act in trying to protect the rights of HIV-infected individuals—patients and providers—while at the same time protecting physicians, employees, patients, and third parties. Within this complicated environment, the issues of serological testing, confidentiality vs. right to know, and discrimination come to bear.

Confidentiality

In a national review of litigation related to HIV/AIDS, Gostin[36] describes how hospitals and health care providers have been held liable for failing to demonstrate proper medical procedures to maintain the confidentiality of HIV test results. Cases have involved the inadvertent or intentional disclosure of a patient's HIV status to family, friends, or employers, as well as to staff members. In the 1991 case of *Behringer v. Medical Center at Princeton*,[11] the court found that the hospital where Dr. Behringer, an HIV-infected otolaryngologist, worked and was hospitalized for *Pneumocystis carinii* pneumonia breached its duty of confidentiality to Dr. Behringer as a patient when it failed to take reasonable precautions regarding his medical record. Among the precautions that the medical center

should have implemented, according to the court, were "securing of the chart, with access only to those health care workers demonstrating to designated record keepers of bonafide need to know, or utilizing sequestration procedures for those portions of the record containing such information."

The Duty to Warn

For centuries, the sacredness of privacy of communication between a patient and his/her physician was considered paramount. In 1976, the case of *Tarasoff v. The Regents of the University of California*[78] was a benchmark decision in which a psychologist was found liable for failure to warn a third party of his patient's intention to murder her. The duty to protect third parties, however, from contracting an infectious disease predates *Tarasoff*, and has been addressed in cases involving smallpox, scarlet fever, tuberculosis, typhoid fever, and septic poisoning.[47,68] Early courts dating back to the turn of the century have cited a need to warn specific individuals in foreseeable danger of contracting an infection and have held doctors responsible to third parties for their failure to advise that a family member has a contagious disease. For the clinician practicing in the HIV/AIDS era, this ethical duty to warn specific individuals has supplanted the traditional code of doctor-patient confidentiality in the greater name of public health and the protection of society.[29,39]

The duty to protect third parties from transmission of HIV arises in relation to specific persons who the physician knows are likely to have an intimate exchange of bodily fluids with the patient. The steps the physician must take to fulfill this "duty to protect" are not entirely clear, but they at least include a threshold obligation to advise the patient to inform close contacts of his/her infection. If the HIV-infected patient refuses to inform others, the physician should consider how to protect the health and welfare of the patient's spouse or other partners. The physician may either notify the partners directly or arrange to have public health officials do so.

In addition, there may arise instances of endangerment or assault where HIV-seropositive persons knowingly expose or infect peers or partners by virtue of their own unethical or malicious behaviors.[76] For situations in which a physician is aware of HIV-seropositive patients who knowingly engage in high-risk sexual and drug-using activity without disclosing their infective status to others, it becomes the ethical responsibility of that physician to determine and inform those sexual partners. In several locales there is statutory legislation that criminalizes such behavior and makes incarceration mandatory for HIV-infected prostitutes who engage in sex with clients, or for any infective person whose continued homosexual or heterosexual activities knowingly endanger the lives of uninformed partners.

It must be noted, however, that the physician's duty to warn is in most instances an ethical and not a legal duty. While many states authorize disclosure of HIV status information by health care providers (e.g., private physicians, health departments) to certain contacts of an HIV patient, and indeed provide civil immunity for doing so (e.g., Pennsylvania), there is no legal requirement in most states to identify, locate, and notify any contacts, and no cause of action shall arise for nondisclosure. Existing statutes, thus, permit but generally do not require disclosure of a patient's HIV seropositivity to his/her sexual partners or others at risk for disease transmission. An exception is *Reissner v. The Regents of the University of California*.[67] In this case, a California appeals court allowed a third party claim against a physician who failed to tell a patient she had AIDS. Jennifer Lawson received a blood transfusion at University of California, Los Angeles (UCLA) at age 12; the day after the transfusion her physician and UCLA discovered that the blood used was infected with HIV, but they did not inform Jennifer or her parents, although the physician continued to treat her. Consequently, she was not warned of the danger of spreading the disease or how to prevent it. Three years later, Jennifer began dating and became intimate with Daniel Reissner. Two years later, the doctor told Jennifer that she had AIDS, and Jennifer told Daniel. Shortly thereafter, Jennifer died and Daniel discovered that he was HIV-infected. Daniel sued the doctor and UCLA for negligence for not warning Jennifer of her HIV status, which, he argued, resulted in his infection. The trial court granted summary judgment for the defendants, holding that no duty was owed to an unidentifiable third party.

The appeals court reversed that decision and, citing *Tarasoff v. The Regents of the University of California*, held that a physician's duty includes a duty to warn others likely to apprise a victim of the danger or to "take whatever . . . steps are reasonably necessary under the circumstances." The court found that Jennifer and her parents were "others" who were likely to warn Daniel of the danger, and that the injury to Daniel was foreseeable. The court held that the duty to warn a contagious patient to take steps to protect others could be extended to a third party not reasonably ascertainable by the physician, but pointed out that the duty would be discharged by the physician warning the patient of the risk to others and advising him/her how to prevent the spread of the disease.

A legal duty to warn has been applied to hospitals as well as to physicians. In a 1993 Pennsylvania case (*In re Milton S. Hershey Medical Center of Pensylvania University*[46]), the Pennsylvania Supreme Court upheld a lower trial court order that permitted two hospitals to disclose an obstetric-gynecology resident's HIV seropositive status to former patients who underwent invasive procedures in which he had been involved. Pennsylvania's Confidentiality of HIV-Related Information Act prohibits disclosure unless "the person seeking to disclose the information has a compelling need to do so."[27] The hospital filed suit under the Act, alleging a compelling need to inform possibly infected patients of their potential exposure and to offer them testing, treatment, and counseling. The Pennsylvania Supreme Court concluded that "the public's right to be informed in this sort of potential health catastrophe is compelling and far outweighs a practicing surgeon's right to keep information regarding his disease confidential." For most hospitals who become aware of HIV-seropositivity within their health professional ranks, the necessity of the "compelling need to inform" the public described above has been questioned and is discussed in the following section.

"LOOK-BACK" INVESTIGATIONS

Current data indicate that the risk of HIV transmission from health care workers to patients is extremely low and not capable of being measured accurately. Despite this low risk, numerous retrospective investigations to notify patients of possible past exposure to HIV-infected health care workers are being conducted with increasing frequency, initiated due to the risk of transmission of disease to patients or, in the absence of incurred risk, because of concerns for the patient's right to know or because of concern for legal liability.[13,21,28,56,69,77] Except for the unusual cluster of cases in David Acer's dental practice in Florida, for which the mode of transmission is still completely unknown, there has not been a documented instance of an HIV-positive physician infecting a patient to date. In formal "look-back" investigations, no instance of nosocomial transmission of AIDS or HIV infection to patients has been documented.

A study from the CDC examined data from hospitals and health departments nationwide, collected in epidemiological look-back studies aimed at determining if HIV-infected health care workers had infected any patient during treatments ranging from dental cleaning to obstetric or orthopedic operations.[69] The data evaluated 64 doctors, dentists, and dental assistants during the period 1987 through January 1995, excluding David Acer; the HIV tests results were available for approximately 22,171 patients treated by 51 of the 64 health care workers. For 37 of the 51 workers, no seropositive patients were reported among 13,063 patients tested for HIV. For the remaining 14 health care workers, 113 seropositive patients were reported among 9,108 patients. Twenty-eight had been infected prior to their treatment by the health care worker, and another 62 patients had risk factors such as intravenous drug use and unprotected sex. Epidemiological and laboratory follow-up did not show any health care worker to have been a source of HIV for any of the patients tested. The CDC researchers acknowledged the limitations of the study, including a lack of antibody test results and complete medical record data for all patients, incomplete knowledge of the invasiveness of the medical procedures performed, and a lack of statistical power needed to detect a low frequency event such as doctor-to-patient HIV transmission. These limitations notwithstanding, this largest study of its kind

found no evidence that patients contracted HIV through medical procedures. The data also supported current recommendations that state that retrospective patient notification need not be done routinely.

The CDC has estimated that a patient's risk of becoming infected by an HIV-positive health care worker to be between one in 42,000 and one in 420,000 surgeries.[17] Based on the number of surgeries in the U.S. and the estimated number of HIV-seropositive surgeons, the CDC has estimated that surgeons could have infected between three and 28 patients as of 1991. However, epidemiological studies have failed to disclose a single case of physician-to-patient infection, and this risk of HIV transmission is so low that hospital health departments should not feel compelled to undertake costly look-back investigations.

In a study conducted by the Veterans Administration Medical Center in Palo Alto, California, and the Stanford and Dartmouth Medical Schools, the universal screening of all U.S. surgeons was analyzed theoretically in terms of cost-effectiveness using mathematical models.[60,77] The study estimated that a one-time national screening program of 141,000 surgeons would cost $8.1 million. Direct and indirect costs of annual testing would be $1.1 million per year of life saved by way of HIV prevention, costs far in excess of medical interventions for other diseases such as hypertension ($12,200 to $42,600 per year of life saved).

The CDC recommendations are the only published guidelines that have addressed the issue of notifying patients cared for in the past by an HIV-infected health care worker. The recommendations state that such efforts should be conducted on a case-by-case basis, given their extremely costly nature in terms of monetary and human resources. Look-back investigations should not be considered standard public health practice or performed merely because of concern for the patient's right to know or because of a concern for legal liability. Following a formal look-back investigation of patients cared for by an HIV-infected family physician, conducted by the Minnesota State Health Department, Danila et al[28] similarly proposed that before a look-back investigation is undertaken there should be a clearly identifiable risk of transmission of the infection, substantially higher than the risk requiring limitation of an HIV-infected health care worker prospectively.

EMOTIONAL DISTRESS FROM FEAR OF CONTRACTING AIDS

Most courts have denied recovery of damages based on the fear of contracting AIDS without proof of actual exposure. The reluctance to award damages appear to stem from a fear of encouraging an "AIDS phobia." The courts seem to find claims of emotional distress with no evidence of actual exposure too speculative. Typical examples of emotional distress cases include those involving needlesticks or other accidental exposures. Health care workers who know they are HIV-seropositive and treat patients without disclosing this fact have also been the subject of numerous emotional distress claims.[33,44]

Exceptions to this trend are seen in the cases *Faya v. Almaraz*[33] and *Kerins v. Hartley*.[49] In *Faya v. Almaraz*, Dr. Rudolf Almaraz, a breast cancer surgeon at Johns Hopkins University, died of AIDS in 1990. Following his death, the hospital sent letters to 1,800 of his former patients offering HIV testing and counseling. Although no former patient tested positive, two patients, Sonya Faya and Perry Rossi, sued the doctor's estate and the hospital for $232 million, claiming emotional distress from fear of contracting AIDS. The trial court dismissed the claims on the grounds that the alleged fear of contracting AIDS was unreasonable as a matter of law without proof of actual exposure. A Maryland Appeals Court, however, reversed the decision, allowing recovery without evidence of documented exposure. It limited the above patients' recovery to "their reasonable window of anxiety," the period from when they learned of the physician's disease to the point when they received their own HIV-negative results. In a similar case, *Kerins v. Hartley*,[49] the California Court of Appeals, Second District, reversed a lower court and held that an HIV-positive physician was liable for a patient's emotional distress because he had performed surgery without notifying the patient of his seropositive

status. The court found that the plaintiff could properly maintain an action for intentional and negligent infliction of emotional distress for the reasonable window of anxiety between the plaintiff's notification of the physician's HIV status and discovery of her own negative test results. Ultimately, however, the Supreme Court of California vacated (i.e., overruled) this decision based on the *Potter et al v. Firestone Tire and Rubber Company*[62] decision in which it had previously held that no damages could be awarded for emotional distress associated with fear of injury or disease unless it is corroborated by reasonable medical and scientific opinion that it is more likely than not that the plaintiff will contract the disease, or that the defendant acted with fraud or malice.

HIV/AIDS AND THE AMERICANS WITH DISABILITIES ACT

Over the past several years, courts have ruled on two main types of discrimination cases involving health care professionals and HIV. The first entails HIV-seropositive patients who have been denied care by health care professionals. The second type centers around health care professionals with HIV, often surgeons, who claim discrimination by hospitals attempting to block their practice because of their seropositivity. The essential issue is that there exists a risk, albeit an extremely low one, that a nearly universally fatal disease will be spread whenever a health care provider performs an invasive procedure in the presence of HIV in either the patient or the provider. There seems to be a trend whereby antidiscrimination laws are understood as obliging providers to perform invasive procedures on infected patients while at the same time denying infected providers the right to engage in procedures involving the chance of transmitting their own blood to patients.

The powerful punitive and discriminatory reactions of society to those with HIV infection contributes deeply and fundamentally to the suffering of HIV-infected patients. This discrimination often leads to loss of home, family, friends, jobs, and insurance, or denial of care.

The Americans With Disabilities Act (ADA) of 1990 was a major step forward. It represents landmark legislation to ban discrimination against persons with disabilities, including persons with HIV infection and AIDS.[4] The eight-member Institute of Medicine-National Academy of Sciences Committee for the Oversight of AIDS Activities concluded that the "fear of discrimination is a major constraint to the wide acceptance of many potentially effective public health measures. Public health programs will be most effective if they are accompanied by clear, strict sanctions to prevent unwarranted discrimination against those who are HIV-infected or at risk for infection."[14] Over the past few years a number of important committee recommendations or legislative documents, both statutory and federal, have arisen to counter discrimination against people with AIDS.

The Duty to Treat

The Rehabilitation Act of 1973[66] expanded on the civil rights antidiscrimination protection legislated by the Civil Rights Act of 1964.[25] Section 504 of the Rehabilitation Act stated that "No otherwise qualified handicapped individual shall, solely by reason of his handicap, be excluded from the participation in, be denied the benefits of, or be subjected to discrimination under any program or activity receiving federal financial assistance. . . ." The question of whether persons with HIV infection qualified for the Rehabilitation Act was addressed by the U.S. Supreme Court in *School Board of Nassau County v. Arline*,[71] a case involving a teacher with tuberculosis. The Court held that a contagious disease was a handicap and that fear of contagion alone could qualify as a handicap under Section 504 of the Rehabilitation Act. The Court limited the protection afforded to individuals with infectious diseases by noting that a significant risk of transmitting the disease would make the individual not "otherwise qualified." The determination of "significant risk" was left to the "reasonable medical judgments of public health officials." The Department of Justice later mandated the application of disability protection to HIV-infected persons under Section 504 of the Rehabilitation Act. In the case of

Doe v. Centinela Hospital,[30] a federal court specifically applied Section 504 to prohibit discrimination against persons infected with HIV in regard to access to health care services. The discriminatory behavior of individual practitioners, however, was not curtailed due to the limited scope of the act.

The U.S. District Court for the District of Delaware ruled in 1995 that claims against health care providers for discrimination based on perceived HIV status were permissible. In the case of *Miller v. Spicer*,[55] the plaintiff sought medical treatment at defendant hospital for immediate surgery due to a lacerated tendon. A defendant physician refused to treat the plaintiff because the plaintiff did not confirm that he was HIV-negative. As a result of the subsequent hospital transfer, the plaintiff suffered apparent permanent damage. The plaintiff sued the defendants for money damages under Section 504 of the Rehabilitation Act of 1973, alleging impermissible discrimination on the basis of his perceived HIV status. The court found the defendant hospital guilty of discrimination under the Rehabilitation Act; the defendant physician was granted summary judgment on this claim because he did not receive any federal funding.

In *Armstrong v. Flowers Hospital, Inc.*,[9,65] the 11th U.S. Circuit Court of Appeals upheld in 1994 the firing of a nurse who, because of her pregnancy, refused to perform the usual nursing duties for an HIV-positive patient. The court said the hospital policies on patient care applied equally to all nurses, and therefore Armstrong could not support her claim that the hospital violated Title VII of the Civil Rights Act and the Pregnancy Discrimination Act of 1978.

The passage of the ADA in July 1990 profoundly affected the long held right of a practicing physician to choose whomever he or she wished to treat. For the first time in federal civil rights history, a physician's office was legally established as a place of public accommodation, and a legal duty to treat patients with disabilities, including HIV infection, was created.[42,61] The ADA expanded the protection afforded disabled individuals under the Civil Rights Act of 1964[25] and the Rehabilitation Act of 1973[66] by broadening the covered entities to include privately-operated public accommodations and by significantly expanding the definition of public accommodations, specifically including the "professional office of a health care provider, hospital, or other similar service establishment."[5] Previously, under both the Civil Rights Act and the Rehabilitation Act, independent practitioners wishing to avoid treating HIV-infected individuals could do so by refusing to accept Medicaid patients (Medicare Part B monies are not considered federal financial assistance to the doctor and, thus, do not subject the practitioner to the provisions of these acts).

In the past, legal challenges to the explicit refusal to treat HIV-positive patients were curtailed by the standard in U.S. case law of the "no duty [to treat] rule." Prior to the ADA, absent a pre-existing professional-patient relationship, a physician was not legally obligated to provide care to any particular patient and could unilaterally withdraw from the relationship if the patient's condition was stable and arrangements were made to assure continuity of care. Exceptions to this rule included contractual obligations (e.g., health maintenance organizations) and emergency room coverage. In the absence of legal imperatives, much of the discussion of a duty to treat HIV-infected patients focused on ethical frameworks and moral tenets of behavior espoused by the medical community. The American College of Physicians, the Infectious Diseases Society of America, and the American Medical Association (AMA) have taken strong positions in support of a duty to treat HIV-positive patients.[3,4,26,34,43] Passage of the ADA, however, has shifted the argument into the legal arena by creating a duty to treat through federal civil rights legislation. The full impact of the ADA will not be determined until the courts more fully interpret it, but decisions in future cases should prohibit discrimination against HIV-infected individuals. A recent example is that of *U.S. v. Morvant*[83] in which an eastern Louisiana U.S. District Court found that a dentist who refused to treat patients with HIV had engaged in unlawful discrimination. It noted that the refusal violated the professional and ethical standards of the American Dental Association, and it referred to the expert opinion of the CDC that universal infection control precautions permitted dentists to safely provide routine dental care to patients with HIV.

HIV-Infected Health Care Providers

The fear of and potential for transmission of HIV from an infected physician has resulted in several important legal decisions addressing whether HIV-seropositive surgeons should be allowed to continue to perform operative procedures. Such cases reflect complex medical and legal issues relating to HIV and AIDS, including effective infection control and anti-discrimination. In 1991, the CDC issued guidelines for the conduct of HIV-infected health care workers. Among other provisions, the CDC requires the identification of "exposure-prone" procedures that present a "recognized risk of percutaneous injury to the health care worker and . . . the health care worker's blood is likely to contact the patient's body cavity, subcutaneous tissues and/or mucous membranes." It stated that HIV-infected physicians "should not perform exposure-prone procedures unless they have been advised by an expert panel under which circumstances, if any, they may continue to perform these procedures."[19] The CDC further recommends that patients be informed of a physician's HIV-seropositive status before undergoing any exposure-prone invasive procedure by the physician. Exposure-prone procedures include those procedures in which a physician digitally palpates the tip of a needle in the patient's body cavity or in which a physician's fingers and a sharp instrument or other objects are simultaneously present in a poorly visualized or highly confined anatomic site. In a minor modification of the guidelines, the CDC eliminated the requirement for listing exposure-prone procedures and referred to them collectively as "invasive procedures."

In *Leckelt v. Board of Commissioners of Hospital District No. 1*,[51] the Fifth U.S. Circuit Court of Appeals in 1990 supported the hospital's firing of a licensed practical nurse who refused to submit the results of HIV testing to his hospital employer so that it could determine the extent of his risk to patients. The hospital knew that he was a member of a high-risk group for HIV. He was a known hepatitis B virus carrier and had a history of syphilis and lymphadenopathy. The court agreed that the hospital reasonably suspected that Leckelt had been exposed to HIV and needed to determine what precautions or restrictions were necessary.

In the earlier mentioned *Behringer v. Medical Center of Princeton* case, a New Jersey trial court upheld the hospital's decision to protect its patients by restricting the surgical privileges of an HIV-infected physician.[11,59,75] Dr. Behringer's estate sued the hospital, claiming that the hospital violated New Jersey's Law Against Discrimination when it restricted Dr. Behringer's privileges to practice surgery and when it required him to obtain informed consent before performing basic procedures. The court considered Dr. Behringer handicapped under New Jersey's Law Against Discrimination, yet it held that the restriction of surgical privileges was permissible because Dr. Behringer posed "a reasonable probability of substantial harm to others" while practicing surgery via potential scalpel cuts, needle sticks, etc. The court ruled that the medical center did not violate the state's anti-discrimination statute when it restricted and later revoked Dr. Behringer's surgical privileges.

Despite the decision in the Behringer case, which "erred" on the side of protecting patients in the face of uncertain risk to patient welfare, there has been considerable disagreement among experts on the kinds of practice restriction, if any, that are appropriate for HIV-infected surgeons. Dispute exists about the amount of risk the patients actually face from an infected surgeon. Based upon a CDC estimate in 1991, the risk of HIV transmission could be as low as one in 420,000[17]—low probability but "seemingly significant" for an almost universally fatal disease such as AIDS. In its ruling, however, the *Behringer* court sought to create a standard of zero risk in regard to HIV in health care settings, choosing to recommend the elimination of all risk of transmission from HIV-infected physicians to patients. Time will tell whether, in future cases, courts will reject this standard of zero tolerance of risk. Subsequent court decisions may defer, as they often do, to the reasonable medical judgment of public health officials in assessing medical risk. It seems likely that hospitals adhering to these CDC guidelines will not be found guilty of unlawful discrimination.

On the controversial issue of informed consent, both the CDC and the AMA have concluded that HIV-infected surgeons may perform significant invasive procedures if they disclose their HIV status to the patient and obtain the patient's informed consent. The impracticality of this approach seems evident, however, because it is highly unlikely that such informed patients would be willing to continue with the services of their surgeon. There is further concern that any practice restriction may deter surgeons from getting HIV-tested or from treating HIV-infected individuals for fear of risking their livelihood through potential transmission. The AMA has addressed this concern by developing a policy that would pay a lump sum disability benefit of up to $500,000 if an insured physician tests positive for HIV. The annual premium for this policy would be no more than $1,000.[2]

Several legal cases have focused on HIV-infected health care workers' claims of professional discrimination based on their HIV seropositivity and violation of the ADA.[8,15,32,45,54,63,73] In these cases, the courts have seemingly assessed "significant risk" of health care worker-to-patient transmission according to the four factors identified in the case of the *School Board of Nassau County v. Arline.*[71,72] The ruling in this case determined whether a person is not "otherwise qualified" under the Rehabilitation Act of 1973, 29 USC 794 according to the following:

1. the *nature* of the risk (how the disease is transmitted);
2. the *duration* of the risk (how long the carrier is infectious);
3. the *severity* of the risk (potential harm to third parties); and
4. the *probability* that the disease will be transmitted.

For example, in *Mauro v. Borgess Medical Center,*[54,80] a U.S. district court in Michigan found that an HIV-positive operating room surgical technician was not "otherwise qualified" under the ADA or the Rehabilitation Act. The medical center learned that the plaintiff might be HIV-positive and asked him to submit to testing. He refused, and when he also refused to accept an alternative accommodating position at the hospital, he was laid off. The court dismissed the plaintiff's claim of discrimination in violation of the ADA and Rehabilitation Act, finding that his HIV-positive condition disqualified him from working as a surgical technician and that he was not "otherwise qualified" to perform this job. The technician acknowledged that his position required him on occasion to place his hand upon and into surgical incisions and that this put him at risk for needle sticks or minor lacerations. The court agreed that there was a real possibility of transmission, and since the consequence of transmission of HIV is death, the nature, duration, and severity of the risk outweighed the fact that the chance of transmission was small. According to the requirements of the ADA and the Rehabilitation Act, the hospital had offered the plaintiff an accommodating position at a similar salary and benefits.

The decision in 1994 of *Bradley v. University of Texas M.D. Anderson Cancer Center*[15] concerned a surgical technician who the hospital learned from a newspaper article was HIV-positive. The employee was reassigned to a position that did not involve patient contact. He then sued the hospital and two supervisors, asserting his reassignment violated both the Rehabilitation Act and his First Amendment rights. The court concluded that while the risk of transmission of HIV was small in the performance of his duties as a surgical assistant, "it is not so small so as to nullify the catastrophic consequences of an accident." A cognizable risk of permanent duration with lethal consequences suffices to make a surgical technician with Bradley's responsibilities not "otherwise qualified." As to the First Amendment clause, the court's position was that it was not his speech—giving the information to the newspaper—but rather his HIV-positive status that laid the basis for the hospital's action. Thus, he was not the subject of retaliatory action for his exercise of First Amendment rights. Of note is that the U.S. Supreme Court has declined to review the decision in *Bradley*.

In *Doe v. University of Maryland Medical System Corporation*,[32] the Fourth U.S. Circuit Court of Appeals in 1995 said a Baltimore hospital acted properly in firing an HIV-positive neurosurgical resident because of the possibility that he might accidentally infect patients during surgical operations. The appeals court unanimously upheld a lower court ruling which had found that Dr. Doe posed "a significant risk to the health and safety of his patients." The appeals court said it would not substitute its judgment for that of the hospital's in assessing the risk to patients, even though it acknowledged that there have been no documented cases of surgeon-to-patient transmission of HIV since the epidemic was first detected in 1981. The decision was the first case in which a federal appeals court ruled on whether HIV-positive surgeons are protected from discrimination under terms of the ADA. In its ruling, the court stated that a hospital is allowed to "err on the side of caution in protecting its patients." The university had suspended the physician's hospital privileges, only to have an expert panel on bloodborne pathogens, which included infectious diseases specialists, the hospital epidemiologist, and consulting neurosurgeons, recommend that Doe be allowed to continue practicing surgery with the exception of a few specific procedures. As such, this recommendation seemed to follow the CDC guidelines of not restricting the practice of HIV-infected physicians, even for most surgical procedures. However, the hospital's senior administrators overruled the panel of experts and instead ended Doe's surgical practice and offered him an alternative residency in nonsurgical fields. When Doe refused, the hospital fired him from its residency program. The lawyer representing the hospital administration cited a study by Tokars and colleagues[79] which determined the incidence of nick or needle puncture injury for operating room surgeons that resulted in bleeding. The study found that surgeons accidentally injure themselves in 6.9% of all surgeries, especially when suturing wounds.

In *Scoles v. Mercy Health Corporation of Southeastern Pennsylvania*,[73,81] a federal district court in Philadelphia ruled in 1994 that the hospital did not violate the ADA or Rehabilitation Act in suspending an HIV-positive orthopedic surgeon and requiring him to tell prospective patients about his condition. Upon learning of the physician's HIV status, the defendant hospital asked the trial court to determine under Pennsylvania's Confidentiality of HIV-Related Information Act that there was a "compelling need" to inform the patients of the plaintiff physician of his HIV seropositivity. The hospital suspended Dr. Scoles' clinical privileges to perform invasive diagnostic or therapeutic procedures. Dr. Scoles sought a hearing under the medical center's bylaws. The center's medical board decided that he should be reinstated with full privileges after an *ad hoc* committee convened by the Board of Directors recommended that his privileges be reinstated under the condition that he inform his patients of his HIV status prior to any invasive procedures. The federal district court ruled that the medical center was entitled to prohibit Dr. Scoles from performing surgery without his patients' consent because his HIV status presented a "direct threat" to his patients.

If patients have a right to know their unforeseen risk of HIV exposure and infection in the health care workplace, then it follows that there may be a doctor's right to know the HIV status of his/her patient. A New York trial court recently ruled that HIV-infected patients have an affirmative duty to inform health care professionals of their seropositive status.[1,31,58] The court stated that although New York laws provide important protection for HIV-infected patients, they are not sufficient to release patients from their legal obligation to disclose their HIV-positive status to their health care providers, particularly when patients are about to undergo invasive procedures.

The above cases reflect the intricate balance between issues of confidentiality, the right to know, and discrimination as they pertain to protection, fairness, and legality in the health care workplace. The risk that infected surgeons and dentists pose to their patients is of a low, but uncertain magnitude. As Dr. Sheldon Landesman, renowned in AIDS clinical research and public policy, has succinctly stated:

> The public health response to a risk of uncertain magnitude is to act. The level of uncertainty at which public health officials are willing to take actions is relatively high. On the other hand, the civil libertarians say that we cannot act, we cannot intrude or limit the rights of the individual until we have a reasonable degree of certainty as to the magnitude and probability of the risk that an individual poses to the population. The severity and certainty of the risk is important to civil libertarians, because only defined risks of a significant magnitude justify curtailment of civil liberties. Risks of uncertain magnitude do not justify incursions by the state in the life of individuals.[50]

Public health and law must continue to find common ground until the AIDS epidemic is past.

REFERENCES

1. AIDS/HIV-infected patient must disclose status to physician. **ECRI.** 1993, pp 12-13
2. **Am Med News.** June 17, 1991, p 7
3. American College of Physicians and Infectious Diseases Society of America: Human immunodeficiency virus infection. **Clin Infect Dis 18**:963-973, 1994
4. American College of Physicians Ethics Manual. **Ann Intern Med 111**:245-252, 1989
5. Americans With Disabilities Act of 1990, 42 USC §12101 et seq
6. Angell M: A dual approach to the AIDS epidemic. **N Engl J Med 324**:1498-1500, 1991
7. Annas GJ: Control of tuberculosis–the law and the public's health. **N Engl J Med 328**:585-588, 1993
8. Appeals court upholds firing of HIV-positive doctor. **AIDS Policy Law 10(9)**:1-11, 1995
9. *Armstrong v Flowers Hospital, Inc,* 33 F3rd 1308 (11th Cir 1994)
10. Bayer R: Public policy and the AIDS epidemic. An end to HIV exceptionalism. **N Engl J Med 324:** 1500-1504, 1991
11. *Behringer v Medical Center at Princeton,* 592 A2d 1251 (NJ Super 1991)
12. Benenson AS: **Control of Communicable Diseases Manual.** Washington, DC: American Public Health Association, 1995
13. Bernat JL: **Ethical Issues in Neurology.** Boston, Mass: Butterworth-Heinemann, 1994, pp 287-310
14. Blendon RJ, Donelan K: Discrimination against people with AIDS: the public's perspective. **N Engl J Med 319**:1021-1026, 1988
15. *Bradley v University of Texas MD Anderson Cancer Center,* 3 F3d 922 (5th Cir 1993), *cert denied,* 510 US 1119 (1994)
16. Brudney K, Dobkin J: Resurgent tuberculosis in New York City: human immunodeficiency virus, homelessness, and the decline of tuberculosis control programs. **Am Rev Respir Dis 144**:745-751, 1991
17. Centers for Disease Control: **Estimates of Risk of Endemic Transmission of Hepatitis B Virus and Human Immunodeficiency Virus to Patients by the Percutaneous Route During Invasive Surgical and Dental Procedures.** Atlanta, Ga: Centers for Disease Control, 1991
18. Centers for Disease Control: Initial therapy for tuberculosis in the era of multidrug resistance: recommendations of the Advisory Council for the Elimination of Tuberculosis. **MMWR 42(RR-7)**:1-8, 1993
19. Centers for Disease Control: Recommendations for preventing transmission of human immunodeficiency virus and hepatitis B virus to patients during exposure-prone invasive procedures. **MMWR 40 (RR-8)**:1-9, 1991
20. Centers for Disease Control: Update: AIDS among women–United States, 1994. **MMWR 44**:81-84, 1995
21. Centers for Disease Control: Update: investigations of persons treated by HIV-infected health care workers–United States. **MMWR 42**:329-331, 337, 1993
22. Centers for Disease Control: Update: mortality at-

tributable to HIV infection among persons aged 25-44 years–United States, 1994. **MMWR 45:** 121-125, 1996

23. Centers for Disease Control: Update: transmission of HIV infection during invasive dental procedures–Florida. **MMWR 40:**377-381, 1991

24. Ciesielski C, Marianos D, Ou C-Y, et al: Transmission of human immunodeficiency virus in a dental practice. **Ann Intern Med 116:**798-805, 1992

25. Civil Rights Act of 1964, 42 USC §2000e et seq

26. Code of Medical Ethics: **Annotated Opinions of the Council on Ethical and Judicial Affairs of the American Medical Association.** Chicago, Ill: American Medical Association, 1992

27. Confidentiality of HIV-Related Information Act, PL 585, No. 148, 1990

28. Danila RN, MacDonald KL, Rhame FS, et al: A look-back investigation of patients of an HIV-infected physician: public health implications. **N Engl J Med 325:**1406-1411, 1991

29. Dickens BM: Legal limits of AIDS confidentiality. **JAMA 259:**3449-3452, 1988

30. *Doe v Centinela Hospital,* 57 USLW 2034, 1988 WL 81776 (CD Cal 1988)

31. *Doe v Roe,* 588 NYS2d 236 (Sup Ct 1992), *modified,* 599 NYS2d 350 (App Div 1993)

32. *Doe v University of Maryland Medical System Corporation,* 50 F3d 1261 (4th Cir 1995)

33. *Faya v Almaraz,* 620 A2d 327 (Md 1993)

34. Ficarra BJ, Dorian AL, Wecht CH: Ethics, in American College of Legal Medicine (ed): **Legal Medicine: Legal Dynamics of Medical Encounters. 2nd ed.** Philadelphia, Pa: Mosby-Year Book, 1991, pp 152-153

35. Gerberding JL, Littell C, Tarkington A, et al: Risk of exposure of surgical personnel to patients' blood during surgery at San Francisco General Hospital. **N Engl J Med 322:**1788-1793, 1990

36. Gostin LO: The AIDS litigation project. A national review of court and human rights commission decisions, part 1: The social impact of AIDS. **JAMA 263:** 1961-1970, 1990

37. Gostin LO: Controlling the resurgent tuberculosis epidemic. **JAMA 269:**255-256, 1993

38. Gostin LO: The HIV-infected health care professional: Public policy, discrimination, and patient safety. **Arch Intern Med 151:**663-665, 1991

39. Gostin LO, Curran WJ: AIDS screening, confidentiality, and the duty to warn. **Public Health Law 77:** 361-365, 1987

40. Gostin L, Curran WJ, Clark ME: The case against compulsory casefinding in controlling AIDS–Testing, screening, and reporting. **Am J Law Med 12:**7-53, 1986

41. Gramelspacher OP, Miles SH, Cassel CK: When the doctor has AIDS. **J Infect Dis 162:**534-537, 1990

42. Halevy A, Brody B: Acquired immunodeficiency syndrome and the Americans With Disabilities Act: A legal duty to treat. **Am J Med 96:**282-288, 1994

43. Health and Public Policy Committee, American College of Physicians, and the Infectious Diseases Society of America: The acquired immunodeficiency syndrome (AIDS) and infection with the human immunodeficiency virus (HIV). **Ann Intern Med 108:** 460-469, 1988

44. HIV-positive surgeon may be liable for patient's emotional distress. **J Health Hosp Law 26:**352, 1993

45. Hospital fires surgeon infected with HIV. **Lawyers Weekly USA 349:**95, April 24, 1995

46. *In Re Milton S Hershey Medical Center of Pennsylvania University,* 634 A2d 159 (Pa 1993), *affirming,* 595 A 2d 1290 (Pa Super 1991)

47. Jenner RK, Schupak S: Liability for HIV transmission. **Trial 28:**24-29, 1992

48. Kalkut G, Catalano MT, Steibigel NH: Tuberculosis, 1993–the captain still commands, in Mandell GL, Douglas RG Jr, Bennett JE (eds): **Principles and Practice of Infectious Diseases.** New York, NY: John Wiley & Sons, 1993, pp 3-22 (Supplement Chapter)

49. *Kerins v Hartley,* 17 Cal App 4th 713, 21 Cal Rptr 2d 621, (Cal App 1993), Cal App 4th 1699a *vacated,* 868 P2d 906 (Cal 1994)

50. Landesman SH: The HIV-positive health professional. Policy options for individuals, institutions, and states. Public policy and the public–observations from the front line. **Arch Intern Med 151:**655-657, 1991

51. *Leckelt v Board of Commissioners of Hospital District No. 1,* 909 F2d 820 (5th Cir 1990)

52. Lo B, Steinbrook R: Health care workers infected with the human immunodeficiency virus: the next steps. **JAMA 267:**1100-1105, 1992

53. Lo B, Steinbrook RL, Cooke M, et al: Voluntary screening for human immunodeficiency virus (HIV) infection: weighing the benefits and harms. **Ann Intern Med 110:**727-733, 1989

54. *Mauro v Borgess Medical Center,* 886 F Supp 1349 (WD Mich, 1995)

55. *Miller v Spicer,* 822 F Supp 158 (D Del 1993)

56. Mishu B, Schaffner W: HIV-infected surgeons and dentists. Looking back and looking forward. **JAMA 269:**1843-1844, 1993

57. The National Childhood Vaccine Injury Act of 1986, 42 USC §300aa-1 et seq

58. New York Supreme Court determines that HIV-infected patient has a legal duty to disclose HIV status to treating physician. **Risk Managers Law Alert 1(9):** 1-2, 1993

59. Orentlicher D: HIV-infected surgeons: *Behringer v Medical Center.* **JAMA 266:**1134-1137, 1991

60. Owens DK, Harris RA, Scott PM, et al: Screening surgeons for HIV infection. A cost-effectiveness analysis. **Ann Intern Med 122:**641-652, 1995

61. Pellegrino ED: Editorial response to Halevy and Brody. **Am J Med 96:**289-291, 1994

62. *Potter et al v Firestone Tire and Rubber Company,* 6 Cal 4th 965, 863 P2d 795, 25 Cal Rptr 2d 550

63. Reassignment of HIV-positive surgical assistant ruled legal. **Hosp Law Newsletter 11(12):**1-2, 1994

64. Reed BS: Testing health care workers for AIDS. **J Contemp Health Law Policy 8:**237- 244, 1992

65. Refusal to treat *Armstrong v Flowers Hospital.* **AIDS Policy Law.** February 10, 1995, p 3

66. Rehabilitation Act of 1973, Section 504, 29 USC §701 et seq

67. *Reissner v Regents of the University of California,* No. B076913 (Cal Ct App 2d App Dist Jan 26, 1995)

68. Risk analysis: AIDS liability. **ECRI.** 1993, pp 1-16

69. Robert LM, Chamberland ME, Cleveland JL, et al: Investigations of patients of health care workers infected with HIV. The Centers for Disease Control and Prevention Database. **Ann Intern Med 122:** 653-657, 1995

70. Rogers DE, Osborn JE: Another approach to the

AIDS epidemic. N Engl J Med 325:806-808, 1991

71. *School Board of Nassau County v Arline*, 480 US 273 (1987)

72. Schulman DI: HIV-infected health care providers: legal rights and protections. **Ann Emerg Med 20:** 1379-1380, 1991

73. *Scoles v Mercy Health Corporation of Southeastern Pennsylvania*, 887 F Supp 765 (ED Pa 1994)

74. Shelton DL: What's in a name. **Am Med News.** Nov 16, 1995, pp 13-14

75. Shuster E: A surgeon with acquired immunodeficiency syndrome: a threat to patient safety? The case of William H Behringer. **Am J Med 94:**93-9, 1993

76. Smego RA Jr, Barranco EA: AIDS legislation needed. **NY State J Med 90:**163, 1990 (Letter)

77. Study finds no HIV infections from health workers to patients. **AIDS Policy Law.** 1995, p 8

78. *Tarasoff v The Regents of the University of California*, 551 P2d 334 (Cal 1976)

79. Tokars JI, Bell DM, Culver DH, et al: Percutaneous injuries during surgical procedures. **JAMA 267:** 2899-2904, 1992

80. US Court in Michigan finds HIV-positive surgical technician not "otherwise qualified" under ADA and Rehabilitation Act. **Harv Law Digest 23**(7):13, 1995

81. US Court in Pennsylvania finds HIV-positive surgeon not "otherwise qualified" to perform invasive techniques and that he cannot sue under ADA or Rehabilitation Act. **Harv Law Digest 23**(1):9, 1995

82. US Department of Labor, Occupational Safety and Health Administration: Occupational exposure to bloodborne pathogens: final rule. 56 **Federal Register** 64004, 64175-64182 (1991)

83. *US v Morvant*, 898 F Supp 1157 (ED La 1995)

CHAPTER 17

PUBLIC HEALTH ISSUES: RADIATION

CHENG B. SAW, PHD, MATHIS P. FRICK, MD, AND LEROY J. KORB, MD

This chapter deals with the impact of radiation on the public health. Radiation is everywhere; it is emitted from the earth and space around us, as well as from artificially produced radionuclides and radiation-generating equipment. It is the latter sources that may cause medical and legal problems. Small amounts of radiation exposure may increase the risk of radiation damage to genetic material of many types of human cells. The damage is due to the ability of ionizing radiation to remove electrons from an atom, which can lead to the breakage of atomic bonds and thus disrupt the functioning of genetic molecules. In biological terms, the damage is cumulative and may express itself immediately in the form of "acute" reactions such as skin redness or diarrhea or in later years result in "chronic" problems such as leukemias or other cancers. Despite the known risks, the medical use of radiation is routine and beneficial, and as such, is an integral part of modern medicine.

The following discussion covers radiological units, background radiation from the natural environment, radiation from medical generating sources, and radiation from industrial projects such as nuclear weapons testing. There is also a review of the biological effects of radiation and risk estimates of radiation injury. Because of the risks associated with radiation injury, advisory boards such as the International Commission of Radiological Protection and the National Council on Radiation Protection and Measurements were formed to recommend guidelines for the safe use of radiation. A brief description of these commissions and their recommendations will be presented. In addition, the regulatory guidelines as adopted in the United States by federal and local government agencies, including the Food and Drug Administration, the Nuclear Regulatory Commission, and the Environmental Protection Agency, will be examined. Even though these regulations are intended to minimize exposure and prevent radiation incidents, adverse events do occur. The impact of these radiation incidents on the public, occupational personnel, and regulatory bodies will be discussed.

RADIOLOGICAL UNITS

The radiological unit of "radiation absorbed dose" is the rad, which equals 100 ergs of energy absorbed in a gram of matter. This unit is used for expressing radiation quantity received by living tissues in a patient or animal. The International System of Units (SI) for radiation absorbed dose is the gray (Gy). For conversion purposes, 100 rad equals 1 Gy. The next radiological unit of dose equivalent or occupational exposure is the rem (acronym of rad equivalent man). This unit is used to express the amount of radiation dose received by personnel working in a radiation environment—occupational exposure. In addition to the physical exposure, the rem also takes into account differences in the biological destructiveness of the different forms of radiation. For example, the thermal neutron, which is biologically more destructive, has been assigned a relative value of 5 while the photon (x-ray and gamma-ray) has a relative value of 1. The radiation dose of 1 rad to a person will be 5 rem from the neutron and 1 rem from the photon. Because of this biological consideration, rem is said to be the unit of dose equivalent. This biological consideration is particularly important to personnel working near nuclear reactors or particle accelerators, who may be exposed to various types of radiation. The SI for dose equivalent is the sievert (Sv). One sievert equals 100 rem. Another radiological unit of radiation exposure is the roentgen (R). This unit is defined in terms of the number of charges or ion pairs produced per unit volume as photons traverse through air. Although the rem, roentgen, and rad have slightly different values, they are assumed to have the same value here to simplify discussion in this chapter. The last radiological unit we will discuss is the curie (Ci), the quantitative description of radioactivity. One curie equals 3.7×10^{10} nuclear disintegrations per second (dps) from radioactive materials. The SI of radioactivity is the becqueral (Bq), which equals 1 dps.

Environmental Radiation

Natural environmental radiation contributes an estimated dose equivalent of 1 milliSv (mSv) annually to the general population.[1,2] The principal sources of natural environmental radiation are cosmic rays from space, terrestrial radionuclides in the soil and bedrock, such as radon-222, radium-226, and carbon-14, and radionuclides internal to all living organisms, such as potassium-40. The radiation exposure from natural sources varies considerably depending on the altitude, latitude, and the difference in radioactivity in the earth's crust. The intensity of extraterrestrial cosmic rays is significantly greater at higher altitudes and higher latitudes (the polar regions). Therefore, travel by airplane exposes crew and passengers to increased cosmic radiation. However, the largest contributor of natural radiation to the population in the U.S. is radon, a radioactive gas. Radon gas is produced through the natural decay of uranium, which is present in trace quantities in the earth's crust. Radon gas emits alpha particles which are helium nuclei. Helium nuclei generally do not penetrate deep into tissues but deposit their energy within a few millimeters of the surface. Radon's main effect relates to the damage of the mucosal region of the lung by alpha particles with the inhalation of the gas.

The primary source of man-made radiation exposure to the public is the medical use of ionizing radiation. The estimated average annual effective dose equivalent is .54 mSv.[1,2] This average value takes into account those persons not receiving any x-ray examinations as well as those receiving several exposures within a year. While health care is the largest source of man-made radiation exposure, one must consider that the benefits derived generally outweigh the risks. Nevertheless, the medical use of radiation must be carried out with prudence to minimize unwarranted radiation exposure to patients as well as personnel. The responsibility for the safe use of radiation falls primarily on the radiologic technologist, radiation therapist, medical physicist, radiation oncologist, radiologist, and nuclear medicine physician.

Other sources of man-made radiation are the testing and use of nuclear weapons, uranium mining, nuclear reactors used to generate electricity, consumer items, and the industrial use of radiation, such as the irradiation of food for preservation. At the height of atmospheric nuclear weapons testing in the early 1960s, nuclear fallout contributed about .05 mSv per year to radiation exposure. Today, the fallout exposure is less than .01 mSv. Nuclear power stations and other industrial applications do not contribute significantly to our radiation exposure. Consumer items such as watch dials, television sets, smoke detectors, and airport surveillance systems including air baggage inspection machines contribute a few millsievert to our annual exposure.

RADIATION INJURY

For many years after their discovery, x-rays and radioactive materials were used with little regard for their potentially harmful biological effects. Many early pioneers in the application of radiation in medicine died from the late effects of x-ray exposure. Madame Curie and her daughter are both suspected to have died from leukemia as a result of their radiation experiments. Early physicians and health care workers also used x-ray-producing equipment that lacked shielding. Furthermore, patients had to undergo lengthy radiation exposure from the low energy x-rays used at that time to obtain an acceptable radiograph from the units. These exposures occasionally led to severe skin burns, loss of hair, nausea, and anemia, as well as, after a time, leukemia and other cancers. Today, exposure to personnel and patients is greatly reduced as a result of better understanding of the biological effects of radiation and better equipment, as well as legal mandates.

The most catastrophic acute result of radiation exposure is death. High-level radiation exposure leading to death within hours, days, or weeks is called acute radiation syndrome. Depending on the dose, there may be hematological death (in weeks), gastrointestinal death (in days), or central nervous system death (in hours). The radiation exposure for hematological death due to bone marrow suppression is in the range of 200-1000 cGy. Gastrointestinal death occurs in the range of 1000-5000 cGy from the loss of gastrointestinal mucosa, leading to fluid electrolyte imbalances. Doses above 5000 cGy result in death due to overwhelming disruption of the central nervous system. Whole-body exposure is typically worse than partial-body exposure, since doses required for biological injury are less for larger volumes. Examples of total-body exposure occurred in the Chernobyl nuclear reactor incident in April 1986, while partial-body exposures are seen with diagnostic x-ray exposure. Thus far, side effects are rare and there have been no reported deaths following diagnostic x-ray exposure.

Daily observations of patients undergoing radiation therapy indicate that significant acute radiation injuries are rare. This is because low-level radiation outside the treatment field often leads only to sub-acute and latent injury. Most litigation occurs after more noticeable events associated with high-level radiation exposure. Because of the regulatory guidelines and the expected training required of radiation workers, these high doses of radiation are viewed as unusual, but do occur in the area of therapeutic radiology[3] and more rarely in diagnostic radiology.

The most common scenario for radiation injury in diagnostic radiology is a prolonged fluoroscopic procedure. This may result when a procedure such as cardiac catheterization or balloon angioplasty is difficult and therefore lengthy. Another scenario is obtaining radiographs of obese patients. These patients typically require several exposures before producing acceptable radiographs, resulting in higher exposures to the patient. In these cases, the skin and other superficial structures receive high doses of radiation. Reactions can range from immediate erythema to delayed breakdown or ulceration which may require plastic surgery to repair.

Radiation injuries are more common in therapeutic radiology, where high doses of radiation are used to treat cancer and the margin of safety is typically much lower. However, radiation injury is well understood in the treatment of cancer and untoward events often can be predicted. Litigation is rare, since most patients realize that there is a trade-off between doses that cause side effects and doses that are effective in controlling disease. Additionally, because no dose can be considered safe for all individuals, adverse effects do occasionally happen at doses considered "safe." Less common is unintentional overdosage caused by technical errors in either treatment planning or execution.[3,9] With the use of high-energy x-ray beams for therapeutic purposes, any injuries that may occur typically involve deeper structures and do not often affect the skin. Depending on the site, severe damage can result in fibrosis, scarring, bowel damage, fistulas, paralysis, or death. However, many of these chronic reactions may take months to years to occur and often cannot be distinguished from the original disease process.

Statutes of limitations may play a significant role in the litigation of chronic radiation reactions that can take years to develop. Each state has a statute of limitations that requires a suit to be filed within a certain period of time, typically 1 to 3 years, after infliction of personal injury. In most states, the courts apply a "discovery rule" to extend the limitations period for injuries that are not readily apparent, so that the limitations period does not begin to run until the plaintiff knows or could reasonably be expected to discover the existence of damage or injury. The limitations period also can be extended or "tolled" on the basis of fraudulent concealment, in which case the limitations period does not begin to run until actual discovery of the injury.[15] In the case of radiation injuries that takes years to develop, plaintiffs may assert that the fact of damage was not apparent or readily discoverable or was actively concealed, whereas defendants will assert that the plaintiffs knew or should have known of the *fact* of injury at some earlier date, even if the *extent* of injury was not immediately known.

A review of the *Medical Malpractice, Verdicts, Settlements and Experts* journal for the years 1995 and 1996 indicates that all but two cases of malpractice litigation related to radiology involved the failure to diagnose.[10,11] The two remaining cases dealt with errors in the administration of radiation.

In *Patient v. Dr. John Doe*,[10] the plaintiff underwent cancer surgery for carcinoma of the rectum in January 1992, followed with radiation therapy. The plan for radiation therapy approved by Dr. Doe consisted of a series of treatments with a specified dose over a specified number of days. The treatments were closely and continuously monitored and checked by the defendants. Three days after the completion of the treatment, the plaintiff was admitted to the hospital with a diagnosis of radiation enteritis. She was readmitted for bowel obstruction 3 days later. Ten days later, the plaintiff was found to have received twice the intended dose of radiation during each of her radiation therapy treatments. The plaintiff claimed that her radiation therapy treatments were negligently administered, specifically in delivering to her twice the daily prescribed dose, and resulted in long-term serious damage to her small bowel. A $1,484,000 settlement was reached between the parties.

In *Adamson v. Wimbush*,[11] the plaintiff received radiation therapy to stop possible ectopic bone growth around a total hip prosthesis. The radiation treatment scheme was to follow that of a Mayo Clinic protocol consisting of 10 fractions of radiation treatment, with 200 rad delivered in each fraction. Instead, all 2,000 rad were administered in a single fraction. The plaintiff sustained radiation burns to the upper right thigh, back, and front. There was damage to the femoral, sciatic, and peroneal nerves. The plaintiff lost all motion of the hip and knee and developed a foot drop. The treating radiologist admitted liability. The radiation technician and the owners of the hospital radiation department denied liability. This case was settled out of court for $1 million.

RADIATION ADVISORY COMMISSIONS

Several scientific and advisory committees have published risk estimates for ionizing radiation. These committees include the United Nations Scientific Committee on the Effects of Atomic Radiation (UNSCEAR), National Academy of Sciences—National Research Council, Committee on the Biological Effects of Ionizing Radiation, National Institutes of Health, International Commission on Radiological Protection, National Council on Radiation Protection and Measurements, and U.S. Nuclear Regulatory Commission. The sources of human exposure data for risk estimation include:

- survivors of the atomic bombing of Hiroshima and Nagasaki;
- children exposed prenatally as a result of abdominal x-ray examination;
- children treated for enlarged thymus glands by irradiation of the thymus or with scalp irradiation for tinea capitus;
- adults who underwent x-ray treatment to the spine for ankylosing spondylitis;
- adults who received radioactive iodine for treatment of thyroid conditions;
- individuals with body burden of radium; and
- uranium miners exposed to high levels of radioactive gases and radioactive particles.

An excellent review dealing with ionizing radiation and public health can be found in the text written by Shapiro.[12]

One of the most recent and widely quoted risk estimates is from Report No. 5 of the National Academy of Sciences Committee on the Biological Effects of Ionizing Radiation (BEIR V), 1990. The BEIR V report used the linear quadratic dose-effect model for leukemia estimates and the linear dose-effect model for all other cancers.[4] The effects of age at the time of irradiation and the time elapsed since irradiation were also considered. There was an assumed latency period of 2 years after irradiation for leukemia and 10 years after for all other cancers. The relative-risk model of cancer incidence as a function of age based on the recent trends in stochastic effects (i.e., the probability of such effects occurring increases with increasing radiation exposure, but not the severity of the effects) among the atomic bomb survivors was also included in the estimation.

To reduce appreciated risks associated with using ionizing radiation, advisory groups were formed all over the world to establish acceptable limits of exposure. Such advisory groups included the American Roentgen Ray Society, the American Radium Society, and the International Commission on Radiological Protection (ICRP), which was formed by the International Congress of Radiology. In 1929, the U.S. advisory committee on x-ray and radium protection, known now as the National Council on Radiation Protection and Measurements (NCRP) was formed to interpret the recommendations of the ICRP for the United States.[6]

The philosophy of these groups was to establish upper limits of radiation exposure, to theoretically minimize the hazards to individuals and the population as a whole but not encumber the beneficial use of radiation. These groups took into consideration social and economic aspects of protection (i.e., shielding materials, monitoring devices, personnel restrictions, and remote control techniques). In practice, the radiation protection principle is to keep the radiation exposure to individuals "as low as reasonably achievable" (also known as the ALARA principle).

In developing acceptable upper dose limits of ionizing radiation exposure to personnel, the ICRP and NCRP divided the population into occupationally exposed individuals and members of the general public (those with no occupational exposure to radiation). The acceptable dose limits of radiation exposure have been revised numerous times. The most recent recommendations of the NCRP *Report No. 116* (1993) are given in Table 1.[6] The effective dose (E) limits do not include the exposures from natural background or medical exposures when the person is a patient. The term "effective dose" is used to imply the same probability of the occurrence of cancer and genetic effects whether the dose is received by the whole body through uniform irradiation or partial body or individual organ irradiation. The effective dose limit for a radiation worker is set at 50 mSv/year, while for the general public the limit is set at 5 mSv/year for infrequent exposure. If a radiation worker is pregnant, the embryo/fetus is subjected to a more stringent requirement than the occupational exposed limit. The total exposure limit to the embryo/fetus should not exceed 0.5 mSv/month. In most instances, when the pregnancy is made known, the duties of the pregnant worker are modified so that the exposure limit cannot be reached. Such measures follow the ALARA principle. The exposure limit for students undergoing educational training is set at 1 mSv per year.

UNITED STATES REGULATORY AGENCIES

The use of ionizing radiation-producing units is governed either by the individual states or the U. S. Nuclear Regulatory Commission (NRC). The NRC regulates all reactor-produced (by-product) materials such as cobalt-60, while the naturally occurring radioactive materials and x-ray producing units (linear accelerators and x-ray machines) are regulated by individual state agencies. Through an agreement with the NRC, some states (referred to as agreement states) are allowed to govern those by-product materials usually regulated by the NRC. The NRC regulations are contained in Parts 20 and 35 of the Code of Federal Regulations.[5,13] Some of these regulations have been enacted in response to problems brought to the attention of the NRC. The NRC has also enacted a quality management program to attempt to minimize

TABLE 1
DOSE-LIMITING RECOMMENDATIONS OF RADIATION EXPOSURE*

Occupational Exposures (annual)	
Effective dose limits	
annual	50 mSv
cumulative	10 mSv × age
Equivalent dose annual limits for tissues and organs	
lens of eye	150 mSv
skin, hands, and feet	500 mSv
Public Exposures (annual)	
Effective dose limit, continuous or frequent exposure	1 mSv
Effective dose limit, infrequent exposure	5 mSv
Equivalent dose limits for tissues and organs	
lens of eye	15 mSv
skin, hands, and feet	50 mSv
Education and Training Exposures (annual)	
Effective dose limit	1 mSv
Equivalent dose limits for tissues and organs	
lens of eye	15 mSv
skin, hands, and feet	50 mSv
Embryo/Fetus Exposure (monthly)	
Equivalent dose limit	0.5 mSv

* Reproduced with permission from the *National Council on Radiation Protection and Measurements Report No. 116.*[6]

or eliminate errors, in particular human errors. Again, this enactment is based on the assessment of past incidents reported to the NRC.

The requirements of notifying either the state or the NRC of any adverse radiation event depends on the severity of the incident. Notification must be immediate for serious events, such as the loss of a radiation source in quantities that are deemed hazardous to the people in unrestricted areas. The notification is followed by a written report within 30 days.[13] The notification must also be immediate if an individual receives: 1) a total effective dose equivalent of more than 250 mSv; 2) an eye dose equivalent of more than 750 mSv; or 3) a shallow-dose equivalent of more than 250 cGy. Less severe events require notification within 24 hours. Notification also must be made in the event of misadministration. Currently there are six categories of misadministrations (Table 2). In the event of a misadministration (i.e., the unin-

tended administration of radioisotopes or radiation from by-product materials), the NRC must be notified within the next calendar day after the discovery. As part of the NRC regulation, the referring physician (the physician who refers the patient to the radiation oncologist, radiologist, or nuclear medicine physician) and the patient also must be informed of the incident within 24 hours unless the referring physician personally informs the authorized user (radiation oncologist, radiologist, or nuclear medicine physician) that either he/she will tell the patient or that, based on medical judgment, telling the patient would be harmful. Furthermore, a written report (which includes a description of the event, why the event occurred, effect on the patient, what improvements are needed to prevent recurrence, actions taken to prevent recurrence, and whether the patient has been informed) must be submitted to the NRC within 15 days.

TABLE 2

Misadministration Classifications (NRC Part 35.2)

1. A radiopharmaceutical dosage greater than 30 mCi of either sodium iodide I^{125} or I^{131}:
   - Involving the wrong patient or wrong radiopharmaceutical, or
   - When both the administered dosage differs from the prescribed dosage by more than 20% of the prescribed dosage and the difference between the administered dosage and prescribed dosage exceeds 30 mCi.

2. A therapeutic radiopharmaceutical dosage, other than sodium iodide I^{125} or I^{131}:
   - Involving the wrong patient, wrong radiopharmaceutical, or wrong route of administration, or
   - When the administered dosage differs from the prescribed dosage by more than 20% of the prescribed dosage.

3. A gamma stereotactic radiosurgery radiation dose:
   - Involving the wrong patient or wrong treatment site, or
   - When the calculated total administered dose differs from the total prescribed dosage by more than 10% of the prescribed dose.

4. A teletherapy radiation dose:
   - Involving the wrong patient, wrong mode of treatment, wrong treatment site, or
   - When the treatment consists of three or fewer fractions and the calculated total administered dose differs from the total prescribed dose by more than 10% of the total prescribed dose, or
   - When the calculated weekly administered dose is 30% greater than the weekly prescribed dose, or
   - When the calculated total administered dose differs from the total prescribed dose by more than 20% of the total prescribed dose.

5. A brachytherapy radiation dosage:
   - Involving the wrong patient, wrong radioisotope, wrong treatment site (excluding, for permanent implants, seeds that were implanted in the correct site but migrated outside the treatment site), or
   - Involving a sealed source that is leaking, or
   - When, for a temporary implant, one or more sealed sources are not removed upon completion of the procedure, or
   - When the calculated administered dose differs from the prescribed dose by more than 20% of the prescribed dose.

6. A diagnostic radiopharmaceutical dosage, other than quantities greater than 30 mCi of either sodium iodide I^{125} or I^{131}, both:
   - Involving the wrong patient, wrong radiopharmaceutical, wrong route of administration, or when the administered dosage differs from the prescribed dosage, and
   - When the dose to the patient exceeds 5 rems effective dose equivalent or 50 rems dose equivalent to any individual organ.

IMPACT OF RADIATION INCIDENTS

As alluded to above, the NRC maintains a reporting system in the event an incident occurs. The NRC generally investigates the event and formulates a report. The report is presented to the authorities of the "offending" institution for further action. Meanwhile, the institutional personnel charged with overseeing the use of the radioisotopes and radiation from by-product materials, typically the radiation safety officer and/or medical physicist, perform their own investigations to determine if there is any weakness of the program which led to the incident. Corrective action is proposed to ensure that such an incident will not recur.[7,9] The final step is either an admission of the weakness in the program, followed by corrective action, or a negotiation with the NRC leading to taking the appropriate steps to ensure the incident will not occur again. Depending on the type and severity of the infraction, a fine may be imposed by the NRC. Since the NRC is obliged to inform the public, the fear and lack of understanding of radiation often leads the public to adopt a fearful attitude towards the use of radiation and increases the risk of malpractice litigation.

Any incident involving x-ray producing units not regulated by the NRC must be reported to the appropriate local government agencies. Procedures identical to those used by the NRC generally have been adopted by the local government agencies. However, the mechanism of reporting incidents often may not have been properly established. Consequently, there are not many documented incidents involving radiation producing equipment cited in the literature.

In addition, the U.S. Pharmacopoeia maintains a medical device and laboratory product problem reporting program. Reports voluntarily submitted by practitioners are forwarded to the manufacturer and the U.S. Center for Device and Radiological Health. This reporting program serves as a method of informing users and/or owners of the possible safety hazards of devices, in particular radiation therapy devices.

In spite of the many regulations and precautions taken, accidents have occurred. Shapiro[12] reviewed accidents associated with: 1) the dropping of atomic bombs over Palomares, Spain in 1966; 2) the crashing of a bomber and its nuclear weapons near Thule, Greenland in 1968; 3) the plutonium contamination of a weapons plant in Rocky Flats, Colorado; and 4) the nuclear plant accident at Three Mile Island, Pennsylvania. The most recent nuclear reactor accident occurred at the Chernobyl nuclear power plant, in Russia, in April 1986. It was the worst disaster in the history of nuclear power, producing the most serious contamination ever recorded.[14] Approximately 1.85×10^{18} Bq of different radionuclides escaped from the power plant, and more than 21,000 sq km of soil was contaminated with levels higher than 3.7×10^{10} Bq/sq km.

With respect to state-regulated radiation producing units, there have been few documented radiation accidents other than those that have been publicized by the media. These include the malfunctioning of the computerized linear accelerator in Tyler, Texas and the reporting of radiation violations by the *Cleveland Plain Dealer*. However, the most eventful medical-related accident occurred in November 1992 at Indiana (Pennsylvania) Regional Cancer Center, involving high-dose-rate brachytherapy. Information on most of the radiation incidents involving by-product materials has been disseminated by the NRC.

Enforcement actions have been taken by the NRC for noncompliance with its regulations. These enforcement actions are published on a quarterly basis in the Nuclear Material Safety and Safeguards (NMSS) Licensee Newsletter and as a Semiannual Progress Report in *NUREG-0940*.[7] *NUREG-0940*, Volume 15, No. 1, Part 3 is a compilation of significant enforcement actions that were resolved during the period from January to June of 1996. Included in the publication are copies of letters, notices, and orders sent by the NRC to material licensees with regard to the enforcement actions. There were 13 civil penalties and orders issued to material licensees within the first half of 1996 (Table 3). The table demonstrates that the dollar amount of penalties can vary significantly depending on the severity of the violations. Out of the 13 civil penalties, five were associated with medically related violations. Three of the five violations dealt directly with quality management programs and related to the administration of radiopharmaceuticals, the training of employees in the administration of brachytherapy, and the identification of correct radioactive sources in the administration of brachytherapy. The largest penalty was handed down to Oncology Services Corporation to emphasize to the licensee, and to the medical industry in general, the importance of meticulous management oversight of the radiation safety program. The action taken by the NRC was based on an event which occurred in November 1992 at Indiana, Pennsylvania, in which a 4.2-Ci iridium source was left inside a patient who was undergoing a brachytherapy treatment using a high-dose-rate afterloading unit. The patient received a very high radiation

TABLE 3

SUMMARY OF PROPOSED IMPOSITION OF CIVIL PENALTIES BY THE
NUCLEAR REGULATORY COMMISSION (JANUARY TO JUNE 1996)

Asford Presbyterian Community Hospital	$2,500
Ashland Petroleum Corporation	$500
B & W Fuel Company	$12,500
Bemis Construction, Inc.	$2,500
Combustion Engineering Inc.	$12,500
Department of Army, Madigan Army Medical Center	$8,000
Department of Navy, San Diego Naval Medical Center	$2,500
Diamond H Testing Company	$8,000
The Duriron Company, Inc.	$2,500
Foley Construction Services	$1,000
Monsanto Chemical Company	$2,500
Oncology Services Corporation	$280,000
Radiation Oncology Center at Marlton	$80,000

exposure and subsequently died. In addition, numerous individuals in the public were needlessly exposed to radiation in this incident. The investigation of this accident resulted in the publication of *NUREG-1480* by the NRC.[8]

Instead of a civil penalty, the NRC may issue warnings to encourage prompt corrective actions by the material licensees. During the first half of 1996, the NRC issued such communications to 19 material licensees.[7]

Besides imposing civil penalties on the "offending" institution, individuals involved in the event may also be penalized. The sanction may prohibit the individual from being involved with NRC-licensed activities for a certain number of years. Names of these individuals are published in the *NMSS Licensee Newsletter*.

To summarize, benefits usually outweigh the risks associated with the medical use of radiation. Today, exposure to staff and patients has been greatly reduced, in part through a better understanding of the biological effects of radiation. A strong and rigorous quality management program would reduce the risk of malpractice due to radiation exposure. Advisory and governing bodies play important roles in the reduction of exposure to individuals. Though radiation incidents do occur, preventive actions continually are being implemented based on past experiences. Failure to comply with regulations can lead to federal or state sanctions, and often civil and criminal actions.

REFERENCES

1. American Association of Physicists in Medicine. Report No. 18. A Primer on Low-Level Ionizing Radiation and Its Biological Effects. New York, NY: AIP, 1986
2. Bushong SC: Radiological Science for Technologists, Physics, Biology, and Protection. 5th ed. St Louis, Mo: Mosby-Year Book, 1993, pp 6-7
3. Cohen L, Schultheiss TE, Kennaugh RC: A radiation overdose incident: initial data. Int J Radiat Oncol Biol Phys 33:217-224, 1995
4. Committee on the Biological Effects of Ionizing Radiation: Health Effects of Exposure to Low Levels of Ionizing Radiation. National Academy of Sciences/National Research Council (BEIR V). Washington, DC: National Academy Press, 1990
5. Human Uses of Byproduct Materials. 35 CFR 1-20 (1994)
6. National Council on Radiation Protection and Measurements Report No. 116: Limitation of Exposure to Ionizing Radiation. Bethesda, Md: National Council on Radiation Protection and Measurements, 1993
7. NUREG-0940. Enforcement Actions: Significant Actions Resolved Material Licensees, Semiannual Progress Report, January-June, 1996. Volume 15, No. 1, Part 3. Washington, DC: US Government Printing Office, 1996
8. NUREG-1480. Loss of an Ir-192 Source and Therapy Misadministration at Indiana Regional Cancer Cen-

ter, Indiana, Pennsylvania on November 16, 1992. Pittsburgh, Pa: US Government Printing Office, 1992

9. Ostrom LT, Rathbun P, Cumberlin R, et al: Lessons learned from investigations of therapy misadministration events. **Int J Radiat Oncol Biol Phys 34:** 227-234, 1996

10. Plaintiff claims twice the daily dosage negligently administered during radiation therapy–radiation enteritis. **Medical Malpractice Verdicts Settlements Experts 11:**45, April 1995

11. Radiologist administers two thousand rads in one segment instead of two hundred rads in ten segments —causes severe radiation burns and permanent disability of one leg. **Medical Malpractice Verdicts Settlements Experts 12:**52, August 1996

12. Shapiro J: **Radiation Protection. A Guide for Scientists and Physicians.** 3rd ed. Cambridge, Mass: Harvard University Press, 1990

13. Standard for Protection Against Radiation. 20 CFR 1-48 (1993)

14. Weinberg AD, Kripalani S, McCarthy PL, et al: Caring for survivors of the Chernobyl disaster. What the clinician should know. **JAMA 274:**408-412, 1995

15. West Virginia Code Chapter 55-7B-4. **Health Care Injuries; Limitations of Actions; Exceptions.** Charlottesville, Va: The Michie Company, 1994, 475 pp

CHAPTER 18

TOXIC EXPOSURES: THE EXPERT WITNESS IN ENVIRONMENTAL TOXIC TORT LITIGATION

ALAN M. DUCATMAN, MD, MS

In "toxic tort" litigation, monetary compensation is sought for personal injury allegedly caused either by toxic chemical substances or by physical or biological agents. Some authors have defined this term more narrowly and limit it to encounters with toxic chemical waste.[4] In this chapter, toxic tort litigation is used in a broader sense, to include poisonings from toxic items in the home, such as childhood lead poisonings, and encounters with ambient phenomena, such as manmade electromagnetic fields. An encompassing definition of toxic litigations includes lawsuits seeking recovery for exposures to toxic waste, to physical hazards incidental to energy production and distribution, and to occupational exposures not addressed by workers' compensation, such as an allegation of intentional injury or an exposure caused by someone other then the employer, consumer exposures, and other environmental exposures.[22]

The right to recover compensation for harm from toxic exposure might be claimed under several legal "theories": trespass, nuisance (devaluing or limiting the use of land), breach of warranty, negligence (implying lack of due care), intentional misconduct, and strict liability (ab-

normally dangerous activity or defective and unreasonably dangerous product). In practice, toxic tort lawsuits are most commonly filed under theories of strict liability, which require only that a dangerous substance was used and that it can be shown to have caused harm. Neither foreknowledge of risk nor unacceptable behavior is required, although awards may be greater if either is present. Toxic tort actions may apply to single individuals such as a lead-poisoned child, to small groups of individuals such as a disease "cluster," or to large groups such as in "mass toxic torts." Examples of mass toxic torts include silicone breast implants for patients and asbestos exposures for workers. This chapter will concentrate on environmental settings (such as asbestos), rather than medical examples. Expanded discussions of legal aspects of litigation are included elsewhere in this book.

Under workers' compensation laws, exposure-outcome issues involve similar problems but take place in a different legal environment. Workers' compensation is designed to be a "no fault," wage-replacement and medical benefits system. When there is litigation, the use of experts is generally less intensive and the burden of proof historically is lower in workers' compensation cases. For example, workers' compensation laws may find in favor of the plaintiff-employee provided that the employer added *any* burden to pre-existing risks or conditions. In toxic tort litigation, the alleged outcome must be substantially related to the alleged cause, and the ability of the agent to cause the outcome is usually required to be well accepted. Toxic tort litigation should also be distinguished from legislated solutions to nationwide exposure problems, such as the federal programs for coal miners and certain veterans exposed to toxic substances.

Physicians may appear in toxic tort litigation either as "outside experts" or "treating clinicians." All physicians are regarded as experts due to education, training, and licensing requirements. National prominence is an additional expectation of "outside experts" but not of "treating clinicians" in toxic torts. There is some thought that treating physicians may be afforded additional credibility by courts because of a perceived lack of bias,[38] but there are no data to support or refute the concept that treating physicians give more meaningful or less biased testimony.

A persistent problem of expert testimony is germane to the role of the testifying expert physician in toxic tort litigation. Courts have great difficulty in determining whether expert testimony is valid in cases involving exposure-outcome allegations. This is understandable since most toxic tort allegations feature experts who provide diametrically opposed opinions. Critical to many courts' acceptance of expert testimony are the *Frye* Rule of 1923 and the critical modern precedent known as the *Daubert Decision*. (See Chapter 4 on trial testimony for references to these cases and a discussion of their significance.) From a clinician's perspective, it appears that the legal standard is that expert testimony be based on valid scientific theories and "trustworthy" data. Issues such as peer-reviewed publications, textbook commentary, repeatability of findings, falsifiability of data, and general acceptance of hypotheses by the scientific community ultimately enter into the court's recognition of reliable scientific evidence. Nevertheless, different courts still interpret the weight and acceptability of evidence in markedly different ways. The responsibility of

the expert physician witness is a consistent need to provide the most presentable opinion. What is the most "presentable" opinion? A colleague, himself the author of several texts, teaches the "grand rounds" rule. The expert will do well in court so long as the position taken is one that would happily be presented to peers during grand rounds at a hospital, or whichever professional venue one chooses, as requiring clinical excellence in the face of informed skepticism. One expert has recommended that testimony be treated as a scholarly endeavor and that expert witnesses first obtain review of their opinions from peers.[7] The mechanisms for doing this are not now clear, however, and the additional costs to all sides in disputes could be considerable.

Role of the Expert and Initial Contact With the Attorney in Toxic Tort Litigation

Why are experts needed when there are disagreements concerning environmental causation? Basically, "outside experts" are needed to define the diagnosis and to establish whether a diagnosis is related to an environmental "insult." These are the central issues for the court, and establishing the truth about them is the job of the expert. In performing these duties, it is essential that the expert provide an honest view of best available medical science. There are several helpful rules that guide expert behavior in this endeavor. First, the experts should give testimony not factually different than if they were appearing for the opposite side in the same dispute. Second, the expert should understand that winning or losing "the case" is the job of attorneys. The job of the expert is to explain the data and tell the truth, including factual data that are inconvenient from the perspective of the expert's "side" in the dispute if a question pertaining to such data is posed. Attorneys point out that experts can honestly focus on different facts depending upon who is asking the questions. This is correct; the expert need not volunteer information, but must not be evasive when questions pertaining to "inconvenient" data are posed. Furthermore, experts can gain credibility by volunteering such information if it is important. To expert clinicians, legal aspects of the case are the attorney's domain. The job of the expert is to be a scholar, not a partisan.[7]

Before that expertise is called upon in formal legal settings, however, the expert must make decisions concerning whether to participate and the circumstances of any participation. Attorneys call on potential experts in toxic tort cases for many reasons. Usually, the reason is to understand if the expert can help. An alternative potential reason for an initial contact is to "neutralize" a witness considered important to the other side's argument. Once a physician has committed to discussion of the merits of a case with one side of a legal dispute, there are potential ethical constraints to activities undertaken on behalf of the other.[16] Therefore, it can be important to consider carefully what to discuss with attorneys seeking support.

For example, in a mass asbestos toxic tort litigation involving thousands of Gulf Coast shipyard workers, the author received telephone calls from opposing attorneys on the same day—each claiming that a published paper concerning quality assurance problems in asbestos x-ray evaluations[15] was vital to their respective cases. The importance of these data diminished when the response to both attorneys was an offer to appear before the judge to explain the findings as a "friend of the court." From the attorneys' perspective, the witness was now efficiently neutralized. No further action was needed, the outcome was satisfactory for all interested in the legal aspects of the case. Each attorney could now prepare for battle without facing the distressing possibility of an opposing witness capable of suggesting that their experts' x-ray interpretations of pneumoconiosis were less reliable than the opponents'.

When is it reasonable to agree to appear in a toxic tort lawsuit? A "treating clinician" can always appear to recount the findings and conclusions that pertain to one or more of his/her patients. A clinician whose expertise is relevant and whose perspective may add something to the evaluation of the case can appear as a witness or can advise attorneys about factual aspects of their case. A clinician who has never or infrequently been involved in legal settings can, nevertheless, agree to appear or advise. In

fact, honest and straightforward opinions from those who do not relish legal encounters are valuable to litigants and to society. They reduce unnecessary litigation and serve to caution litigants about clinical realities of their cases.[5] Motivations for appearance include obligation to patient(s), respect for truth, professional satisfaction, advocacy of economic or social needs, and personal gain.[12] Some of these are better motivations than others. For all motivations, experts need be prepared to swear to tell the truth. It is important to remember that one can be helpful and still decline participation if the facts of the case sound tenuous at the outset or become tenuous as the case progresses, if the expert is too busy, or even if the issue does not particularly interest the clinician. Once engaged in the process, the expert has several responsibilities: verify with attorneys that the records reviewed are complete; always let attorneys know when it is appropriate that there be discussions between experts; be cautious concerning activities which may decrease objectivity, such as strategy sessions with attorneys.[16]

Issues for the Expert

There is substantial literature concerning *legal* aspects of toxic tort litigation, but few practical guides to *physician* expert behavior. The expert witness in toxic tort cases alleging a health outcome may clarify several issues concerning causation. These are:

1. Does the patient have a condition? (In the case of a population, are there physiologically related conditions?)
2. Is the condition the same as alleged?
3. Was the patient or population exposed to a hazard?
4. Does the condition follow reasonably from exposure events, with appropriate temporal sequence (temporal plausibility)? Are there other population issues that increase or decrease the plausibility that the condition follows from exposure?
5. Is the toxicology or physiology of exposure plausibly related to the outcome ("qualitative plausibility")? Is the extent of the exposure within the range of the hypothesized or known relationship ("quantitative plausibil-

ity")?

6. Is toxic exposure a more likely cause of the condition than other possible alternative causes?

7. Do epidemiological or other data link the exposure(s) to the outcome of interest? What is the strength and consistency of the relationship? If there are no epidemiological data, is there an accepted, known association anyway?

Toxic tort litigations are often decided in favor of plaintiffs when critical features of this cascade are in place. This does not mean that all features must be present. Recognition of exposure-outcome relationships need not always be accompanied by physiological understanding or epidemiological characterization. Unfortunately, decisions are also rendered in favor of the plaintiff when requisite conditions are absent and an etiological relationship unlikely.

A physician expert may be called to testify about any or all of the critical issues listed above. An additional role of certain experts may be to advise attorneys concerning the testimony of opposing experts. This expert has a role very close to the legal, adversarial aspects of the case and may wish to avoid appearing in court.

An early responsibility of an expert physician is to assist the interested attorneys to appropriately define the expert role. For example, the treating physician may be an expert yet limit testimony to stating how the patient came to his/her attention, whether the patient is ill, whether the condition is the one alleged and how its diagnosis follows from specific, enumerated findings, and whether the temporal sequence relating outcome to exposure is plausible. In contrast, an expert physician who has not cared for the patient may be called to testify about the known toxicology and epidemiology of exposure of interest in relationship to the patient's condition. Experts may also serve both roles. It is the responsibility of the testifying physician to limit testimony to appropriate areas of expertise.

Clinicians are taught to think in terms of symptoms, physical findings, laboratory data, and treatment. The expert witness should also think like an autopsy pathologist, working both forward and backward between outcomes and causes. Some steps to help in the process are discussed in the following.

Does the Patient Have a Condition?

In order to receive tort compensation, patients generally must have a condition. Courts resist compensation for concepts such as "reasonable fear" of illness or "increased risk" unless there is some present manifestation of the deleterious results of exposure.[28] Plaintiff populations may sometimes be granted financial access to routine medical surveillance when increased risk is documented. This medical surveillance award is not the same thing as compensation for fear of illness,[4] and claimants rarely are given other awards if risk of disease is the only issue. A critical introductory question when examining environmental torts is, therefore, whether the patient has a diagnosis. Although this sounds simple to physicians, it is a persistent issue in toxic tort litigation. Controversy concerning the presence or absence of illness occurs in several settings. Most legal writing concerning toxic tort litigation focuses on pitfalls and interpretations of epidemiology. In practical experience, the presence and nature of the disease entity may be as important.

One example of controversy (among many that could be featured) involves claims of immune suppression, immune activation, or immune complex disease following chemical exposure. [The alleged problem is sometimes called "immune dysregulation."] Untold thousands of patients have been told that they are ill following substantial or trivial chemical exposures, supported partly on the basis of batteries of allegedly abnormal immunological tests. Testing has frequently included antismooth muscle, antiparietal cell, anti brush border, and antimitochondrial antibodies, as well as interleukin levels and T-cell subsets. Once patients were told that their immune systems were altered, many legal actions were initiated. Occupational physicians seeing the same patients on a referral basis reported anecdotally, but consistently, that these laboratory results were not reproducible. (The cost of repeating such testing can be substantial.) Furthermore, physical examinations did not show any consistent pattern of findings referable to the immune system other than disconnection between symptom description and observable signs.

The issue of "immune dysregulation" reached

a climax when the most popular laboratory providing the testing was sent blinded specimens under experimental conditions. Authors from this laboratory had published a series of peer-reviewed reports demonstrating immune abnormalities in patient populations with alleged chemical sensitivity. These reports were technically sophisticated, but it was not clear that they were based on interpretation of blinded specimens. Once adequately blinded, the laboratory diagnosed *more* immune abnormalities in back pain patient controls than in the group diagnosed by treating clinicians to have immunological abnormalities following chemical exposure.[34] Laboratory findings once cited to support clinical diagnosis of immune dysregulation and legal claims for compensation are now rarely mentioned in legal settings, although other concerns of the same population (including neuropsychological responses to odors) are under active scientific investigation.

A federal appeals court subsequently supported exclusion of expert testimony concerning the allegation of illness in patients with one of the syndrome beliefs featuring immune dysregulation, "multiple chemical sensitivity." The U.S. Court of Appeals for the Seventh Circuit ruled that the opinion of experts concerning the cause of this syndrome was subjective and speculative.[3] The courts were not saying (and cannot say) that the patients were well. Rather, the decision stated that the burden of proof for a specific diagnosis had not been met. Since then, the focus of research (and legal) attention on this group of patients has evolved rapidly from immunological assertions to other issues. Two lessons from the rash of immune toxicity claims were that trivial differences from laboratory reference ranges did not have much significance in the context of human immunological disease, and that courts should not consider tests to have diagnostic significance if they cannot be repeated.[13] It is, nevertheless, doubtful that the last salvo in this legal battle has been fired or that courts will react to available evidence in predictable ways.

Rejection of offered testimony in the case described above was based in large measure on concerns about validity of claims concerning the existence of an outcome. Refutation of expert testimony is not a trivial undertaking, however. A Portuguese-descended toddler was exposed to lead paint from her apartment. She eventually required four courses of chelation therapy treatments for lead poisoning. When she was old enough, educational and neuropsychological testing revealed substantial, persistent deficits. The plaintiffs' attorney presented medical witnesses from several disciplines who described a number of developmental and educational impairments, attributed in substantial part to lead. Expert defense witnesses for the landlord countered that there was no illness or impairment; the child was merely bilingual and therefore expected to perform poorly. The child's teachers had testified previously that they planned to retain the child in second grade. During this testimony, evidence was presented that most of the child's class was also bilingual. The jury rejected bilingualism as an alternative diagnosis for lead poisoning and found for the plaintiff. Triple damages were awarded.[23] The explanation of a deficit implicit in bilingual status, especially when pertaining to a child failing in a class of more successful bilingual children, was insufficient to reverse the concept of harm to this child. Expert opinion that illness does or does not exist must be based on convincing data.

Is the Condition the Same as Alleged?

These are critical questions for illness or death attributed to a known cause, especially if there is a potential competing cause. Asbestos-related disease may provide the most common historic example.

Potentially compensable diseases due to asbestos exposure include asbestosis (parenchymal fibrosis of the lungs, a pneumoconiosis), pleural fibrosis (thickening of the lung lining) especially if associated with respiratory impairment, lung cancer (all cell types), and malignant mesothelioma (cancer of the lining around lung and gut). Other potential outcomes of asbestos exposure are less frequent subjects of litigation. Controversy can exist in legal settings when any of the asbestos-related diagnoses are made. This is particularly the case because several of the asbestos-related outcomes, such as respiratory problems attributed to asbestosis and lung cancer, have an important alternative/contributing cause (i.e., cigarette smoking).

For example, the diagnosis of asbestosis can be made with relative certainty at autopsy (if done by an expert) but rests on clinical judgment before death.[33] The less severe the disease, the more judgment is an issue. A "significant" occupational exposure is essential, as are appropriate latency from initial exposure and radiographic demonstration of bilateral small irregular lung parenchymal opacities in the lower lobes and often associated with pleural charges. Spirometry may sometimes be distinctive, but most commonly shows abnormalities which are neither specific for asbestosis nor able to rule it out.[33] In the face of these uncertainties, radiographic findings most often are given credence by courts when differentiating the effects of asbestos from those of smoking alone in the asbestos-exposed patient with a history of smoking. Asbestos is a characteristic radiographic appearance. Diagnoses are often based on the International Labor Office (ILO) system for codifying radiographic severity of pulmonary opacities;[27] this system was designed for epidemiological use but finds most of its U.S. application in impairment and indemnity assignments.[2] Physicians who pass a certification examination in ILO interpretations are relied upon by attorneys for opinions. More than 700 certified interpreters perform this service,[31] but some may not get enough practice to stay expert.[36] The ILO system of severity has four major categories of severity (range 0 (normal) to 3 (severe)) and minor gradations between. A problem for courts is that certified interpreters are supposed to provide consistency, yet they often disagree about severity, sometimes dramatically. It is not unusual when reviewing a record to have one certified opinion that the level of parenchymal abnormality is 0/0 (no findings suggestive of pneumoconiosis) and another that it is 2/2 (moderately severe findings). Epidemiological studies of quality assurance persistently describe differences between observers,[14] and it is reasonable to believe that the legal environment increases the likelihood of disagreement.

The ILO system is based on training designed to produce normative behavior; the toxic tort litigation environment may create advocacy incentives which act as a "polarizing lens" from normative behavior, encouraging diagnostic opinions at opposing extremes.

Asbestos radiographic interpretation is but one example of how attorneys may have incentives to find the least normative observers who will pass muster with the court or assigned indemnity agents. The courts and indemnity systems set up by the courts may therefore need additional means to deal with subjective interpretations of experts chosen by opposing attorneys. The issue in some cases is presence or absence of illness, while in other cases it is whether the existing illness is a compensable one, such as asbestosis. Most pulmonary impairment in our society is due to causes other than asbestos, so the integrity of funds set aside for asbestos victims depends in part on accurate diagnosis. In this instance, courts and assigned guardians of indemnity funds may be unable to interpret the numerical diagnosis of severity by certified readers chosen by attorneys unless confirmation by experts independent of either party can be obtained. Neither defense nor plaintiff attorneys are comfortable with the concept of independent readings, although plaintiff attorneys appear more uncomfortable. There are other technologies for making the same diagnosis, such as high-resolution computed tomography. They can increase diagnostic sensitivity, but they do not address the legal need to eliminate subjectivity. This generic problem leads to frequent scientific recommendations that courts obtain their own independent experts.[6,26] However, courts rarely exercise their power to do so.

The need for accurate diagnosis in the context of toxicants pertains to individual cases as well. A young worker with a childhood history of asthma performed a repetitive task mounting radar nonreflective parts for a highly technical military application. Metal inserts were unacceptable for this purpose, so a toluene di-isocyanate (TDI)-based glue was employed. TDI has been known since 1951 to commonly cause asthma.[21] Its ability to less commonly cause hypersensitivity pneumonitis was recognized in 1976.[8] The worker performed this job in a workroom setting with open containers in proximity to his breathing zone and without specific ventilation or personal protective equipment. He was possibly unaware of the nature and significance of his exposure, because of the secrecy of the process. He developed asthma, almost certainly related to his exposure.

After he was removed from the workplace, he

improved initially, but then developed a complex series of pulmonary problems following an episode of what may have been pulmonary coccidiomycosis. Over several years, he was maintained on a high dosage of steroids. He showed signs of immunosuppression and ultimately died while awaiting a lung transplant. Treating and outside expert clinicians provided opinions for the plaintiff that clinical and histopathological evidence showed that death was due to implacable progression of allergic alveolitis due to isocyanate exposure, possibly complicated by immunosuppression by high-dose steroids required to treat the alveolitis. One other isocyanate case had been reported previously to progress to death, although the plaintiff's case would be the first mortality reported after the worker had shown initial improvement upon removal from the hazard. Shortly after the patient died, his stored blood tested positive for human immunodeficiency virus. On the advice of a reviewing expert, lung tissue was re-evaluated and found to be laden with *Pneumocystis carinii.* Histopathological lung findings were also reinterpreted in that context. The case was settled out of court for an undisclosed sum. Even experts can overlook alternative diagnoses, and it is important to review a case comprehensively.

Was the Patient or Population Exposed to a Hazard?

Measurements of environmental exposures are performed most often by industrial hygienists, health physicists, and environmental engineers. Physicians, nevertheless, are entitled to provide three essential types of opinions concerning exposure to hazards: 1) whether the patient was exposed; 2) whether exposure preceded the outcome with appropriate temporal latency; and 3) whether the exposure was sufficient to explain the outcome, in the context of other risk factors pertaining to the patient.

The clinician's tools for establishing a historical impression of exposure are described in journals,[24] in texts concerning environmental disease,[20] and in government publications.[19] Training, experience, keen interest in exposures, and adequate time with the patient or patient records are prerequisites for performing this function expertly. All clinicians can and should obtain some information about exposure.[19,20] The following examples illustrate exposure estimates of a type accessible to any clinician.

1. A 63-year-old former shipyard worker now has a job as a heat and vent mechanic at a hospital. He was never an insulator or an asbestos worker per se. In his early days as a sailor and then as a shipyard worker, he performed numerous operations requiring that he remove insulation around boilers, plumbing, and other insulated fixtures. He believes asbestos was common in the areas where he worked, but he never thought about this when working. He states that he performed these operations intermittently, sometimes for days on end, sometimes only once or twice a month. He never used a respirator. He wore his own work clothes on the job. It was common for him to be covered with dust at the end of a work day. Some operations, such as replacing or sawing through transite (asbestos) boards, were extremely dusty.

2. A younger colleague at the hospital actually performs asbestos removal, and has done so as his primary function for the last three years. He knows how to set up enclosures and glove bags. Each job is authorized by an inspector before starting and rechecked upon completion. He has been fit-tested for and trained to use a respirator, as well as other protective clothing. He states he always uses his protective equipment.

Based on these histories, the clinician may consider the older worker to have a substantial exposure history, but the younger worker to have potential but little actual exposure. The younger worker has a job title reflecting his career in asbestos removal; the older worker has no such designation but does have actual exposure.

In courtroom discussions of exposure impressions, the point may be made that the clinician does not have actual exposure measurements or even that such measurements do not exist. Workers may further be unable to recall all of their potential exposures, and the employer may not have complete historical information. The clinician's reliance on the history provided by the patient(s) may also be mentioned, with a clear implication or statement that a misleading history by the patient(s) would also mislead the clinician. Of course, patients may mislead physicians in any number of ways. The patient history is nevertheless the essential element of medical diagnosis. In a practical sense, the argument that no one can now reconstruct precisely what an employer or polluter did to an environment makes a fairly unconvincing defense. ("We didn't hurt the victims because no one can figure out what we did.") The obligation of all concerned is to make the best possible reconstruction with available data, which frequently comes directly from individuals who were in the environment of concern. This is no different from any other aspect of medical history taking. In the same vein, limitations of available data should be discussed and accepted frankly.

Exposure histories and environmental measurements should be presented in the context of real health outcomes. If sloppy practices might easily have caused lead poisoning but blood lead levels are near population norms, then the salient point for a toxic tort is that lead poisoning is not demonstrated, although there may still be important legal issues in a regulatory framework. If the eight-hour time-weighted air sampling averages are all well within acceptable levels but three welders using a new Teflon coating process which produces 300 brief puffs of smoke per hour show classic signs of polymer fume fever, then a belief in short-term peak exposures not revealed by long-term sampling procedures may be justified. Other limitations of environmental exposure measurements relate to susceptible individuals (such as those who have allergies), exposures to additional agents whose toxic activities may be potentiating, and to skin exposures. Substantial skin exposure and absorption may occur in the absence of abnormal air measures. A similar limitation exists for hand to mouth contamination when hygiene practices are poor. Experience and good history taking skills are key aspects of clinician exposure assessments.

Is the Temporal Sequence Plausible ("Temporal Plausibility")?

Several considerations influence the analysis of temporal sequence. The first is pre-existing conditions. Just as accurate diagnosis is a primary responsibility of experts, so is accurate depiction of pre-existing conditions. It should be reiterated that the mere presence of a pre-existing condition is not disqualifying. In a previous example, an individual with a past history of asthma nevertheless sustained an additional burden from what all experts agreed was occupational asthma. The perception may change when the condition appears unremitting and precedes the diagnosis. Individuals who have had hepatitis may become worse following solvent exposure (and may therefore require protection), but attribution of liver damage to environmental toxins obviously should be made with great caution in a patient with pre-existing hepatitis C infection.

A second consideration is latency, which relates to the known toxicity of the agent. Asbestos-related diseases generally have a long latency period, often decades. An exception may be benign pleural effusions, but this manifestation is rarely a subject of litigation. In contrast, highly toxic irritant gases such as chlorine, phosgene, or phosphine will produce dramatic pulmonary effects acutely, subacutely, or both. Any concern about an outcome that was distant from the phosphine exposure event would have to account for outcomes expected at or near the time of exposure. For acute toxins, it is prudent to be cautious about chronic outcomes in the absence of acute symptoms. The general concept of latency is properly broken down into components. First is an "induction period," from exposure to disease onset. A "latency interval" follows, from disease onset to disease detection.[10] Further subdivisions relating to times of exposure are possible. Both induction time and latency intervals may be critical to expert discussions when temporal plausibility is an issue.

Some of the most obvious offenses against latency considerations involve inappropriate selection of laboratory testing or temporally irrelevant laboratory results. The metabolic half lives of most organic solvents within the human body range from hours to days. Solvent levels may be ordered well after the exposure period by inexperienced providers or requested by unknowing attorneys. Current solvent or metabolite levels in blood or urine most often bear no relationship to distant past exposure. Additional claims of solvents found in hair or under nails add further complexity to this issue. Patients often are unable to correctly discern the value of laboratory testing that they undergo. It is not surprising that this testing can lead to unnecessary legal friction.

It is equally unfortunate when present circulating levels are invoked inappropriately to negate past exposures. While it is sometimes possible to find evidence of distant past exposure to mercury, cadmium, or even lead in blood or urine, present tests may be normal or near normal despite substantial distant past exposure. To the degree that these toxicants are still present, they are likely to be in less accessible tissues. On the other hand, a blood lead level is a sensitive and relatively specific marker of recent exposure, within up to several half lives of the red cell. Elevated blood lead levels can be found well after this time, but the relationship to recent exposure becomes less clear. Confounding issues include: circulating lead from previous exposures, stored in bone and other integument in equilibrium with blood levels; higher absorption rates in susceptible groups (e.g., iron-deficient children); higher circulating levels in those with conditions causing high bone turnover such as Paget's disease; differences in excretion; and even differences in genetic subtypes for certain enzymes. An understanding of the physiology of human exposure is a critical part of evaluating the temporal significance of human biological monitors of exposure.

Is the Toxicology or Physiology of Exposure Plausibly Related to the Outcome ("Quantitative and Qualitative Plausibility")?

There are two sequential toxicology causation questions in many toxic tort lawsuits. The first is the "threshold" question. Can the exposure in question cause the type of harm alleged by the plaintiff? The second question is whether the outcome found actually did result from exposure.[37]

It is reasonable to believe that there are many as yet undiscovered exposure-outcome relationships, but it is unreasonable to bring new hypotheses into court without considerable supportive data. It sometimes is clinically acceptable for physicians to leave open the *possibility* that vague symptoms or even well-defined conditions may be due to unsuspected exposure(s) or exposures not known to cause the outcome of interest. This acceptance of remote possibility can be comforting to certain patients and even improve recovery. Furthermore, new etiological hypotheses serve a potential public health function; other clinicians can respond affirmatively if they believe that a similar exposure-outcome relationship has been seen elsewhere. It is unreasonable for attorneys (and especially for clinicians) to turn an acceptable clinical statement admitting that we have much to learn into a legal assertion that we have learned something. New hypotheses are just that—hypotheses. "Causal chain reasoning" is the most common fallacy. Clinicians are trained not to blindly accept yesterday's encounter with a black cat as a cause of today's illness. It is disconcerting that some clinicians will accept yesterday's toxin as a cause of today's illness even if the dose, route of exposure, symptoms, and laboratory data have no known relationship to the alleged outcome. This harks back to the "grand rounds rule." Toxicological exposure-outcome relationships supported or rejected in court should be the same as relationships defensible in grand rounds, even if "our side" finds the impartial opinion uncomfortable. An alternative, more likely cause of immune suppression and death was found in the previously presented isocyanate case, but defense experts advised defense attorneys that reappearance of asthma in the deceased patient was very plausibly due to isocyanates. This was potentially unwelcome advice, but defensible in grand rounds and therefore acceptable in court.

Toxicological thinking relies on four types of evidence: structure activity relationships, cell or system biological assays (often for genetic damage), animal studies, and human outcomes. The concept that all human outcomes must be confirmed by well-designed epidemiological studies appears in some literature at this point, but is manifestly an exaggeration. Many accepted toxic outcomes were well characterized in the era before epidemiological design was understood,[9] such as hepatotoxicity from carbon tetrachloride. The recognition of an excessive incidence of respiratory cancer in miners by Hessing and Hartung as early as 1879 was valuable and correct,[9] although it occurred in a pre-epidemiological setting. The results of other toxic outcomes are evident from single or several modern outbreaks in small populations. Isocyanate asthma, peripheral neuropathy from dimethylaminopropionitrile, and malignant mesothelioma from erionite are but three of numerous examples of exposure-outcome relationships accepted before the appearance or still in the absence of a designed population study. It is reasonable to hope that we will never do well-designed epidemiological studies on human outcomes of MPTP (1-methyl-4-phenyl-2, 5, 6-tetrahydropyridine), the contaminant in a designer drug that gave us a human and animal model of parkinsonism. The absence of a well-designed population study does not diminish our certainty about the outcome or of the harmfulness of such exposure.

Dose is also important. Hepatic damage following exposure to a number of solvents such as carbon tetrachloride[1] and central nervous system damage following exposure to lead are well-described in workers exposed to large doses, but they are less plausible in school teachers who work down the hall from the chemistry laboratory. When there is documented exposure following poor hygiene and without adequate protection, an absence of more compelling alternative causes, and objective support for an outcome, the prudent expert may assert or concede that a cause-effect relationship appears likely. If exposed populations and not just solitary individuals show an established outcome, then the level of certainty may increase.

The consideration of toxic outcomes also should include route of exposure. Toxicity of small quantities of ingested ethylene glycol is very different from inhaled ethylene glycol. Skin is impervious to lead, except for organic lead compounds. Yet lead on the skin of the fingers may be ingested quite easily, especially by small children. Workers who eat in the workplace may also create an oral route of exposure for surface contaminants. Ingested metallic mercury is not nearly as hazardous as inhaled metallic mercury because of the difference in absorption. The potential examples are endless. The point is that toxic outcomes must be based on real exposure, known toxicity (qualitative plausibility), or else on convincing new data of toxicity, and adequate exposure (quantitative plausibility).

Is There Alternative Causation for the Condition?

Alternative causes of a diagnosis generally relate to pre-existing medical conditions, complications or side effects of treatments for conditions, accidents, or life-style considerations, including smoking, alcohol use, or even hobbies related to exposures of interest. Acknowledgment of the presence of an alternative cause is an essential function of the honest expert. For example, it is often unwise to attribute an individual case of hepatotoxicity to workplace solvent exposure if the exposed worker is also an alcoholic or has a history of hepatitis C. It is important to recognize, however, that the existence of plausible alternative explanations does not necessarily rule out the alleged relationship. Smokers get obstructive lung diseases but they also get silicosis when exposed to silica. A population exposed to hepatotoxins is likely to include some obese individuals and some alcoholics; the alcohol and obesity might also cause liver abnormalities in individual cases but does not rule out the etiological contribution of an environmental liver toxin. This is particularly important if an exposed population appears to have more than an expected prevalence of an outcome. Similarly, a weekend at the rifle range does not necessarily exonerate a defective product containing lead. Consideration of medical and environmental aspects of alternative causation requires a sense of population outcomes, environmental health expertise, and common sense.

Do Epidemiological Data Support the Assertion?

Many published discussions of the role of the expert witness start at this point, perhaps reflecting academic perceptions of toxic tort litigation. These discussions miss an essential point. While epidemiological interpretations are often critical to allegations of previously unknown or still legitimately disputed mass exposure-outcome relationships, many tort allegations involve well-established relationships. It is recognized that there may be holdouts against a strong scientific consensus. Attorneys (on either side) who seek "hold-out" experts may not be doing their clients a service. Cases involving well-established outcomes frequently settle before they reach a courtroom, especially if experts have been careful to advise attorneys concerning the clinical aspects of the case, including diagnosis, exposure, and toxicology. Cases involving allegations rejected by expert consensus often are dropped before enormous, futile expense is incurred.

New etiological allegations grab headlines and may be controversial. It is not uncommon for controversy to revolve around some aspect of epidemiological interpretation. The apparent controversy can be magnified because epidemiology is a discipline designed, in part, to quantify uncertainty in population research. The scientific quantification of statistical uncertainty carries natural limitations in the search for legal truth.

Epidemiologists and, therefore, attorneys on all sides of epidemiological controversies are able to point to technical points of disagreement, or possible areas for improvement, in virtually any study. This reality also pertains to many other aspects of causation, including modern developments in forensic science. It certainly is not unique to epidemiological studies. A generic problem is that scientists and lawyers have different concepts of standards of proof. Scientists typically work toward consensus through open hypothesis testing. In epidemiology, this process permits attribution of risks for an outcome to many different causes simultaneously. For example, heart disease can be due to heredity, several aspects of diet, personal habits, a number of chronic diseases, a host of measurable biological parameters such as lipid levels, and these are related in part but not wholly to other factors, and possibly to personality type and stress. It is typical of the complex web of causation that all factors may contribute. Courts, on the other hand, sometimes are impatient with the concept that a single outcome has numerous potential causes and generally require that a cause be a "substantial contributing cause." Courts may also retain older, single-concept "but for" approaches to causation. This implies that the victim would have been whole "but for" the exposure of concern. Imagine trying to understand heart disease in this context! Courts, in their effort to accept or reject "substantial contributing" or "but for" causes, may even distrust scientific population thinking and

prefer causal-chain reasoning.[5] Again, causal-chain reasoning is a prescientific concept that something unusual that happened yesterday must have caused today's outcome. While this is sometimes true, the logic is comparable to a belief in bad outcomes from broken mirrors and black cats. It is unfortunate that courts and legislatures are the places in our society where scientific thinking sometimes can be refuted without data. Furthermore, attorneys on opposite sides of legal disputes naturally may seek standards of proof which are either much less or much more than scientists accept—depending on client needs. Scientific developments probably have always had an uneasy home in the courtroom, and statistical sciences with their characterization of uncertainty may be extremely troubling to juries. Epidemiology is an extremely powerful tool for public health, but its application by courts has a spotty record. To be clear, this is a problem of the courts, not of the science. The legal use of epidemiology is nevertheless improving markedly as courts gain experience with probabilistic thinking.

Straightforward presentation of epidemiological data for courtroom use follows a number of rules which have been discussed in several papers. The following data should be presented: strength of association, consistency of association, specificity of association, and population (as opposed to individual) dose-response relationships. Also important is avoidance of detection bias, which is a common problem pertaining to comparison between groups that are not comparable.[17] (Other aspects of data presentation, such as temporal association, intervention trials, or toxicological analogy, are discussed elsewhere in this chapter.)

Stronger associations generally are more convincing than weak ones. One measure of association is relative risk. For example, relative risk of lung cancer following asbestos exposure to World War II-era insulators was two to five times unity; the relative risk of lung cancer following asbestos exposure *and* cigarette smoking was many times that (and higher than either risk alone). The presentation of relative risk should acknowledge the "confidence interval" and whether it includes unity. Confidence intervals that include unity do not rule out chance as a statistically possible cause. The role of asbestos in both circumstances is clear, although it is less potent than the role of cigarettes in a straight-up comparison. Sometimes, the role of an epidemiological study is to deny the existence of an excess risk. When this is the case, the ability of the study to find the risk, assuming its existence, should be defined. "Power calculations" should be presented when no excess risk (confidence interval includes unity) is the outcome. It is important to note that real risk factors can be missed in epidemiological studies if the population is too small or if the study contains bias. Poorly designed or preliminary studies may also exaggerate risk.

Courts have been most comfortable making causal attributions when relative risks are greater than two (double the risk),[4,5,16] and may sometimes require this burden before accepting a risk factor as a "substantial contributing cause." A doubled risk comports with one intuitive interpretation of the legal requirement, "more likely than not." Improvements in epidemiological studies permit reliable detection of small relative risks as well. Accepted relative risks of only slightly above unity can now be detected for certain risk factors in large enough populations. Whether courts will choose to accept or reject environmental causation in the face of a reliable relative risk of between one and two (less than doubling) should be a matter of both legal perspective and effective testimony. A relative risk of 1.5 can reasonably be cited as a probable contributing risk factor to a known outcome. The expert's job should be to present the information in a way that attorney, judge, and jury can understand. The "but for" or "more likely than not" concept of causation is based on a concept of one risk at a time which may not accurately model real-life exposures. Whether courts accept or reject "robust" (well-accepted) risks of less than two is probably outside the domain of the physician expert. When understanding of a risk factor is based primarily on epidemiological study, one job of the expert is to accurately address relative risk even if less than two, without exaggerating or diminishing the finding.

From a physician's perspective, a more essential epidemiological issue is consistency of association. Plausibility is high when some outcome follows consistently from exposure. Consistency is most easily visualized by lay audiences when outcomes follow exposures in quick succession. Anoxic events from numerous chemical exposures induce death quickly; lawsuits following such exposure events are often settled with so little dispute about physiology or epidemiology that they may not even be recognized as toxic tort actions.

When outcome follows exposure after a latent period, however, as in the appearance of lung cancer or parenchymal lung fibrosis following asbestos exposure, it is often important to discuss the consistency of the association in populations. Consistency can be of two types. One is confirmation of a similar outcome when similarly exposed populations are studied at other places. Another is consistency with animal studies, a less important but still fundamental issue. Sometimes, consistency with animal toxicology data can be hard to establish. Population concepts of asbestos carcinogenesis were well established in humans before good animal models were developed.

A third principle of epidemiological presentation is consideration of alternative causal factors. This relates to the specificity of a relationship. Most malignant mesotheliomas in the U.S. construction and shipyard workers are due to asbestos exposure. This is a fairly specific relationship. A host of workplace toxins cause peripheral neuropathy, but a wide variety of common chronic diseases do so more commonly. For the individual worker with neurotoxin exposure and peripheral neuropathy, competing causes must be considered. These should be considered for each individual in the context of who else is sick in the same environment. A workplace epidemic definitely should increase environmental suspicions. Incidentally, it may be that certain types of outbreaks are seen less commonly than in the past. This is due to appropriate substitution of less toxic chemicals in modern workplaces. Substitution for the hepatotoxin carbon tetrachloride is an example. It is rarely found in modern workplaces. We nevertheless know with certainty from numerous historic disease outbreaks that it is a potent human hepatotoxin, even in the absence of large-scale, recently designed studies.

The complexities of dose-response are an important consideration in epidemiological studies. These are discussed briefly in another part of this chapter. The presence of dose-response data provides strong confirmation for a hypothesized or known causal relationship. Absence of dose-response data may be because the hypothesized relationship really does not exist. Alternatively, absence of dose-response data may be because the measurements simply are not taken or not taken appropriately, or the measurements are taken at the wrong time, or the susceptible subpopulation is not identified within a larger population, or the mechanism is partly independent of dose (allergy), or the measurements were taken correctly but not in such a way that they related to the physiology of the problem (sampling data measured an 8-hour time weighted average but the risk was contained in very brief peak excursions), or the route of exposure is misunderstood (air is measured and skin is exposed). Of potential limitations to understanding dose-response, the absence of good measurement is the most common.

A misunderstanding of dose-response is that operation within historic regulatory standards proves absence of dose-response. Genuine outbreaks of disease can occur even in the presence of well-performed and apparently benign sampling data, for a host of reasons. The presence of a substantial body of benign environmental sampling data is nevertheless of critical importance to the defense of toxic tort allegations and serves to raise the burden of proof for health outcome findings in individuals or populations, especially if intentional misconduct is alleged.

The purpose of epidemiology in the setting of a toxic tort is to infer or rule out causal association. The following are minimum criteria for inference when epidemiology is the relevant science: 1) the outcome of interest is more common in the exposed population; 2) association is unlikely to be due to chance (confidence interval); 3) the association is unlikely to be due to confounding or other bias; and 4) findings are consistent. When substitutes are found for the offending agent, the health outcome should decrease in frequency. More complete taxonomies of epidemiology applied to toxic tort litigation exist within published literature,[30] but these four issues remain the essential points. Their purpose is to evaluate a "reasonably exclusive factual connection" from exposure to human outcome.[11] Finally, the assertion that there must be support-

ing, designed studies for any exposure-outcome relationship is a misunderstanding of the history and limits of epidemiology. Sometimes, there is no relevant designed study, yet the case reports are consistent and represent the best available evidence. The expert is then entitled to discuss the strengths and weaknesses of the best available clinical data.

DEPOSITION AND TRIAL BEHAVIOR OF AN EXPERT WITNESS

The expert witness usually is expected to provide an up-to-date curriculum vitae. Subpoenas from opposing counsel often may require that the expert bring certain things to the table. In some instances, this may include the contents of all material ever read or considered, a demand that would require a moving van if taken at face value. This is impractical. Eaton and Kalman[16] point out that experts are permitted to testify from their experience and should bring the literature most directly relevant to their opinions. Copies should be created for material that the expert wishes to keep.

The number of times an expert has previously appeared in court and the nature of appearances are important to attorneys. Experts should expect intensive questioning about this. Opposing attorneys may also ask when the expert was contacted about the case and the circumstances. It is important to do one's best to recall such events, although it is not imperative that exact dates be remembered. A common and puzzling request by attorneys may be the exact date and sequence from which particular information about the case was reviewed. It is flattering that attorneys imply that physician experts remember not only what they read, but also the date and sequence in which they read it. If you do not remember, however, it is best to acknowledge that.

Eaton and Kalman have also provided the most useful summary of physician behavior in the toxic tort courtroom environment. Helpful hints from Eaton and Kalman include:[16]

- Speak, do not nod.
- Be courteous and professional, yet calm

and confident. Do not be sarcastic.

- Answer responsively, but do not volunteer information.
- Do not guess.
- Do not allow an attorney from the opposing side to put words in your mouth. Do not accept paraphrasing of data unless completely comfortable with it.
- Stand by your statement, but avoid being argumentative.
- Do not be distracted by arguments and objections between attorneys. In depositions or filmed testimony, a judge will rule later about objections. The experts' job is to provide honest, accurate answers, without worrying about what will later be included or excluded. Refrain from answering questions only when directed to not respond.
- If a jury is present, speak directly to the jury. If filmed, speak directly to the camera.
- Avoid jargon.
- If using charts and graphs, be sure they are large and clearly presented.

Finally, Eaton and Kalman point out that honest testimony, from reputable experts, can represent a real public service.[16] This positive view has to be balanced against the negative "hired gun" image, which is often invoked by opposing attorneys and which certainly applies to some participants in certain circumstances. Again, the decision to appear or not ought to be predicated on allegiance to the best available science, regardless of other motives. For this reason, the author expresses concern about the pervasive concept that the expert should not "volunteer" information. Public-spirited education of the attorneys, judge, and jury is a potentially valuable role of the expert.

Public Health Significance of Environmental Toxic Torts

Toxic tort litigation addresses public health issues indirectly. The direct outcome of each suit is about the possible transfer of wealth from an alleged injurer (or insurer) to victims who have been harmed. However, it has been pointed out that a substantial percentage of recoveries from settlements and verdicts may go to attorneys.[35]

There are two secondary outcomes of public health significance. First, toxic tort lawsuits are expensive. They may add to the cost of a variety of useful manufactured products. Affected sectors include manufacturing, mining, construction, health care, and utilities. Increased cost may make useful products inaccessible to some consumers. Fear of toxic tort litigation may even delay entry or bar introduction of new products or cause existing products to be removed unnecessarily from the marketplace. The morning sickness drug Bendectin is said to have been removed because of litigation.[18] Strong opinions have been voiced that this move was not in the public interest.[29] There is also the concern that the judicial process operates without adequate documentation of evidentiary standards, leading to inconsistent and untenable conclusions.[30] Certainly, it is clear to all concerned that litigation can be resolved by settlement or trial and product decisions made in the absence of good science. This risk is inherent in the adversarial process. It has been argued that fear of toxic tort litigation is also a barrier to innovation and development. This perspective pertains to much of tort law, not just toxic tort action.[5] Much of the cost to a consumer of a ladder, of health care, or of a recreational trip on a raft through river rapids relates to liability. Insurance economists identify torts (of all types) as a contributing cause of a nationwide insurance liability crisis.[25]

A second perspective concerning indirect outcomes of toxic torts relates to public protection. Toxic tort lawsuits create incentives and a climate that sometimes generates funds for compensation of needy victims. Each verdict for plaintiffs is a reminder to potential offenders of the economic and public costs of introducing toxic products or releasing toxic by-products. The fear that drives up the cost of some products and makes others inaccessible may also provide powerful incentives for positive innovations. A host of other products now substitute for asbestos, even in some areas where it might

TABLE 1

ON-LINE OR CONSULTING SERVICES

Resource	Sponsor
Chem ID	National Library of Medicine
Chemline	National Library of Medicine
Hazardous Substances Data Bank	A Toxnet Data Resource
Integrated Risk Information System	A Toxnet Data Resource
Medline, Medlars	National Library of Medicine
National Institute of Occupational Safety and Health Technical Information Center (on CD-ROM)	National Institute of Occupational Safety and Health
Registry of Toxic Effects of Chemical Substances	National Institute of Occupational Safety and Health
Tomes Plus	Micromedix
Toxic-Chemical Release Inventory	National Library of Medicine
Toxline	National Library of Medicine
Toxnet	National Library of Medicine

best be used. The extent to which toxic tort precedents promote safety is an empirical question. The impact on public health is difficult to assess; studies done on this topic have been inconclusive.[35] There is no foreseeable mechanism for accounting putative savings from unknown disasters averted by the effect of litigation on product stewardship and waste handling. In the face of incomplete evidence, expert medical-legal opinion on the topic has suggested that toxic tort litigation will persist so long as other means of deterrence (including regulation and regulatory enforcement) remain inadequate.[4]

Many suggestions for reform have been made, including "no fault" taxpayer subsidized insurance pools. Other approaches include the recommendations for financial ceilings on "pain and suffering" settlements and subtraction of other benefits such as social security and insurance from verdicts.

SOURCES OF INFORMATION FOR CLINICIANS IN ENVIRONMENTAL TOXIC TORTS

For most toxic allegations, the key documents for the clinician are the medical record, the occupational and environmental exposure history that should be within the medical record (but is often missing), and other related data concerning exposure, including material safety data sheets (for workplace exposures) and environmental measurements. The occupational and environmental health literature has experienced recent growth, and there are a variety of excellent texts at many levels of detail and historical completeness. These include texts on toxicology, environmental epidemiology, environmental health, and occupational medicine. Chemical agent-specific publications prepared by the Agency for Toxic Substances and Disease Registry are both detailed and readable.

Some on-line services are listed by resource in the accompanying table (Table 1). A list of sources accessible to treating clinicians is also available in an excellent review concerning occupational illness.[32] The expansion of accessible information progresses so rapidly that the list will be woefully incomplete by the time of publication.

REFERENCES

1. Agency for Toxic Substances and Disease Registry: **Toxicological Profile for Carbon Tetrachloride (update)**. Washington, DC: US Department of Health and Human Services, 1993 (TP-93/02)
2. Balmes JR: To B-read or not to B-read. **J Occup Med** 34:885-886, 1992 (Editorial)

3. *Bradley v Pickens Brown*, 42 F3d, 434 (7th Cir) 1994
4. Brennan TA: Environmental torts. **Vanderbilt Law Rev 46**:1-73, 1993
5. Brennan TA: Untangling causation issues in law and medicine: hazardous substance litigation. **Ann Intern Med 107**:741-747, 1987
6. Brennan TA: Would a federal judicial science board improve toxic tort litigation? **Am J Indust Med 17**:761-771, 1990
7. Brent RL: The irresponsible expert witness: a failure of biomedical graduate education and professional accountability. **Pediatrics 70**:754-762, 1982
8. Charles J, Bernstein A, Jones B, et al: Hypersensitivity pneumonitis after exposure to isocyanates. **Thorax 31**:127-136, 1976
9. Checkoway H, Pearce N, Crawford-Brown DJ: **Research Methods in Occupational Epidemiology.** New York, NY: Oxford University Press, 1989
10 Checkoway H, Pearce N, Hickey JLS, et al: Latency analysis in occupational epidemiology. **Arch Environ Health 45**:95-100, 1990
11. Christoffel T, Teret SP: Epidemiology and the law: courts and confidence intervals. **Am J Public Health 81**:1661-1666, 1991
12. Cole P: The epidemiologist as an expert witness. **J Clin Epidemiol 144 (Suppl 1)**:35S-39S, 1991
13. Cornfeld RS, Schlossman SF: Immunologic laboratory tests: a critique of the Alcolac decision, in: **Toxics Law Reporter.** Washington, DC: Bureau of National Affairs, 1989, pp 381-390
14. Ducatman AM: Variability in interpretation of radiographs for asbestotic abnormality: problems and solutions. **Ann NY Acad Sci 643**:108-120, 1991
15. Ducatman AM, Yang WN, Forman SA: "B-readers" and asbestos medical surveillance. **J Occup Med 30**:644-647, 1988
16. Eaton DL, Kalman D: Scientists in the courtroom: basic pointers for the expert scientific witness. **Environ Health Perspec 102**:668-672, 1994
17. Feinstein AR: Scientific standards in epidemiologic studies of the menace of daily life. **Science 242**:1257-1263, 1986
18. Foster KR: Science in the courtroom: What is valid evidence? **Health Environ Dig 8**:1-3, 1994
19. Frank A: The environmental history, in Brooks S, Gochfeld M, Herzstein J, et al (eds): **Environmental Medicine.** St Louis, Mo: CV Mosby, 1995
20. Frank A: Taking an exposure history, in Balk SJ (ed): **Agency for Toxic Substances Disease Registry: Case Studies in Environmental Medicine 26.** Washington, DC: US Department of Health and Human Services, 1992
21. Fuchs S, Valade P: Étude clinique et expériementale sur quelques cas d'intoxication par le desmodur T (diisocyanates de toluyène 1-2-4 et 1-2-6). **Arch Mal Prof 12**:191-196, 1951
22. Gaines SE: A taxonomy for toxic torts, in: **Toxics Law Reporter.** Washington, DC: Bureau of National Affairs, 1988, pp 826-831
23. *Gibau v Vicente.* Civil No. 92-06782, Mass Sup Ct, Suffolk Co, 1994
24. Goldman RH, Peters JM: The occupational and environmental health history. **JAMA 246**:2831-2836, 1981
25. Harrington S, Litan RE: Causes of the liability insurance crisis. **Science 239**:737-741, 1988
26. Holden C: Science in court. **Science 243**:1658-1659, 1989
27. International Labour Office: Classification of radiographs of the pneumoconioses. **Med Radiogr Photo 57**:2-18, 1981
28. McElveen JC Jr, Beck T: Legal and ethical issues, in McCunney RJ (ed): **A Practical Approach to Occupational and Environmental Medicine.** 2nd ed. Boston, Mass: Little, Brown, and Co, 1994, pp 20-36
29. Mills JL, Alexander D: Teratogens and "litogens." **N Engl J Med 315**:1234-1235, 1986
30. Muscat JE, Huncharek MS: Causation and disease: biomedical science in toxic tort litigation. **J Occup Med 31**:997-1002, 1989
31. National Institute for Occupational Safety and Health, Division of Respiratory Disease Studies: **List of NIOSH Certified Roentgenographic Interpreting Physicians: B-Readers by State.** Washington, DC: US Department of Health and Human Services, February 1, 1995
32. Newman LS: Occupational illness. **N Engl J Med 333**:1128-1134, 1995
33. Rom WN: Asbestos related diseases, in Rom WN (ed): **Environmental and Occupational Medicine.** 2nd ed. Boston, Mass: Little, Brown, and Co, 1992
34. Simon GE, Daniell W, Stockbridge H, et al: Immunologic, psychological, and neuropsychological factors in multiple chemical sensitivity. A controlled study. **Ann Intern Med 119**:97-103, 1993
35. Sugarman SD: The need to reform personal injury law leaving scientific disputes to scientists. **Science 248**:823-827, 1990
36. Wagner GR, Attfield MD, Kennedy RD, et al: The NIOSH B reader certification program. An update report. **J Occup Med 34**:879-884, 1992
37. Whitehead GM, Espel LD: Legal proof of causation in toxic tort litigation, in: **Toxics Law Reporter.** Washington, DC: Bureau of National Affairs, 1988, pp 1040-1047
38. Widess E: Toxic tort litigation and United States occupational and environmental legislation, in Rosenstock L, Cullen MC (eds): **Textbook of Clinical Occupational and Environmental Medicine.** Philadelphia, Pa: WB Saunders, 1994, pp 84-91

CHAPTER 19

FOOD AND DRUG ADMINISTRATION: DRUGS AND DEVICES

ROBERT F. MUNZNER, PHD

The responsibility for enforcement of the Federal Food, Drug, and Cosmetic Act of 1938 is delegated to the Food and Drug Administration (FDA). This chapter identifies ways in which enforcement of the Federal Food, Drug, and Cosmetic Act (hereafter referred to as the "Act") can impact directly on the physician. This Act requires that the FDA assure that drugs and medical devices (among other things) are safe and effective. At first glance, this would not appear to burden the physician; however, if we consider that this law creates the potential for illegal products (more precisely adulterated or misbranded products) to exist, the physician, as the learned intermediary, is forced to assume some responsibility for recognizing devices that do not conform to the law and assuring that the patient is properly informed.

On May 28, 1976, the medical devices amendments to this Act were enacted. Because of a "grandfather" provision for devices marketed prior to this, the task of identifying the legal status of devices is made more difficult by the complexity of the law that establishes classes of products which may be marketed without FDA approval.

Before tackling the complexities of market-

ing status, one must be familiar with the legal definitions of drugs and devices; therefore, a discussion of definitions is included to assure that the critical nuances of "labeling" and "intended use" are understood.

There are special provisions in the law for undertaking research with products that have not been shown to be safe and effective for use, but utilization of these provisions brings additional responsibility to the physician-investigator to assure that the rights, safety, and welfare of research subjects are protected. The regulations in this area are very specific and detailed; therefore, a large section is devoted to these specific requirements.

The topic of "custom devices" also has been included because of problems for physicians that have arisen from these provisions due to misinterpretation (i.e., a more liberal interpretation than the FDA will allow).

The process of interpretation is critical to understanding how the FDA and other regulatory agencies go about enforcing the laws which the United States Congress has enacted; therefore, it is necessary to consider how the words in the law are translated into actions, both by the Agency and by the courts.

LAWS ADMINISTERED BY THE FDA

The Federal Food, Drug, and Cosmetic Act of 1938 established a legal framework for regulating the production of food, drugs, and cosmetics. It has subsequently been amended, expanded, and augmented by other legislation. The legislation that pertained to drugs was, at least in retrospect, rather general. This allowed the FDA a great deal of latitude for interpretation in the creation of regulations to implement and enforce the law. FDA regulations and policies, which have evolved over a period of nearly 60 years, have often been tested in the courts and upheld. The FDA was also delegated the authority to enforce the Biologics Act, which had been enacted in 1902, and which provided the basis for regulation of vaccines and human blood products. In 1968, the FDA was given the additional responsibility for enforcing the Radiation Control for Health and Safety Act. Again, this legislation granted very general regulatory authority.

The 1938 Act introduced the requirement for approval of certain new drugs, primarily to assure consumer safety. The Act was amended several times to strengthen and broaden this requirement. The most important amendments were passed in 1962 and prohibited the marketing of a new drug unless the FDA has approved a New Drug Application (NDA) that include reports of studies to show that the new drug is effective. The 1962 amendments introduced the requirement that the FDA withdraw approval of an NDA if new data showed a lack of evidence of effectiveness.

Prior to 1976, the authority to regulate drugs was also applied to many medical devices. This interpretation and extension of the law could be argued reasonably for such things as sutures and implanted devices, but the authority for regulating such things as diagnostic laboratory products was unclear. Amendments to the Act in 1976 not only gave clear authority to regulate medical devices, but it also provided exhaustive, detailed specific requirements to the FDA for implementation of the regulations. The general provisions of the law, such as the prohibition of "adulteration" and "misbranding," applied to both drugs and devices. Products (drugs and devices) that are adulterated or misbranded are subject to seizure. Persons who commit any of the prohibited actions (e.g., the introduction of an adulterated product) can be punished by fine and imprisonment.

Included in the 1976 amendments was the implementation of a three-tier regulatory approach for those medical devices which had been marketed prior to enactment of the amendments. A device introduced after enactment of the amendments would be included in this three-level approach only if the FDA determined that the device was "substantially equivalent" to pre-amendment devices. The lowest level of regulatory control, class I, required only that the device conform to the general provisions of the Act. The next level, class II, provided for mandatory performance standards. The device amendments of 1990 subsequently redefined class II to provide for "special controls," which included performance standards. Class III provides for premarket application (PMA) approval, a process analogous to the NDA approval process.

To understand the classification of devices, it is essential to recognize that the process of classifying pre-amendment devices had no immediate effect whatsoever on the introduction of devices to the market. The implementation of performance standards required a complex rule-making procedure to become effective; thus, there was virtually no difference between class I and class II. Approval of a premarket application could not be required for pre-amendment (or equivalent) devices until 30 months after classification, and then only through the formal rule-making procedure to establish an effective date.

The primary impact on the marketing of medical devices was the requirement that all manufacturers notify the FDA 90 days before introducing any device; this is known as "510(k)." The FDA then had an opportunity to evaluate the device prior to marketing and determine whether it was substantially equivalent to pre-amendment devices or whether it should be classified as a new device. If it was determined to be a new device, the law required that it be assigned to class III and that it could not be marketed before approval of a PMA. The most significant criterion affecting marketing, therefore, was pre-amendment status (or "equivalence") not classification. Classification, however, has established a long-term regulatory agenda which is gradually affecting the marketing of medical devices.

Medical device classification is sometimes confused with the classification of radiation-emitting devices because of regulations previously written under the authority of the Radiation Control for Health and Safety Act. Unfortunately, the terminology of classes of I, II, and III was also used when classifying regulations to designate the level of risk of injury to the eye by light sources. In this classification system, the order of severity is reversed, with class I having the highest risk and being the most restrictive and class III having the least risk and the least control of exposure.

Interpretation of Federal Law

Interpretation of the law occurs at three distinct levels: the reading of the law enacted by the U.S. Congress; the writing of the rules (regulations) by the FDA that interpret the law and add essential detail; and the writing of orders (letters) by the FDA that make specific determinations in applying the rules. Interpretation at any of these levels can be contested judicially. Consequently, it is often difficult to say with certainty which interpretation will prevail unless a specific judicial ruling has been made and upheld in the appellate courts. Such tests of the interpretations are few in number; therefore, the statements we make concerning what is "legal" must be hedged according to the limits of the interpretive data that are available. Throughout this chapter, the phrase "current policy seems to indicate" should be inserted before any statement of legal interpretation.

The Federal Food, Drug, and Cosmetic Act, as amended, is primarily based on the federal authority to regulate interstate commerce. (Note: the codified version of the act as currently amended is published in Title 21 of the United States Code, Chapter 9, beginning with Section 301.4.) The FDA's principal mandate with regard to medical products, as expressed in the Act, is to assure that these products are reasonably safe and effective.

The authority of the FDA to assure effectiveness was tested in court when a petitioner argued that the FDA should not require a device to be shown effective before reclassifying it from class III to class I if that device did not present an unreasonable risk of illness or injury. The U.S. District Court of Appeals cited several references in the legislative history, and stated: "These general statements, many of which are unqualified, emphasize that Congress's primary concern was to prevent the marketing of devices not both safe and effective."[10]

The FDA's interpretation of the law, as a matter of policy, generally avoids regulatory actions that interfere with the practice of medicine; however, some mandates of the law conflict with this policy. For example, the requirement that the FDA assure that drugs and devices are effective implies that there must be at least one proven use for each product before it is approved. If there is no scientific evidence to support effectiveness for any use, a new product cannot be legally marketed and, therefore, is not legally available to most practitioners.

The FDA policy generally dictates that law enforcement be directed at those persons who distribute devices, not at the user. However, there are exceptions. In the case of *Drown v. U.S.*[8] in the 1950s, a physician who built his own device was found to be engaged in interstate commerce because the cancer patients that he treated traveled from other states to seek treatment from him. More recently, in September 1990, EAV Dermatron devices were seized at the Century Clinic in Reno, Nevada, and the appropriateness of the action was reaffirmed in U.S. District Court.[12]

Should the physician be interested in rules that are directed at the manufacturers and the importers? Physicians who wish to advance the state of the art may also wear the inventor's hat, and in that role they may become a manufacturer by modifying a device or creating a device; therefore, the legal responsibility they assume in this role must be appreciated. Most importantly, one should recognize that using a device obtained from any source other than the domestic medical product marketplace conveys additional responsibility. Discussion of these responsibilities is therefore included under "use of unapproved devices" below.

Definition of a "Drug"

The Act[4] defines (not verbatim) drugs as articles recognized in the United States Pharmacopoeia, the official Homeopathic Pharmacopoeia of the United States, or the official National Formulary, or any supplement to any of them; and articles intended for use in the diagnosis, cure, mitigation, treatment, or prevention of disease in humans or other animals; articles (other than food) intended to affect the structure or any function of the body of humans or animals; and articles intended for use as a component of any of the three aforementioned articles.

Definition of a "Device"

The Act, as amended in 1976, defines (not verbatim) a device as an instrument, apparatus, implement, machine, contrivance, implant, in vitro reagent, or other similar or related article, including any component part or accessory which meets any of the criteria for a drug given above, and which does not achieve any of its principle intended purposes through chemical action within or on the body of humans or other animals, and which is not dependent upon being metabolized for the achievement of any of its principle intended purposes.

Other Definitions

It is most important to recognize the use of the word "intended" in these definitions. It is also important to appreciate how broad these definitions are. Drugs and devices are primarily defined by "intended use" and only secondarily, and very broadly, as a physical entity. For this reason, product labeling that specifies the intended use is critical to drug and device regulation. Note that the word "labeling" as used by the FDA means all written or graphic matter accompanying the product, as well as any associated advertising material.

APPROVED DRUGS

As can be seen from the definition of a "drug" given above, the law recognizes that many drugs are not new drugs. A new drug cannot be marketed without an approved NDA. To determine whether or not a drug requires an NDA, the manufacturer must request an advisory opinion from the FDA.

The FDA's responsibility for assuring the safety and effectiveness of drugs under the very general provisions of the law that have prevailed for many years has resulted in an extensive body of rules that are incorporated in Title 21, Code of Federal Regulations, Parts 300 to 499. These rules are described in about 1,000 pages of text and are not amenable to summary here; however, Part 329[1] may be of interest to the physician because of its impact in other spheres of the law.

Part 329 designates particular substances as "habit forming" and requires special labeling for their distribution. These substances are chemical derivatives of the parent substances barbituric acid, cannabis, bromal, carbromal, chloral, cocaine, codeine, heroin, morphine, opium, paraldehyde, and sulfonmethane. The regulation also designates specific concentrations of particular substances which are exempt from prescription labeling.[2] For example, preparations containing no more than one-fourth grain of morphine per fluid ounce may be exempted.

Although the regulations for marketing new drugs directly impact only the manufacturers and importers, there is an indirect effect on the physician, in that new chemical entities are made generally unavailable. The FDA policy usually interprets the phrase "valid scientific evidence that assures safety and effectiveness" to mean that favorable results from a well-controlled clinical trial are required before marketing is approved. This position has often been criticized by various industry and public interest groups who believe that the introduction of new drugs is delayed unnecessarily by the FDA review process.

The commissioner of the FDA recently replied to this criticism in the *Journal of the American Medical Association*[11] by presenting a rigorous comparison between the introduction of new drugs in Great Britain, Germany, Japan, and the United States for the period between January 1990 and December 1994. The approval rates for the U.S. and Great Britain are shown to be comparable to each other and to significantly outpace both Germany and Japan. Also, there are FDA initiatives underway to expedite the approval of new drugs, and the time required for FDA review has been declining steadily. The willingness of the FDA to allow the marketing of a product when its benefits outweigh the risks of significant adverse effects does allow increased availability; however, the product labeling must convey the risk and benefit information to the physician who has the responsibility of "learned intermediary" with regard to the individual patient.

APPROVED DEVICES

Fewer than 5% of the medical devices being marketed have gone through the FDA's PMA approval process, which requires that the manufacturer submit a PMA and that this application be approved by the FDA before the product can be available commercially, as is required for new drugs through the NDA process. Most devices are otherwise "legally marketed" as described below. Technically speaking, the FDA does not approve devices—it is only applications to market devices that are approved by an "order" (letter) from the FDA. Approval may also be withdrawn by order. Devices that have been subjected to the rigorous PMA approval process are, of course, subject to the greatest scrutiny and the strictest controls by the agency. The labeling for these products, which must specify the intended use (or "indications"), becomes a part of the approval record and cannot be modified without supplemental approval.

"LEGALLY MARKETED" DEVICES

Most medical devices (i.e., the other 95%) that enter the market do so on the basis of a determination by the FDA that they are substantially equivalent to devices that were marketed prior to May 28, 1976, the enactment date of the medical device amendments to the Act. The amendments specified that there would be no immediate effect on devices being marketed at the time of enactment, and that manufacturers who intend to introduce similar competing products should "notify" the FDA 90 days in advance. This notice to the FDA is commonly referred to as a "510(k)," which corresponds to the section of the Act that imposes the notification requirement. As a consequence of the special pre-amendment statutory provision, there are many medical devices presently being legally marketed for which the FDA has had no official notice of introduction simply because these devices were marketed prior to enactment of the device amendments and have never been significantly modified. However, the current regulations do require all manufacturers to report their place of business (registration) and to identify the devices they are marketing (listing), and the Agency periodically inspects these establishments and their records.

The determination of "intended use" by the FDA for pre-amendment devices is subject to some uncertainty due to a lack of precise knowledge about the intended uses for which these devices were promoted. Although device labeling must now specify the uses for which the device is being promoted, pre-amendment devices often lacked definitive labeling because there was no regulatory requirement for such labeling.

How can the physician be assured that a product is legally marketed? Generally, the physician can presume that any product purchased in the U.S. that is accompanied by labeling promoting it for some medical purpose is safe and effective. Based on this presumption, the Act prohibits any drug or medical device from being labeled as "FDA approved" or "reviewed by FDA" because such statements imply some degree of endorsement by the government. Ironically, any product promoted with such labeling is automatically illegal!

If the legal status of a device is suspect, a definitive answer almost always can be obtained by contacting the FDA's Division of Small Manufacturer's Assistance by telephone (800-638-2041) or by e-mail (dsmo@fdadr.cdrh.gov), provided that the name of the manufacturer and the trade name of the device are known. A database is maintained which allows the FDA staff to determine whether or not a device is "equivalent" or approved, but access is not available to the public because much of the data is proprietary. Data files which list many 510(k)s are available to the public by Internet access (http://www.fda.gov/cdrh/510khome.html), but a failure to find a device in the Internet files cannot be interpreted as reliable evidence that the device was not legally marketed.

Off-Label Use

Considering that the intended use for PMA-approved devices is very strictly defined, any other use is clearly outside the scope of the legal approval. As noted above, one cannot specify with any certainty the limits of the law until interpretations are made and upheld by the courts. However, one can look back at the history of enforcement to get a sense of the strictness with which the law has been interpreted. Generally speaking, it has not been agency policy to seize devices because they are not being used in accordance with approved use. There are, however, many examples of legal actions taken with regard to promotion of devices for unapproved use. Again, this reflects the general agency policy to exclude regulation of the practice of medicine, as long as regulation of commerce is not compromised. The distinction between enforcement policy and precise legal authority would be academic, except for the fact that policy is subject to change without an act by the U.S. Congress.

Reporting Adverse Events

The Act, as amended in 1990 and 1992, requires that device-related deaths, serious injuries, and serious illnesses be reported by distributors and user facilities to the FDA, to the manufacturer, or both. User facilities must also submit semi-annual reports to the FDA, listing all adverse events that have been reported to both the FDA and the manufacturer. In November 1991, the FDA[6] published a "tentative final rule" specifying that user facilities must report deaths to both the manufacturer (if known) and to the FDA within 10 working days of the time the facility becomes aware of information that reasonably suggests that a device has caused or contributed to the death of a patient. Serious injuries or illnesses caused by a device must be reported to the manufacturer, or to FDA if the manufacturer is not known, also within 10 days.

"User facility" is defined in the regulations as a hospital, an ambulatory surgical facility, a nursing home, or an outpatient diagnostic or outpatient treatment facility that is not a physician's office.

The Act provides for civil penalties to be imposed on user facilities that fail to report adverse events.[9] The rule allowing the FDA to assess civil penalties became effective on November 4, 1994, but this sanction has not yet been exercised. According to one source, ". . . user penalties are likely to be imposed only for violations that are significant or knowing. Such penalties would be specifically appropriate for repeat offenders."[14]

The FDA maintains a voluntary program, "MedWatch," for reporting adverse events and product-related problems noted by physicians and other health care professionals who are not working in a hospital or other facility. Telephone reports can be made (800-FDA-1088) and written reports can be submitted (use FDA Form 3500 and forward it to MedWatch, 5600 Fishers Lane, Rockville, Maryland 20852-9787, or by fax to 800-FDA-0178. This form is available on the final page of the *Physician's Desk Reference.*) Other than user facilities which are required to report, physician reporting remains voluntary in most cases, with the exception of special categories of adverse reaction to vaccines.[7]

INVESTIGATIONAL NEW DRUG APPLICATIONS

The approval of an "investigational new drug" application (IND) allows the legal distribution of new drugs that otherwise would require an approved NDA for distribution. Note that the legislative history for drugs predates the amendments for devices; therefore, the rules for drugs, although parallel to those for devices, differ substantially.

The requirements for informed consent which apply to both INDs and Investigational Device Exemptions (IDEs) are promulgated in 21 CFR 50; however, only the responsibilities of the investigator are addressed in this rule. The

IND rules also provide for clinical investigations by an individual "sponsor-investigator" as defined by 21 CFR 312.3. Additional responsibilities for the sponsor and the institutional review board with regard to informed consent for device investigations are given in the discussion on IDEs below.

Labeling

An investigational new drug intended for human use must bear a label with the statement: "Caution: New Drug—Limited by Federal (or United States) law to investigational use." The labeling must not represent the device as being safe and effective for the purposes for which it is being investigated.

Prohibition of Promotion and Charging

Promoting or representing an investigational new drug as safe or effective for the use for which it is being investigated is prohibited. Charging for a drug being used in clinical trials under an IND is also prohibited, unless the FDA gives prior written approval.

IND Phases

The clinical investigation of a previously untested drug is divided into three phases, which may overlap. Phase 1 includes the initial introduction into humans, either patients or normal volunteer subjects, to study the metabolism and pharmacological actions, the side effects associated with increasing doses, and other data needed to design well-controlled, scientifically valid Phase 2 studies. Phase 2 includes controlled clinical studies to evaluate effectiveness when used for specific indications, and to determine the common short-term side effects and risks. Phase 3 studies are performed after preliminary evidence of effectiveness has been obtained to gather further evidence of effectiveness using both controlled and uncontrolled trials with large numbers of patients. The data obtained in Phase 3 are used to evaluate the overall risk-benefit relationship and to provide a basis for physician labeling.

Sponsor Responsibilities

The sponsor, the person who initiates the investigation, is responsible for selecting qualified investigators, providing them with what they need to conduct an investigation properly, ensuring proper monitoring of the investigation, ensuring that the investigation is conducted in accordance with the general investigational plan and protocols contained in the IND, maintaining an effective IND with respect to the investigation, and ensuring that the FDA and all participating investigators are promptly informed of significant new adverse effects or risks with respect to the drug. The specific responsibilities associated with an IND are summarized below, but it is essential that sponsors and investigators read and be familiar with the actual rules as published in 21 CFR 312 before undertaking a clinical investigation.

Assuring an IND is in Effect

The sponsor may commence the clinical investigation as soon as the IND is in effect. The IND is in effect 30 days after receipt by the FDA, or sooner when authorized by the FDA. An IND may be obtained by executing the form FDA 1571 ("NDA Application"), which can be obtained from the FDA Center for Drug Evaluation and Research, Executive Secretariat Staff, HFD-8, 5600 Fishers Lane, Rockville, Maryland, 20857, or by calling (301) 594-1012. For sponsor-investigators, the process is further simplified by also including a form FDA 1572 ("Statement of Investigator") that replaces some of the detailed information required by form FDA 1571.

The rules (21 CFR 312.42) also provide for a "clinical hold" to delay the proposed investigation by FDA order. Although, the rules specify that an IND is "in effect" 30 days after receipt, the FDA routinely contacts the sponsor by telephone or letter before the 30-day period expires to assure the sponsor that he/she may begin; therefore, it would be unwise to commence without this assurance.

Selecting Investigators and Monitors

The sponsor is responsible for the selection of persons who are qualified to be investigators and monitors for the investigation. The sponsor must select a monitor who is qualified to monitor the progress of the investigation.

Review of Ongoing Investigations

If the sponsor discovers that an investigator is not complying with the signed FDA 1572 (Statement of Investigator) or the investigational plan, the sponsor must either secure compliance or discontinue shipment of the drug. The sponsor must review evidence of safety and effectiveness obtained by the investigators. If the sponsor determines that the investigational drug presents an unreasonable and significant risk to subjects, the sponsor must, within 5 days, discontinue the investigations that present the risk and notify the FDA, all institutional review boards, and all investigators of the discontinuance.

Providing Information to Investigators and the FDA

Before an investigation begins, the sponsor must give all investigators a copy of a brochure that includes a brief description of the drug, a summary of the pharmacological and toxicological effects of the drug, a summary of the pharmacokinetics and biological disposition of the drug, a summary of information relating to the safety and effectiveness in humans obtained from prior clinical studies, and a description of possible risks and side effects to be anticipated and any special monitoring needs.

Records

The sponsor must maintain records showing the receipt, shipment, or other disposition of the investigational drug, including the name of the investigator to whom the drug was shipped, the date, quantity, and batch or code mark. The sponsor must also retain reserve samples of any test article and reference standards used in bioequivalence or bioavailability studies. If the drug is a controlled substance, additional records are required under the Controlled Substances Act administered by the Drug Enforcement Agency of the U.S. Department of Justice. The sponsor is also responsible for the secure storage of controlled substances.

Reports

The sponsor must promptly inform the FDA and all participating investigators of significant new adverse effects or risks with respect to the new drug. The sponsor must also submit any records or reports requested in writing by the FDA.

Investigator Responsibilities

The investigator must ensure that the investigation is conducted in accordance with the signed investigator statement, the investigational plan, and all applicable regulations. The investigator is responsible for the protection of the rights, safety, and welfare of the subjects and for obtaining informed consent from the subjects in accordance with 21 CFR 50. The investigator is also responsible for control of the drugs under investigation.

Records

An investigator is required to maintain records of investigational drug disposition and subject case histories. Disposition records must include dates, quantity, and use by subjects. The investigator must prepare and maintain case histories designed to record all observations and other data pertinent to the investigation for each individual treated with the investigational drug or employed as a control in the investigation. Records must be retained for a period of 2 years following approval of the NDA corresponding to the investigation; if the NDA is not approved, records must be retained for 2 years after the investigation is discontinued and the FDA is notified.

Reports

The investigator must provide progress reports, safety reports, and a final report to the sponsor. Safety reports must be made promptly of any adverse effect that may reasonably be regarded as caused by, or probably caused by, the drug. If the adverse effect is "alarming" (the word used in 21 CFR 312, without definition), it must be reported immediately.

INVESTIGATIONAL DEVICE EXEMPTIONS

The basic law prohibits distribution of devices that are not safe and effective; therefore, "exemptions" are needed to allow legal distribution of unproven or experimental products for purposes of research and testing. The legislative history shows that the U.S. Congress intended this part of the law to encourage the development of new technology by reducing the burden on device investigators to the greatest extent possible without infringing on the rights, safety, and welfare of the study subjects. The manufacturer of an investigational device is exempted from numerous provisions of the Act; however, other responsibilities are applied to sponsors, institutional review boards (IRBs), and investigators. Usually, the manufacturer is the sponsor. However, the investigator becomes a "sponsor-investigator" for studies that are being conducted without the manufacturer's sponsorship or for studies of devices designed by the investigator. The sponsor-investigator, of course, assumes the responsibilities of both entities.

The principal purpose of the requirements imposed by the IDE rules is to assure that the rights, safety, and welfare of the study subjects are protected. FDA policy has also recently emphasized the need for a rigorous study design and protocol that will provide for valid scientific evidence.

Sponsor Responsibilities

The sponsor must have an approved application for an IDE and approval by the IRB before allowing the study to commence, and must answer to the FDA for any violation of the rules. Proposed and final rules are published in the Federal Register and are codified annually (in April) in Title 21 of the Code of Federal Regulations (CFR). Part 812[3] of the code contains the IDE rules. The primary sanction that the FDA uses to enforce the IDE rules is withdrawal of approval of the IDE. The IRB also has the

authority to halt a study. The rules are outlined below, but sponsors and investigators must read and be familiar with the actual rules as published in 21 CFR 812 before undertaking a study.

Approved Application

Except for "nonsignificant risk" studies, the sponsor must apply to the FDA for an exemption and must provide all of the information specified in 21 CFR 812.20. The FDA always sends a reply letter to the applicant within 30 days that either approves, conditionally approves, or disapproves the IDE application. The law requires the FDA to respond in 30 days; otherwise, the application is automatically approved. If the application is disapproved, the FDA also must specify the data that the sponsor needs to obtain an approved application.

If the IRB concurs with the sponsor that the investigation does not expose the subjects to significant risk and meets the other applicability criteria stated in Section 812.2(b) titled "Abbreviated Requirements," the sponsor is considered to have an approved IDE without applying to the FDA. In this situation, responsibility for oversight and control of the investigation is vested in the local IRB.

Labeling

The device labeling must have the information specified in 21 CFR 812.5, primarily the statement: "CAUTION—Investigational device. Limited by Federal [or United States] law to investigational use." The labeling also must identify all relevant contraindications, hazards, adverse effects, interfering substances or devices, warnings, and precautions.

Prohibition of Promotion

Promoting, selling for profit, and representing an investigational device as safe or effective for the use for which it is being investigated are prohibited acts for any person.

Monitoring the Conduct of the Investigation

The sponsor is responsible for the selection of persons who are qualified to be investigators and monitors for the investigation. The sponsor must select a monitor who is qualified to ensure that the investigation is conducted in compliance with FDA rules, the investigational plan, and the signed investigator agreement.

Providing Information to Investigators and the FDA

The sponsor must provide all investigators with a copy of the investigational plan and a report of prior investigations. The investigational plan must specify the purpose of the study, provide a written protocol, a risk analysis, a detailed description of the device, monitoring procedures, copies of all labeling, consent materials, IRB data, a list of other institutions involved in the study, and a description of the records and reports that must be maintained. The report of prior investigations must include all prior clinical, animal, and laboratory testing of the device. The report also must include a bibliography of all relevant publications, whether adverse or supportive, and a summary of available unpublished data relevant to the safety or effectiveness of the device.

Records

The sponsor must maintain accurate, complete, and current records of:

- correspondence with an IRB, any other sponsor, a monitor, an investigator, and the FDA, including all required reports;
- shipping and device disposition, including: name and address of the consignee, type and quantity of device, dates of shipment, identification codes, and the disposition of returned devices;
- signed investigator agreements; and
- complaints and adverse effects, both anticipated and unanticipated.

If the study is being conducted under the abbreviated requirements for a nonsignificant risk investigation (i.e., under Section 812.2(b)), the sponsor must maintain consolidated records for each investigation that include the name of the device and its intended use, the objectives of the investigation, a brief explanation of why it is not a significant device investigation, the name and address of each investigator and each IRB, and a statement of the extent to which good manufacturing practice rules will be followed.

Reports

The sponsor must prepare and submit reports of:

- unanticipated adverse effects, to the FDA, the IRBs, and all investigators;
- withdrawal of IRB approval, to the FDA, other IRBs and investigators;
- withdrawal of the FDA approval, to IRBs and investigators;
- current list of investigators, to the FDA;
- progress reports, to the FDA;
- requests that an investigator return, repair, or dispose of devices, to the FDA and IRBs, and with a statement of why the request was made;
- completion or termination of the study (final report), to the FDA, all IRBs, and investigators;
- use of a device without informed consent, to the FDA; and
- a determination by any IRB that a device investigation involves significant risk when the sponsor had proposed that risk was not significant, to the FDA.

Investigator Responsibilities

It is the responsibility of the investigator to ensure that the investigation is conducted in accordance with the signed agreement, the investigational plan, and all applicable FDA regulations and conditions of IDE approval. The investigator must also ensure that informed consent is obtained using materials that conform to 21 CFR 50 and that no subject is allowed to participate in a study before FDA and IRB approval is obtained. The investigator controls access to the device and must not allow it to be used outside of the investigation, and must dispose of unused devices as directed by the sponsor.

Records

An investigator must maintain accurate, complete, and current records of:

- correspondence with the IRB, the sponsor, the monitor, the FDA, and any other investigator;
- device disposition, including dates of receipt, quantities, identification codes, persons possessing devices and device disposition, devices returned to the sponsor, and the reason for any disposal;
- case histories for each subject exposed to the device; and
- the protocol, changes, and deviations.

Reports

The investigator must prepare and submit reports of:

- unanticipated adverse effects, to the IRB and the sponsor;
- withdrawal of IRB approval, to the sponsor;
- deviations from the investigation plan, to the IRB and sponsor;
- use of a device without informed consent, to IRB and sponsor;
- annual progress, to the IRB, the sponsor, and the monitor;
- completion or termination of the investigation, or the investigator's part of it, along with a final report, to the IRB and the sponsor; and
- information on any aspect of the investigation requested by the IRB or FDA.

The Use of Unapproved Products

Drugs and devices that are used for purposes not identified in the product labeling are, strictly speaking, not approved for that use. However, by serendipity, physicians often discover that drugs and devices have uses that are not included in labeling, and this situation has historically posed a dilemma for the FDA.

Although important new uses are being discovered for medical products, often these "discoveries" do not withstand the tests of valid scientific evidence. For example, methotrexate was first marketed only for treating cancer, but was used for years by physicians to treat psoriasis

before the FDA approved it for that use. On the other hand, in retrospect, the serious adverse effects experienced with off-label use of chloramphenicol makes its widespread use now seem tragic.[13] Consequently, rules limiting the availability of investigational new drugs and devices were promulgated and the medical device amendments require an IDE when a device is being investigated for a new use.

Investigational New Drugs

A drug which has entered, or completed, Phase 3 clinical trials may be used to treat patients who are not in the clinical trials, provided that the criteria specified in 21 CFR 312.34 are met. In some cases, a drug in phase 2 might also be used for treatment. The term "compassionate use" is sometimes used by the public in this context; however, there is no formal definition of this term in the regulations. The term "treatment IND" is used, as explained below.

The investigational drug may not be used unless the following criteria are met:

1. The drug is intended to treat a serious or life-threatening disease.
2. There are no comparable and satisfactory drugs or therapies.
3. The drug is, or has been, under investigation in a controlled clinical trial.
4. The sponsor is diligently pursuing marketing of the drug.

The FDA may require the sponsor to submit a protocol for a "treatment IND." Any licensed practitioner who receives an investigational drug for treatment use under a treatment protocol is an "investigator" within the meaning of the rules and must assume all the responsibilities of an investigator.

Investigational Devices

Devices for which there is no pre-amendment status, no finding of substantial equivalence through the 510(k) process, no order of reclassification into class I or class II, and no approved PMA are described as "investigational," whether or not there is an actual investigation in progress. Investigational devices are not assured to be safe and effective. The term "unapproved device" has been used synonymously by the FDA in the Federal Register notice discussed below. Marketing and promotion of unapproved devices is clearly prohibited and can be a felony. Also, such devices can be considered misbranded or adulterated within the meaning of the Act and are subject to seizure.

The IDE provision in the law establishes a means by which the distribution of unapproved devices for purposes of research is made legal; however, situations often emerge in which the patient's health is in jeopardy and the physician can find no reasonable alternative to using an unapproved device. To alleviate this situation, the FDA published a **Federal Register** notice in 1985[5] formalizing the agency policy to "exercise discretion" when enforcing provisions of the Act under which devices might be considered adulterated, misbranded, or otherwise subject to seizure.

This notice informs physicians that they may use an unapproved device in a situation in which a patient is in danger and there is no reasonable alternative. This notice also suggests criteria for assuring that the action is a bona fide emergency. These are:

1. The patient has a life-threatening condition that needs immediate treatment.
2. No generally acceptable alternative for treating the patient is available.
3. Because of the immediate need to use the device, there is no time to use existing procedures to get FDA approval (an IDE) for the use.

Since the publication of this notice, changes in FDA policy have allowed a broadening of these criteria. Conditions other than "life-threatening" have been considered adequate justification, but all reflected extremely serious health consequences. In addition, the early interpretation of this notice by the FDA limited "emergency use" to a single occasion, but later interpretation removed this restriction. However, repeated "emergencies" may bring an order from the FDA requiring an approved IDE for any additional use.

The "emergency use" notice also recommends that the physician employ the following procedures to assure that the patient's rights are protected:
1. Obtain an independent assessment by an uninvolved physician.
2. Obtain informed consent from the patient or the patient's legal representative.
3. Where institutional policies apply, obtain permission from the institution.
4. Obtain the IRB chairperson's concurrence.
5. If an approved IDE is in effect, obtain permission from the sponsor.

Note that no contact with the FDA is required prior to an emergency use! However, in the situation where the device is not immediately available to the physician and it is necessary to have it shipped from the manufacturer, the person authorizing the shipment should notify the FDA by contacting the IDE staff in the Office of Device Evaluation. (The current telephone number is 301-594-1190.)

Following the emergency use, the physician must report the use of the device to the FDA if the device was not obtained under an existing IDE. If the device was obtained under an existing IDE, the use is reported as a protocol deviation, in accordance with the IDE rules. For details, a copy of the Federal Register notice cited above should be obtained and consulted.

THIRD-PARTY REIMBURSEMENT AND INVESTIGATIONAL DEVICES

The Act requires that the FDA evaluate medical products to assure safety and effectiveness, but there is no mention of cost considerations in these evaluations. However, many third-party payors, including the Health Care Financing Administration (HCFA), which administers the Medicare program, use FDA decisions concerning marketing and labeling as a basis for their reimbursement decisions.

These decisions, in the past, did not usually distinguish between devices that were new and unproven and those representing only refinements of existing technology that have not yet been marketed. Nonpayments that were attributed to the use of the latter type of investigational device imposed a hardship on persons participating in these studies and also caused difficulty for manufacturers who needed to evaluate new refinements to "old" devices. It also has been noted that some studies were adversely affected because the patient population did not include the proper demographic proportion when persons unable to pay could not participate.

To help correct this situation, a memorandum of understanding between the FDA and HCFA has established criteria by which the FDA Office of Device Evaluation determines whether each investigational device is a "first-of-a-kind" or whether it is based on proven technologies. The FDA will report this determination to HCFA so that they can use this information in making reimbursement decisions. HCFA will make these data available to the IDE sponsor, so that it may be released to the public (i.e., other third-party payors) insofar as this is possible without divulging proprietary information. This should assure that the use of devices such as new aneurysm clips or new shunt valves that are being clinically evaluated will not jeopardize reimbursement for treatment.

CUSTOM DEVICES

Section 520(b) of the Act (custom devices) states that Sections 514 (standards) and 515 (premarket approval) do not apply if the device:

1. is not generally available in finished form for purchase or for dispensing upon prescription and is not offered through labeling or advertising by the manufacturer, importer, or distributor thereof for commercial distribution; and

2. is intended for use by an individual patient named in such order of such physician or dentist (or other specially qualified person so designated) and is to be made in specific form for each patient, or is intended to meet the needs of such physician or dentist, and is not generally available to or generally used by other . . . physicians. . . .

Section 812.3 of the IDE regulation adds the two following criteria to the definition:

1. . . . necessarily deviates from devices generally available or from an applicable performance standard or premarket approval requirement in order to comply with the order of an individual physician or dentist;

2. . . . is not generally available to, or generally used by, other physicians or dentists.

The general idea seems to be that a special device may be manufactured to fit the needs of a particular patient or physician without going through the FDA approval process. The need for this special manufacture is apparent in such things as orthopedic braces and dental appliances. However, some persons believe that the "special needs of the physician" could be interpreted to include devices being used by that physician. The FDA has taken exception to this interpretation many times; therefore, it appears this interpretation is not consistent with FDA policy. The production of multiple devices or identical modifications of a device for a single physician will likely bring a letter from the FDA ordering that an IDE be obtained.

REFERENCES

1. 21 CFR 329
2. 21 CFR 329.20
3. 21 CFR 812
4. 21 USC §321(h)
5. 50 **Federal Register** 42866-42867 (1985)
6. 56 **Federal Register** 60024-60039 (1991)
7. American Medical Association: Report of AMA's Council on Ethical and Judicial Affairs. **Food Drug Law J 49:**362, 1994
8. *Drown v US*, 198 F2d 999 (9th Cir 1952), *cert denied,* 344 US 920 (1953)
9. **FDC Law J 46:**166-169, 1991
10. *General Medical Company, Petitioner v US Food and Drug Administration, et al,* Respondents (No. 83-2298, DC Cir 1985)
11. Kessler DA, Hass AE, Feiden KL, et al: Approval of new drugs in the United States. **JAMA 276:** 1826-1831, 1996
12. Legal Corner: **FDA Quarterly Activities Report. First Quarter.** Rockville, Md: US Food and Drug Administration, 1992
13. Merrill RA, Hutt PB: **Food and Drug Law.** Mineola, NY: The Foundation Press, 1980, p 462
14. Sheehan JM: Final civil penalties rule published. **Food and Drug Administration User Facility Reporting.** Fall 1995

CHAPTER 20

ISSUES IN PHYSICIAN LICENSURE

GRACE J. WIGAL, JD

Health care reform. Everyone talks about it, and everyone seems to have a slightly different proposal for how to address the issues embodied in health care reform. Yet most people tend to agree that a new health care system must encompass (1) quality care (2) rendered by competent physicians (3) in a convenient location and (4) at an affordable cost.[40,98,109] Physician licensure is implicated in each of these four goals.

Physician licensure, which is the process by which the government authorizes an individual to engage in the practice of medicine,[78] reflects two common beliefs about consumers. The first is that consumers are incapable of evaluating the quality of the medical services they receive, so they must be protected from fraud and harm at the hands of incompetent and unethical practitioners.[33] A second belief is that consumers should be able to trust in the highly-trained medical professionals who make complex medical decisions about their health care.[7]

These beliefs help explain the three most-often stated purposes of physician licensure: enhancement of patient safety, improvement of public confidence, and protection of professional welfare. The first purpose targets the patient and reflects a desire to improve quality of care by eliminating quacks, charlatans, and incompetents and thereby diminishing the occurrence of injuries related to health care.[14,38]

The second purpose reflects both the patient's desire to establish a physician-patient relationship built upon trust and the historical desire of all professions to improve public confidence.[48] The third purpose focuses on the physician and reflects the profession's desire to protect its status by limiting the number of persons who enter the profession.[37,43,89,94] Thus, while licensure protects patient health, it also protects the professional's job security and income.

Although many 20th century commentators have criticized medical licensure's ability to improve the quality of care to the public,[37,43] consumers generally have favored licensing of their medical professionals for a number of reasons. Consumers believe that a government licensing agency helps assure competence and quality by screening out applicants for medical licenses who do not possess the knowledge and skills necessary to enter the practice of medicine, by periodically reviewing each licensed physician's practice performance, by requiring all physicians to stay abreast of new medical developments related to their practices, and by rapidly identifying and efficiently disciplining licensed practitioners who develop problems that affect their ability to practice medicine competently or ethically.

Nevertheless, some consumers recently have become skeptical about the success of licensure.

During the 1980s, when stories proliferated about rogue physicians who malpracticed with little professional censure,[3] consumers began to ask whether the profession actually can police itself and assure both competence and quality of care.[13,29,34] Specifically, consumers now ask whether doctors are receiving the right kind of training in medical schools, whether a pencil and paper licensing test is related to competence in practice, and whether physician-dominated licensing boards have the motivation to screen out incompetent license applicants or to discipline incompetent physicians.[10] Furthermore, consumers have observed licensure's inability to provide of convenient and affordable health care to all citizens of the United States.[66,109] Because consumers realize that physician licensing affects access to and cost of care by limiting the number of persons who are permitted to become physicians,[18] it is not surprising that many of the current health care proposals suggest providing routine health care more inexpensively and conveniently through licensed health care professionals trained to work under a physician's supervision.[67]

Physicians also are becoming concerned about new developments with licensing and are beginning to realize that the current licensing mechanism may be losing some of its ability to protect the profession.[11] Since the early 1900s, physicians in the U.S. have enjoyed a health care system that permitted them to both define and monitor the quality of physician care. Further, through professional administration of medical school accreditation, licensure, certification, and professional discipline, physicians have controlled access to and regulation of the profession.[35] Recent health care reform initiatives, however, have challenged that professional autonomy. For example, both private and government entities acting as third-party payors in private or government health plans have begun reviewing physicians' performance and disciplining "nonconforming" physicians by withholding payment or by denying them the right to continue treating patients who participate in a private or public health plan. Furthermore, while only a physician can be licensed to practice medicine under existing licensure law, non-physician employees of third party payors are indirectly participating in the medical decision-making process by defining which treatments and procedures will be covered for a particular patient. In addition, as explained later in this chapter, physicians have seen governments act to direct the number of physicians entering specialty practices,[100] as well as to tie the physician's medical license to an ultimatum to serve particular kinds of patients. Thus, physicians are questioning whether professional licensing will continue to offer the kind of benefits and security it has provided in the past.

This chapter focuses upon these and other current licensing issues. Some issues are patient-centered, while others focus upon physician concerns. All are relevant to the discussion of how to structure a new health care system that can meet the needs of both patients and their physicians.

HISTORY OF LICENSURE

The state historically has been involved in controlling who could serve the public's health needs. For example, the Code of Hammurabi established both patient fees and punishment for negligent treatment in Babylonia about 4,000 years ago.[43,65]

Furthermore, because education has always been tied to practice requirements, access to education has regulated who practiced the healing arts. In early Greece and Rome a distinction based on education determined who served the masses and who served the elite.[43] Temple priests who were formally educated served the aristocracy, while common practitioners with less formal medical education served the needs of community members who could afford to pay fees for service. Finally, the indigent were served by folk practitioners, primarily women, who cultivated their healing herbs and learned from each other the secrets of healing. In fact, women were barred for centuries from reading books and attending lectures, thus prohibiting them from entering the recognized practice of medicine.[43]

The requirement of formal medical education continued into 13th-century Europe, when the elite continued to be served by physicians trained and licensed by university-related medical schools. Of course, demand for medical services among the masses assured that women (sometimes known as "witches") and other self-trained practitioners continued to provide aid to the public. In response, merchant guilds began to form in Europe to fill the need for trained practitioners who could meet the masses' needs. The guilds provided medical training to members who were then given the right to practice medicine upon completion of the training. Thus, for a time, both avenues to the practice of medicine, university education and guild membership, required formal training.

By 1422, however, the English Parliament had outlawed apprenticeship programs and required university graduation of all practitioners. A hundred years later, Parliament created the College of Physicians and Surgeons, which was an agency charged with making licensing decisions. Of course, this model of university education and government agency licensing could not readily be transferred to colonial America. In fact, since no medical institutions existed in this country for about 150 years after the first settlements, an apprenticeship tradition of training developed.

The early licensing laws adopted in the colonies reflected a general lack of concern about regulating who practiced medicine. For example, the first physician licensing statute in the U.S., which was enacted in Virginia in 1639, merely controlled the fees charged by medical practitioners.[48] The other colonies seemed to follow Virginia's lead in the years that followed, because the various colonial practice acts included no practice restrictions and instead focused on prohibitions against excessive fees. Thus, for the next 100 years, anyone who set up a medical practice and inspired confidence was welcomed as a community practitioner. This led one physician in 1753 to comment that "there is more Danger from the Physician than from the Distemper."[101]

In the mid-1700s, however, both medical schools and medical societies began to proliferate in response to the need to organize and educate practitioners. One of the first medical schools was begun in Philadelphia in 1765. Its founder, Dr. John Morgan, had hoped to establish a college that would conduct examinations and grant licenses. However, his request for licensing authority was refused by the British government, and his school had to be content with merely educating the physicians who would practice in accordance with the existing colonial practice acts.

However, in the second half of the 18th century, the various medical societies were more successful in advocating for regulation of the profession, and the colonies began to include practice restrictions in their medical practice acts. In 1772, the colony of New Jersey passed the first comprehensive medical practice act, which included a licensing requirement and created a board to regulate the practice of medicine. This regulatory board was given the authority both to examine a physician before granting a license and to levy fines against those who were practicing without a license.[101] For the first time in America, a licensing requirement appeared to be enforceable.

During the period of the Revolutionary War and thereafter, other states followed New Jersey's lead, but instead of creating medical boards, other states tended to rely upon the medical societies to regulate the profession. Thus, by the year 1800, 13 of the 16 existing states had given their state medical societies the authority to both examine and license university-trained and apprentice-trained practitioners.

As envisioned by John Morgan, some states then established a second mechanism for obtaining a license. In 1803, Massachusetts decided to permit Harvard Medical School to license its graduates. Other states also began to permit their medical schools to license their graduates, and this alternative pathway to a medical license encouraged the rapid proliferation of medical schools that began to occur in the early 1800s. Unfortunately, the level of competency of the graduates of these schools continued to be questionable. Those who entered the medical schools often were not required to have a high school education,[18] and some of the medical schools provided no more than a few months of training before licensing their graduates. Furthermore, most schools provided no clinical training.

A rather startling change of events occurred after 1800. Perhaps in response to a growing population and an expanding country that began to expound upon democratic ideals surrounding the capabilities of the common man, the practice of medicine was deregulated during the first half of the 1800s. This period saw the growth of new schools of thought about how to practice medicine. Lay healers, bone setters, botanic Thompsonians, homeopaths, eclectics, and others began to offer medical services,[18] and these "new schools" of medicine rapidly produced practitioners for the masses. States began to repeal licensing laws, and by 1849, only New Jersey and the District of Columbia had laws that set out anything close to a regulatory scheme.[48] Commentators disagree about the effect of this period of deregulation on the practice of medicine, but history reveals that the public began to accuse its healers of quackery, and countless medical malpractice lawsuits were filed against physicians.[30]

Recognizing that the problems in both medical training and the practice of medicine were damaging their professional status, physicians practicing traditional medicine began to seek ways to standardize the practice of medicine and to assure that traditional practitioners met the standards. In response to the New York State Medical Society's call for a national meeting of medical societies, the American Medical Association (AMA) emerged in 1847.[101] One of the AMA's first actions was to accept a code of ethics that distinguished traditional doctors from "new school" doctors.[65] During the latter half of the century, state medical professional societies also organized to establish practice standards that could be used to assess competence and improve professional reputation in the eyes of the public.

At least partially in response to physician demands, "the first modern medical practice act was passed in Texas in 1873," and by 1905, 39 states were again licensing physicians.[43] Twenty-two of these states required practitioners to pass a licensing examination.[47]

Although the licensure acts were challenged in courts because the new laws deprived many existing and potential "new school" practitioners of their right to practice medicine, the 1889 U.S. Supreme Court case of *Dent v. West Virginia*[28] established that the state has a duty to protect the health, welfare, and safety of its citizens, and that as long as the licensing acts were rationally related to this state duty, they would be upheld. The plaintiff in the *Dent* case challenged a licensing law that West Virginia had enacted in 1882. The law required every medical practitioner to get a state board of health certificate attesting to graduation from a reputable medical college, or to continuous West Virginia practice for 10 years prior to 1881, or to a passing score on the medical examination. Illegal practice of medicine was made a misdemeanor punishable by fine, imprisonment, or both. Mr. Dent appealed his case all the way to the U.S. Supreme Court, which ultimately said that a state has the power to provide for the general welfare of its citizens, especially to protect them "against the consequences of ignorance and incapacity, as well as of deception and fraud."[28] The Court said the law of West Virginia was "intended to secure such skill and learning in the profession of medicine that the community might trust with confidence those receiving a license under authority of the state."[28] This decision, of course, opened the floodgate to professional licensing, and almost immediately 10 professional occupations[43] were made subject to licensure. By 1920, the list had expanded to at least 30 occupations,[43] and by 1977, 35 health care professions were licensed in various states.[18]

The modern medical practice acts, which required graduation from medical school, now placed the licensing function in state agencies, and medical schools no longer could license their graduates. But medical schools also began to improve their curricula in the early part of the 20th century as the schools came under the scrutiny of both professional bodies and state agencies. In 1904, the AMA adopted an "ideal standard" of medical education, which it began to use to rate medical schools. In 1907, the AMA inspected and rejected 32 schools and conditionally approved another 46.

A scathing report in 1910 by Abraham Flexner of the Carnegie Corporation led states to put pressure on medical schools to change the direction of medical education.[101] Flexner's report, written for the Foundation for the Advancement of Teaching, evaluated the nation's medical schools and recommended that many be closed because of inadequate programs. The report recommended that all medical programs more closely resemble the first modern medical school, which was established in 1893 at the Johns Hopkins University. Because Johns Hopkins offered a clinical practice component to its students, many medical schools began to standardize programs by including specific science courses[72] and clinical training. They also began to seek accreditation in an effort to validate their programs.

Thus, the early years of the 20th century mark the beginnings of both medical education and licensure as we know it today. Only a person who graduates from an acceptable school is permitted to apply for a medical license. The physician who is licensed under a state medical practice act is permitted to practice medicine in that state, and that practice is virtually unlimited in scope. However, the unlicensed practitioner can be punished by fine and imprisonment.

QUALIFICATIONS FOR LICENSURE

The theory that licensure protects the public from incompetent and unethical professionals is valid only if the licensure mechanism truly screens out the incompetent and unfit applicant. Thus, three universal qualifications for medical licensure are recognized: 1) a high moral and ethical character; 2) graduation from an approved medical school; and 3) a passing score on the licensing examination.[23] Because an "approved" school is usually defined as a nationally accredited school, and because a single licensure test is used nationwide, the medical profession is now close to having a "national" licensure system that provides geographic mobility to licensed practitioners. However, because of its power to provide for the general health and welfare of its citizens, each state retains the authority to define precisely how it will license physicians within its borders.[28] In cases where unlicensed practitioners have challenged the state's licensing requirements, courts have said that no one has an unqualified right to practice medicine and that a state can restrict the practice of medicine to only those who have met the licensure requirements as long as the requirements are related directly and substantially to medical practice.[105] The state also may require applicants to pay a licensing fee and obtain a statutorily specified amount of malpractice insurance coverage before practicing medicine.[58,93]

The state may delegate to a board its authority both to license physicians and to discipline physicians by revoking or suspending their medical licenses. The licensing board typically is given a myriad of administrative tasks including the following: administering statutory requirements, including eligibility of applicants for licenses, setting standards of ethical conduct; disciplining unethical and incompetent practitioners; and assessing the qualifications of applicants who are licensed in another state or country.[78]

The composition of the board usually is described by statute, which commonly dictates that members are to come from the profession and are to be chosen by gubernatorial appointment from a list of persons suggested by leaders of the state professional association. Of course, this mechanism for selecting members has been criticized because it looks much like the fox is guarding the henhouse door when members of the profession determine who is admitted to the profession and who is disciplined. However, numerous court decisions have upheld the state's authority to describe the composition of the board,[82] apparently requiring only that the board *actually* not be biased.[93]

Nevertheless, many states have begun to include laypersons on the board in an effort to hear consumers' points of view. The number of laypersons on boards remains small, however, because of the perceived need to have the board staffed by persons with the qualifications to make the kind of policy and technical decisions that must be made in this highly sophisticated arena.[78]

CONSUMER QUESTIONS ABOUT THE LICENSING PROCESS

The process of licensing described above has raised a number of commonly asked consumer questions that are related to quality of care, competence, cost of care, and access to care. These questions are set out below with responsive information.

1. *The competitive nature of the accredited medical schools' admission processes probably means that many persons who are not admitted are the very persons who would be willing to practice in undesirable locations or for lower fees. To assure more equal care, shouldn't we let*

graduates of non-accredited schools practice if they can pass the licensing exam?

Critics of accreditation and licensure point out that restricting licensure to graduates of accredited schools gives the medical profession control over physician supply, and thereby also gives the profession too much control over its economic interests. However, the answers to questions of cost and access in today's health care environment probably do not lie in graduating more physicians, because we already are in a situation of physician oversupply in the U.S.[84,110] Although additional primary care physicians may be needed in some areas of the country, the excess in the specialty areas is now well-documented.[100,110] In fact, a recent study by the Pew Health Professions Commission predicted a "glut" of physicians in the medical market as the U.S. rapidly moves to managed care in the 1990s. The Commission recommended closing medical schools because fewer physicians will be needed.[113] Thus, the answers to the access and cost questions lie, in part, with convincing medical students and existing practitioners that the profession must better address the needs of society with fewer physicians.

One commentator has noted that a health care system as massive as that found in the U.S. cannot be changed without changing how physicians are educated in the ethics of providing medical care to those who need it at a price they can afford.[106] Not surprisingly, both consumers and physicians have encouraged an educational model that stresses the development of professional ethics and clinical skills by relying less on rote learning and by incorporating more problem-based activities and evaluation of students through use of group interaction, computer-based instruction and simulation, standardized patients, and actual clinical experience. Realizing that practitioners of the future must be able to address "problems such as coping with diversity, working in teams with other professionals, and providing care in managed settings," a modern educational program also should provide students the opportunity to work in the communities the medical schools serve.[17,83,91]

While attending an accredited medical school does not assure that one will become a competent practitioner, accreditation of the school is designed to achieve two generally recognized purposes. First, it establishes for the public, which has little expertise in evaluating technical training programs, that the medical school has met and continues to meet minimum standards recognized by the profession as a whole. Second, in assuring the quality of the school's training and services,[61] accreditation also assures that the graduates of the institution are well-grounded in the study of medicine.

Accreditation is a two-part process. First, the accrediting body must establish standards that will be used to evaluate program quality. Second, a review team from the accrediting body must determine on a regular basis whether each institution has complied with the standards. This two-step process for accreditation by a continuing, established committee of medical professionals satisfies the following attributes of the effective regulatory mechanism: 1) ongoing oversight, supervision, and evaluation of the schools' programs of study; 2) evaluation by a body regularly in place and operating with procedures that are designed to provide an integrated body of interrelated information; 3) a specific process for identification of problems and assistance with rehabilitation when problems are noted; and 4) a review mechanism that assesses quality based upon standards reflecting the shared values of those in the profession.[43,54-57]

On the other hand, accrediting a school that provides an opportunity to become well-grounded in medicine does not mean its graduates actually *are* competent. After all, predicting competency on the basis of a curriculum review is much like complementing the chef on the menu without tasting the food. However, an examination of recent changes in the accreditation process demonstrates how an accrediting body can direct educational programs toward assuring high-quality graduates and becoming responsive to the needs of society. In fact, the Liaison Committee on Medical Education (LCME), the accreditation committee that accredits the 124 medical school educational programs leading to the Doctor of Medicine degree in the U.S.,[8] sponsors a yearly retreat to consider important medical education issues, such as how to assess educational outcomes and how the LCME can encourage schools to promote educational innovation and address social change. Further, the LCME is well aware of the challenges that face the medical profession in demonstrating that it is accountable to the public during an era of reform.

A common complaint from consumers has been that physicians are not trained in basic clinical skills, nor in how to communicate with patients and relate empathetically to patients' needs.[59,62] The LCME responded in 1991 to the public's concern about clinical and communication skills by imposing new accreditation standards that call for schools to:[99]

- establish a variety of educational outcome objectives;
- measure and evaluate their graduates according to those outcome objectives;
- measure their educational outcomes;
- assure that students' educational experiences and evaluation are similar to the experiences and evaluation of students at all other medical schools; and
- observe students performing core clinical skills.

Commentators close to the medical education process have noted that accreditors' pressure for change has led to the following developments in some schools: fewer lecture hours, increased use of small interactive learning groups, more problem-based learning sessions, more integration of clinical courses, more exposure to ambulatory and primary care, and greater emphasis on ethics, communication skills, preventive medicine, and health maintenance.[55] Furthermore, statistics show that between 1988 and 1992 clinical faculty in medical schools increased by 23% when compared to a 9.5% growth in the basic science faculty, another indicator that additional faculty are being used in settings other than the typical classroom. In fact, in some schools, teaching and evaluation of clinical skills are receiving more attention with use of standardized patients and objective standardized clinical examinations.[55,115]

While the LCME obviously has taken steps to assure that medical students graduate with an acceptable level of medical competence, critics of self-regulation contend that medical schools would respond better to public pressure for change if they were unregulated and not subject to accreditation standards.[7] Further, the medical school accreditation process is solely in the hands of medical professionals and provides no actual means for consumer input. The critics argue that since consumers do not participate in the accreditation process, the LCME can pick and choose the issues that it wants to address and can screen out those issues that the medical profession simply does not want to examine. Thus, consumers must go elsewhere to effect important changes. For example, the accreditation process has not addressed the problems associated with having 70% of the combined graduates entering specialty practices and locating in areas where other specialists practice. As a result, 21 schools now are subject to state policy or legislation that stipulates the desired specialty mix of graduates.[8]

Critics also charge that self-regulation through accreditation can stifle innovation in the education and training of practitioners,[31,49] because only current approaches to the practice of medicine tend to be recognized and taught. Thus, even though innovative variations in medical practice ultimately might prove beneficial and desirous to patients,[6] diverse approaches to health care could be discouraged by accreditors who favor more traditional training.[102] For example, recent data suggest that needle biopsies could replace surgical biopsy for diagnosing breast cancer. Nevertheless, because surgical biopsy is still regarded as *the* standard for diagnosis, the far less traumatic, less costly, and less disfiguring (but far more tricky) needle biopsy procedure might not be taught in medical school. A second example might be a school that placed an extraordinary amount of emphasis on intangible aspects of quality of care (e.g., patient communication) and that trained physicians to devise treatment plans that include recommendations of alternative forms of health care such as acupuncture. Would that school run into trouble with the accreditation teams who might disagree with an "unscientific" approach to healing?[1]

Despite such concerns, most medical professionals strongly believe that the traditional rigorous and technical training programs demanded by the accreditation standards, coupled with the professional socialization process that occurs during the course of medical education, provides a mechanism that produces medical professionals who will deliver high-quality care.[16,59]

Medical schools, in fact, do attract extremely bright applicants (the mean premedical grade point average for new students in 1991 was 3.42 on a 4.0 scale) who are carefully tested and screened both upon admission and throughout their school careers.[24] The medical student of today also is evaluated on more than "book learning." In addition to the traditional third and fourth-year clinical clerkship opportunities, many schools use standardized patients to assist faculty in assessing the clinical performance of students.[8] Moreover, traditional medical training "socializes" students by encouraging them to internalize a work ethic that focuses upon the patient and that incorporates "diligence, honesty, carefulness, and fidelity to . . . medical responsibilities."[59] As one AMA committee report stated, "[G]raduation from a medical school is substantial evidence of good character and a solid background in the science of medicine."[88]

Because medical professionals strongly believe in medical education and its ability to adapt to societal demands, the licensing requirement of graduation from an accredited school likely will remain unchanged for years to come. This does not mean, however, that schools will not be subject to state mandates to cap enrollments, change curriculum, or reach a desired graduate specialty mix.[27,111] It also does not foreclose future controls upon resident training programs to control physician distribution.[100] Because most residents locate permanently in the geographic area where they receive residency training,[92,100] it makes sense that residents be trained in nonhospital, community settings rather than urban areas where most hospitals are located and where most residency training now occurs. In fact, the Council for Graduate Medical Education has supported placing residents in alternative settings to acquire skills to meet the public's needs in a particular community.

2. *Doesn't a multiple-choice licensing test merely find out who has memorized material rather than who has acquired enough clinical competence to practice medicine?*

Some form of examination requirement for licensure has been a prerequisite to the practice of medicine for at least a thousand years. An examination requirement was in place in 931AD in Baghdad, which had a board that handled both the examination and licensing of physicians.[8] Roman law also penalized the practice of medicine without a license, which could not be obtained without an examination by a teacher of medicine. As explained in this chapter's section on "History of Licensing," colonial America for some time permitted physicians to be licensed either by passing a test or by graduating from a medical school. But by the early part of the 20th century, the additional requirement of a medical examination was firmly ingrained in the general requirements for physician licensure.

Until recently, the national licensing examination was a multiple-choice achievement-type examination that came in two formats: 1) National Board of Medical Examiners (NBME) Parts I, II, and III—a national examination for graduates of schools in the United States, and 2) Federation Licensing Examination (FLEX)—a special test for graduates of foreign medical schools.

Critics of licensing by examination pointed to a number of reasons why this multiple-choice achievement examination should not be the threshold to a license to practice medicine.[73] First, they noted that a test's validity is measured by two factors: 1) whether its content represents important knowledge or skills, and 2) how well performance on the test relates to performance in practice.[27] They then argued that the licensing tests measured "book" or rote learning and therefore did not assess clinical competence. They also argued that the tests were unfairly race- and culture-biased;[27] and that the licensure test impeded physician movement because various states established different test requirements for obtaining a license.

To make the licensing examinations better predictors of clinical competence and to create a single test that would be the pathway to all state licenses,[80] the NBME began studying testing in the 1980s. A new test was devel-oped through a joint program of the NBME and the Federation of State Medical Boards, and in 1992, the U.S. Medical Licensing Examination (USMLE) began to replace the NBME and FLEX tests. Although the old tests already had a fairly high correlation to the medical school instructors' evaluations of students' clinical performance with standardized patients, test developers designed the USMLE to better assess a student's acquisition of clinically relevant subject matter and ability to solve patient problems.[9] The USMLE includes a three-step examination, each of which must be passed for licensure. The USMLE test materials clarify that "[t]he three Step examinations that comprise USMLE are designed to assess the examinee's understanding of and ability to apply concepts and principles that are important in health and disease and that constitute the basis of safe and effective patient care."[77]

The USLME focuses on the content necessary for the general practice of medicine and assesses the student's ability to solve problems using that content. The test is designed to resemble simulations in that it asks the student to perform the kind of decision-making that a physician must conduct when presented with a patient's problem. For example, the test is written with longer descriptions of the patient's health history and current problems, and this description is often followed by test items calling for extended matching of up to 26 options. The traditional true-false questions have been abandoned, but the test usually also includes the typical five-answer option questions about the patient's problem.

Step 1 of the new test usually is taken by students at the end of the second year of medical school, when the basic science education is completed. The test covers basic biomedical concepts in a 700-question multiple-choice format, usually based upon patient descriptions. Step 2 is taken during the fourth year of study and assesses the medical knowledge necessary to provide clinical care under supervision. Again, the test has about 700 multiple-choice questions. Step 3 is supposed to be taken during postgraduate education and assesses the kinds of biomedical knowledge and clinical knowledge that will be used in a general practice. It does not test an area of specialization.

While preparing the USMLE, the Board and the Federation also have been studying testing through computer-based examination and the use of standardized patients in live or electronic simulations.[63] These formats for testing ultimately may be incorporated into the USMLE, because they may easily and accurately evaluate clinical competence.

The use of the new USMLE extended matching options and the potential use of computer simulations and standardized patients created curriculum questions for medical schools. Because the licensing test is built upon the information and problem-solving skills that a student must possess to be a competent practitioner, the issue is whether medical schools will begin to focus on improving skills through classroom methods that differ from the traditional lecture or discussion. Furthermore, medical schools must decide whether they will establish programs that provide students the opportunity to become familiar with testing formats and objectives, such as the use of standardized patients to test physician competence. Those that do not may find that their students do not perform well on the new tests.

As explained in the preceding section, however, many medical schools have responded to this challenge in a number of positive ways. Approximately 73 schools now use computer-based simulations to teach and evaluate diagnostic or therapeutic decision-making.[8] Furthermore, about 75 schools use standardized patients in evaluation of student performance in basic courses, and approximately 90 schools also now offer some type of ambulatory care experience in the first and/or second year.[8] In other words, many medical schools have begun to value instruction and evaluation conducted through simulation or use of standardized patients, believing that these techniques better prepare their graduates both for the USMLE and for the practice of medicine.[90] At the same time they are addressing consumers' concerns about training.

3. *One of the state licensing boards' functions is to monitor physician competence after licensure to make sure that physicians admitted to practice remain competent and up-to-date. How can boards encourage and assess continuing competence when medicine is changing so rapidly?*

The real challenge to state licensing boards is to develop mechanisms for periodically assessing the competence of practicing physicians in a manner that truly assesses their practice skills. In fact, the licensing boards' failure to assure the continuing competence of practicing physicians was the consumer issue of the 1980s, as horror stories were told of incompetent physicians who malpracticed in one state, were "slapped on the wrist," and then moved on to do the same in another state. The public's concern about licensing boards' inability to control the incompetent physician was part of the impetus for the 1986 Health Care Quality Improvement Act, which established the National Practitioner Data Bank (Data Bank) to collect malpractice and licensure action information about every practicing physician in the U.S. (See Chapter 21 for further explanation about the Act and the Data Bank.)

When a physician receives a medical license, the license is awarded for life and qualifies the physician to practice in all areas of medicine. The license is subject only to the physician's ability to continue to practice ethically and competently. This licensing strategy assumes that the physician will acquire new information and expertise through a quest for knowledge precipitated by the treatment of patients.

Both consumers and professionals, however, now recognize two things: 1) that practitioners must make more formal efforts to keep up with new information and advancements in technology, and 2) that practice skills should be reassessed regularly. Without doubt, acquiring information about new technological advances can be a problem for all physicians in today's increasingly technological practice setting, and it can be particularly difficult for the older practitioner[36] or the practitioner living and working in a very rural setting. Furthermore, many physicians have little time or opportunity to assess whether their skills are improving as they should. For these and other reasons, formal continuing medical education courses are now required in many states to maintain the physician license.[81]

Continuing Medical Education

At least 26 states require physicians to participate in Continuing Medical Education (CME) on a regular basis to retain their medical licenses.[38,75] Most of these states require approximately 150 hours of CME every 3 years, and a third to a half of those hours are required in programs accredited by the Accreditation Council for Continuing Medical Education. However, physicians practicing in states without CME requirements also are taking both non-accredited and accredited courses to maintain standing in professional organizations. Therefore, most physicians in the U.S. rely to some extent upon CME to stay abreast of new treatments and to improve their treatment skills.

The mandates for CME are coming from both professional groups and from individuals, many of whom prefer CME to periodic examinations because traditional CME programs are fairly easy to organize, administer, and attend. Nevertheless, little evidence exists that traditional CME can provide the kind of experience necessary to maintain competence in the clinical setting.[25,26,74] A formal review of CME programs in the U.S. resulted in a report that the programs were plagued by "disjointed delivery, driven by the largesse of drug companies and the request of physicians, and plagued by doubts about and relatively little evidence for its own effectiveness . . ."[25] The reviewers concluded the report with the rather obvious statement that although most CME programs are based on ineffective conferences and meetings, CME need not be so ill-designed. In fact, medical professionals have recognized for years that the CME programs should be based upon individually tailored educational experiences in order to affect physician practice and patient outcomes.[19,25,68] To that end, the Alliance for Continuing Medical Education (ACME) recently announced plans to become more responsive to practicing physicians, especially since so many doctors are adapting to managed care settings.[75] Furthermore, advocates of CME have proposed a national CME requirement to encourage nationwide changes in physician behavior.[75] Nevertheless, many physicians remain skeptical of the effectiveness of traditional CME and believe specialty recertification is the better avenue for assuring continuing physician competence.

Physician Certification and Recertification

Certification is the process by which a nongovernment agency or association grants recognition of competence to an individual who has met certain predetermined qualifications specified by that agency or association.[78] The award of the credential gives the practitioner the right to use that credential, which attests to the competence of the individual while engaged "in the relevant scope of practice."[78] Certification is an entirely voluntary process whereby the applicant agrees to complete the certifying agency's education, training, and competency requirements.

Most medical school graduates enter residency training for the graduate study of medicine and later seek certification from a specialty board. Although certification is not required by law, it often is required in order to perform certain treatments and tests in the hospital setting. Furthermore, the individual practitioner usually wishes to establish his or her credentials as a specialist.

Today, the American Board of Medical Specialities (ABMS) consists of 24 member boards (e.g., internal medicine, obstetrics and gynecology, orthopedic surgery, radiology, surgery, and urology) that organized to assist each other in the evaluation and certification of specialists.[15] Each member board requires the certification applicant to pass a written examination, and over half the boards also require the applicant to pass an oral examination. Often, the boards demand that the applicant complete a certain number of years of graduate training before sitting for the written examination. For example, the American Board of Orthopaedic Surgery requires five years of graduate training before the exam may be taken. Applicants who pass the written exam may then take the oral test, which is a two-hour examination on six oral cases with protocols developed by the examination committee.[15]

Today, at least 16 specialty boards either have instituted or have plans to institute a time limit ranging from 7 to 10 years on their certifications.[81] The boards believe that time limits on certification prompt practitioners to document their competence, promote self-improvement by encouraging continuing education, promote collective improvement through individual improvement, prompt the profession to set standards for the practice of medicine, and promote maintenance of an expanding body of knowledge about the practice of medicine.[4]

On the other hand, many practitioners oppose recertification requirements and argue that because the tests are unrelated to the actual practice of medicine, the tests do not guarantee competence.[73,80] They further argue that practitioners learn throughout their careers from their patients, which is better assurance of competence than any written or oral test. In addition, they say that the costly process of recertification is unreasonable when the efficacy of certification is unclear.[4]

Recertification has become an important issue for all physicians in light of the 1986 Health Care Quality Improvement Act (HCQIA). Under the HCQIA, any board or society that withdraws membership on the basis of competence must report that action to the state licensing board.[45] This requirement is of particular concern to older physicians, because studies have shown decreased performance on most written examinations beginning 10 to 15 years after training.[4] It is unclear whether this is the result of the physicians' inability to keep up with the changes in medicine or the test's inability to reflect questions pertinent to an evolving practice. Therefore, boards have been reluctant to fail many older candidates and have changed the standards on the tests for older candidates in order to avoid the problem.[4] This precedent for creating different standards for different physician populations may be unwise in that it gives fuel to critics of self-regulation who say that physicians will devise ways to protect their own.

Medical Societies

In addition to board certification, most physicians seek membership in medical societies at the state and local level. In fact, states may require a physician to become a member of a state or local society as a condition of licensure. The societies police themselves through various kinds of voluntary controls but for many years had a history of lackadaisical assessment of competence.[108] Yet societies are beneficial as a regulatory mechanism in that mandatory societies must report negative membership decisions to state licensing boards.[97] In addition, the HCQIA requires all societies conducting peer review to report any negative membership decision made on the basis of quality of care.[45] Thus, although a society may have no direct way to keep an incompetent practitioner from practicing medicine, its adverse membership information will be reported to a licensing board, which can then investigate and take action against the practitioner if necessary.

Outcomes Assessment

A relatively new mechanism for assessing clinical competence has developed with outcomes assessment and management, which focuses on monitoring over a period of time the effect of medical care delivered to a patient.[61] Outcomes management contemplates obtaining data about each patient's clinical condition, functional status, and satisfaction with care, and then comparing this individual data to local, regional, or national outcomes information about similar patients.

Proponents of such research say that outcomes data provide information that can assist health care organizations in cutting costs and in assuring that physicians in the organization are rendering high-quality care. Hospitals, for example, are extremely interested in outcomes assessment because they believe such data can assist them in taking corrective action when a physician's practice may be sub-par or excessively costly for the hospital. Furthermore, a hospital might use aggregate data to revise practice guidelines for all physicians.

Government health care programs also are interested in outcomes research. For example, Medicare is implementing a computerized audit system that ultimately will publish reports about individual physicians and hospitals. Where performance is below acceptable standards, Medicare will work with providers to develop mutually acceptable quality improvement programs. Thus, advancing technology and improved ability to collect and analyze data has led to another mechanism for assessing quality of care in a manner that is readily reportable to state licensing boards. The only drawback is that there often is little agreement about what constitutes quality of care.[66]

4. *Isn't it true that medical boards really are doing very little about disciplining incompetent and impaired physicians?*[76]

The state, through its licensing body, has the authority to revoke or suspend a license that has been granted.[46] However, because the right to practice medicine under a license is a property right, the state must use "due process" procedures for restricting that right.[93] Further, the state must base the restriction on one of the grounds found in its revocation statute, which must clearly and specifically set out the conduct that constitutes grounds for revocation. "A typical statute will include many, if not all, of the following as grounds for revocation: fraudulent procurement of a medical license, abandonment of a patient, drug addiction, habitual drunkenness, fee splitting, incompetence, gross malpractice, dishonest or deceptive behavior, the filing of false medical reports or records, unprofessional or immoral conduct, conviction of various crimes, and assistance of an unlicensed medical practitioner."[93] Because the revocation statute sets out the exclusive reasons to revoke a physician's license, the state cannot go beyond these reasons in revoking the license.

The interesting thing about the various states' revocation statutes is that they vary so widely about the kind of conduct that should result in a disciplinary action. Most statutes, however, include five general categories as grounds to act against the license:[32]

1. license-related offenses;
2. crimes: conviction of a felony or misdemeanor involving moral turpitude;
3. physical and mental debilitation;
4. incompetence; and
5. unprofessional conduct, which is usually seen as one of two kinds of conduct—that which hurts the public (such as overcharging) and that which hurts the profession (such as unprofessional advertising).

However, no one ground is found in all of the statutes![88]

Despite continuing problems with understaffing and underfunding, licensing boards are now doing a better job of disciplining physicians. The Federation of State Medical Boards, which among other things tracks licensure actions, found that in 1993 a total of 3,081 prejudicial actions were taken against problem physicians, with this number representing almost a 15% increase over the preceding four years.[69]

The Federation has decided that its information reveals that two kinds of boards are the most efficient in monitoring and disciplining physicians: 1) autonomous boards having comparatively more staff per 1,000 physicians, and 2) boards in smaller states that oversee the lowest number of physicians.[69] Other studies have shown that boards "are significantly more effective . . . in states where medical boards are characterized by nonphysician dominance, where medical boards are small, where income per capita is low, and where the population is relatively well educated."[32] However, of all these characteristics, the most significant may be that board effectiveness is inversely related to the degree of physician power characterizing the board.[32]

While the Federation is impressed by the statistics that reveal heightened board activity in disciplining physicians, consumers may not be so impressed. For example, a 1993 report by a Washington, D.C. consumer group criticized the number of disciplinary actions taken by state medical boards and stated that with 150,000 to 300,000 Americans being injured or killed each year in hospitals, more should be done to protect the public. Consumers also note that professional boards have "strayed from the primary purpose of protecting the public and have become strong lobbyists for professional interest."[20,47] For instance, consumer groups perceive that boards often are more interested in rehabilitating impaired physicians (the board members' medical colleagues) than in protecting the public.[21] The consumer groups do agree, however, with the Federation's viewpoint that boards in some states are doing a better job of protecting patients from unfit practitioners. Therefore, they also recommend increased funding and staffing for state medical boards, routine information-sharing among the boards, and public revelation of disciplinary actions.

In fact, boards now routinely share information about disciplinary actions. All actions taken by a medical board are reported both to the Federation and to the national Data Bank, which was created by the HCQIA.[45] The Federation then disseminates the licensure reports among the states' boards, and under HCQIA law the boards also may directly query the Data Bank for information about physicians. However, as explained in Chapter 21, the public does not have access to Data Bank information.

Physician Questions About the Licensing Process

Changes in the practice of medicine, as well as new governmental attempts to scrutinize physician competence, have prompted physicians to begin asking questions about their rights under a government license and their ability to continue to exercise control over their profession. Some of those questions follow.

1. *What are my rights when defending an adverse licensure decision against a state licensing board?*

The process of obtaining a license is outlined by statutory law in all states. The statutes generally delegate to a public board the state's power to grant the license to practice medicine. The process may vary from state to state, but all licensing statutes require the prospective physician to demonstrate his or her qualifications and competency to practice medicine.

The Fifth and Fourteenth Amendments to the U.S. Constitution, which guarantee that government will not deprive a person of life, liberty, or property without due process of law, protect the applicant in the license application process. An applicant who has studied medicine with the expectation of practicing upon the completion of training has acquired a property interest in a vocation. Therefore, the Constitution says the state licensing board must follow fair procedures and give the applicant an opportunity to be heard if the board is inclined to render an adverse licensing decision. Yet, the right to practice a profession is not absolute, for the state has the obligation to regulate the health care profession in order to protect the public.[86] Therefore, a licensing board must always carefully weigh the rights of the public against the rights of the individual who wishes to practice medicine.

Once the license is granted, the Constitution also guarantees a physician fair procedures in a subsequent proceeding conducted by the licensing board for revocation, suspension, or other curtailment of the individual's license to practice medicine.[39] State statutes generally designate the grounds upon which a license can be revoked or suspended. Those grounds must be clearly stated and must be related to the protection of the public's health and safety.

Furthermore, the Constitution guarantees that the procedures used by the board in revoking or suspending a license will be fair. The constitutional requirements of due process are satisfied if the physician is afforded prior notice of the charges and given a formal hearing on the matter, the right to counsel, prehearing discovery, and the opportunity to affirmatively present his or her case and cross-examine witnesses.[60] However, Constitutional due process is not limited to such a list, for due process calls for procedures that the particular situation demands in order to preserve fairness.

A licensing board also is usually subject to a state's administrative procedure statutes and regulations, which delineate the rights of the physician and the procedures to be used by the boards in rendering decisions. While each state's statutes and regulations differ somewhat, the state's administrative law usually entitles the physician to the following rights and procedures in revocation and suspension actions:[42]

1. A verified complaint that contains enough information to allow the physician to prepare an adequate defense. The complaint should include the reasons for the proposed action, the issues raised, the statutes and rules at issue, and any particular information that has come to the attention of the initiating party that would support granting the agency action sought.

2. A hearing free from fraud, prejudice, and oppression.

3. Timely notice of the hearing setting forth specific information such as time, place, and date of the hearing.

4. Legal representation throughout all proceedings.

5. Discovery mechanisms that may include:
   a) notice of the names and addresses of witnesses known to the party, including but not limited to those the agency intends to call for testimony at the hearing;
   b) a right to inspect and make copies of the statements of all witnesses;
   c) a right to all writings that the agency proposes to offer in evidence or that are relevant and would be admissible in evidence;
   d) a right to investigative reports; and
   e) a right to take depositions.

6. A right to subpoena witnesses, both for deposition and the hearing.

7. A right to testimony under oath, confrontation and cross-examination of witnesses, and introduction of expert testimony in support

of denying the recommended disciplinary action.

8. A formal written decision.

9. A right of appeal.

A complaint against a physician can be filed with a medical board by any number of sources, including patients and employers. In addition, the board may file its own complaint. For example, the HCQIA requires hospitals and professional societies to report all adverse physician membership decisions made in regard to concerns about quality of care (see Chapter 21, which discusses the HCQIA reporting requirement). Such reports may prompt a medical licensing board to file its own complaint against a physician.

Next, the board must decide whether to initiate an investigation. If the complaint was not filed by the board, the board must determine whether the complaint is authentic and sufficient to warrant investigation. "What showing will suffice to meet this burden varies from case to case. It may relate to the reliability of the complainant or the substance of the complaint. Specific detail as to the identification of the complainant, some evidence of the complainant's good faith or reliability, a disclosure of the complainant's knowledge of the substance of the allegations contained in the complaint, and the date of the event will generally suffice."[42] If an investigation is authorized, it is normal procedure for the board to turn the case over to investigators; if the board believes the case may be jeopardized by contacting the physician, the physician may not be informed about the filing of the complaint.

The investigators will set the parameters of the investigation and ultimately may do any of the following as a result of the investigation:[42]

1. Recommend that the case be closed.

2. Recommend that the licensee be monitored by the board where a question exists about the licensee's ability to practice medicine competently.

3. Recommend a disciplinary hearing (thus triggering the rights listed above). In this event, the investigators may:
   a) request additional investigation; and
   b) seek subpoenas for persons, records, and documents for discovery purposes.

4. Refer the case for summary suspension of the license because of immediate danger to the public health (an expedited disciplinary procedure that permits the board to act quickly in an emergency situation and to conduct the formal hearing within a statutorily-prescribed time period following the summary suspension).

5. Refer the case for a warning or consultation (this is not a disciplinary action triggering due process concerns).

If the investigation subsequently leads to formal board action against a physician, the board must notify the physician of the complaint. The complaint usually will be considered sufficient to begin judicial administrative proceedings if it both clearly identifies the nature of the alleged wrongs (most complaints use statutory language to identify the problem(s)) and cites particular instances of the problem(s). In other words, the complaint is sufficient if it gives the physician enough information to know the nature of the allegation and to prepare an adequate defense.[86]

The physician is entitled to the same kind of presumption of innocence accorded criminal defendants, which places the burden of proof on the party seeking revocation. States vary as to whether the standard of proof for the proceedings is a "preponderance of the evidence" (more likely than not that the wrongs were committed) or "clear and convincing evidence" (a higher standard of proof that the wrongs were committed). However, no state requires the complainant to prove the problem with the physician "beyond a reasonable doubt" (the criminal burden of proof).

Both the physician and the complainant may offer expert testimony about the standard of conduct. The licensing board will consider any expert testimony in reaching its decision, even though most members of the board are physicians who presumably are qualified to make their own determinations about standards of care and breach of those standards. For this reason, some courts have held that expert testimony is not necessary in a hearing to revoke or suspend a license.[52]

Additionally, the physician should be prepared for a relaxed standard of admissibility in presenting evidence at the hearing.[86] Because revocation hearings are seen as administrative actions and not criminal or civil actions, the proceedings are more summary and informal. Thus, evidence that might not be admissible in a court of law (e.g., hearsay evidence) can be admissible in revocation hearings.

The physician who receives an adverse license decision next may appeal to a court designated by that state's administrative plan, and that court will review the record of the hearings to determine whether the board's decision was based upon sufficient evidence presented during the hearings, whether the board acted within its scope of authority, whether the physician was afforded due process, whether the board made an error in law or abused its discretion, or whether the board made an arbitrary or capricious decision. Because courts show a great deal of deference to the expertise of the medical boards where facts are in dispute or where inferences can be drawn, most board decisions are upheld by courts if the board has carefully followed the state administrative procedures.[86] Thus, it is important for a physician to present a thorough and adequate defense during the hearings.

2. *If I fail a certification or recertification test, will this affect my chance to win a subsequent medical malpractice lawsuit?*

A license to practice medicine is unrestricted in that it permits a physician to perform any treatment or service that he or she is competent to perform, even though the treatment or service might normally be provided by a specialist physician who is board certified. The license to practice medicine therefore places a duty on the nonspecialist physician to assess his or her competency and make a referral in cases where he or she is not competent to render a specific treatment or service.[103]

As a practical matter, most practitioners want to obtain board certification in at least one specialty area even though certification is not a prerequisite to delivery of specialty services. This is true because physicians are interested in certification's ability to assist them in continuing their personal development and in maintaining specialty standards in their practices.[79] On the other hand, consumers are more interested in certification's ability to identify and screen out physicians who are not qualified or competent to practice in a specialty area. Thus, consumers would cast a wary eye upon a physician claiming specialty status if the physician had not been able to acquire either initial certification or recertification. This also means consumers would probably view with the same wary eye a specialist who permitted his or her specialty certification to expire. Knowing this, a plaintiff's attorney representing a patient in a medical malpractice case generally looks carefully at whether a defendant physician failed to obtain initial certification or recertification in specialty areas relevant to the treatment at issue in the malpractice case. The information could be used to sway a jury's verdict.

To fully understand how failure to obtain certification or recertification might be used against a physician in a medical malpractice case, one must understand the four elements a plaintiff patient must show in order to win the case:[85,103]

1. The applicable medical standard of care (physician's duty).
2. Breach of the standard of care (negligence).
3. Damages to the plaintiff.
4. A causal connection between the breach and the damages.

Thus, in order to prove negligent treatment, the plaintiff patient's critical first step is to establish the physician's standard of care under the circumstances existing at the time of the alleged negligence.

The standard of care usually must be established through expert testimony. For this reason, the plaintiff with an injury must find a physician who is familiar with the nature of the physician defendant's practice and is willing to testify as an expert in the case. Plaintiffs usually choose to use board-certified specialists as experts, believing that the expert's qualifications as a specialist make the expert's opinions more believable to a jury. At trial, the expert witness will explain his or her specialty status before explaining to a jury the standard of care that applies in the case and offering an opinion about whether the standard was breached. As the following example shows, certification becomes relevant to the expert when establishing the standard of care and opining about whether breach occurred.

Suppose a nonspecialist physician is confronted by a patient who chose not to see a costly specialist for a rather serious eye injury. Also suppose that the nonspecialist physician has had some specialty training in ophthalmology, but has not received board certification in ophthalmology. The nonspecialist physician is faced with three options with the eye injury patient: 1) refer the patient to a specialist, 2) treat the eye because the situation does not call for knowledge and skill beyond those of a general practitioner (who admittedly might need to consult with the specialist before proceeding), or 3) treat the eye because the physician believes his or her limited specialty training prepared him or her to render the necessary specialty treatment.

If the nonspecialist provides the treatment or service to the patient's eye and a problem results that causes the patient to file a lawsuit, the nonspecialist's actions will not be judged by a board-certified specialist's standard of care. Instead, in most courts the nonspecialist will be judged by medical standards that apply to a nonspecialist physician in a similar kind of community with similar medical resources and educational opportunities.[72] Some of the relevant factors in establishing the nonspecialist's standard of care are the nature of the medical facilities available in the defendant's practice area, the number and kind of medical practitioners in the area, the availability of medical training and equipment, and the defendant physician's actual training and experience.[72]

On the other hand, the nonspecialist may tell the patient with the eye injury that referral will not be necessary because he or she has specialty training to treat the eye. If this representation is made, then the nonspecialist probably will be held to the specialist's national standard of care in subsequent litigation. The specialist's standard of care will be dictated by the kind of treatment that a certified doctor would have been trained to perform and would have been tested upon in the certification process. In other words, specialty standards are national standards.[72] If the specialist's standard of care dictates a treatment or service that differs from that provided by the defendant physician's, then the defendant's failure to certify or recertify as a specialist is extremely relevant.

As explained above, the expert in the eye injury case will not note the specialist's standard of care where only a generalist's skills and knowledge were necessary and the defendant never claimed to be a specialist. However, if the plaintiff's expert witness is aware that the defendant physician was unable to obtain certification or recertification in the specialty related to the treatment at issue in the case and nevertheless claimed to be a specialist, the expert could use this evidence to help show that the defendant physician was negligent. The expert would first testify to the specialist's standard of care and would explain what the specialist would have done differently. In establishing breach of that standard (negligence), the expert would emphasize that the defendant did not possess specialty certification and that the defendant did not conform to the specialist's standard of care despite the defendant's assertion that he or she was competent to perform the treatment or service. Thus, lack of certification or recertification would be evidence of the defendant's failure or inability to acquire the specialist's knowledge and skills and a general incompetence to provide the eye treatment at issue. Next, the expert would testify that this breach of the standard of care to a reasonable degree of medical certainty (the required causal connection in medical cases) caused the damages that the plaintiff alleges.[85] Finally, the plaintiff would present evidence that actual damage occurred.

Thus, testimony about failure to obtain or renew certification can be relevant in assessing the physician's qualifications and competency to perform the specialty treatment at issue in the case. The jury will weigh this information with all other evidence to determine whether the defendant physician breached the appropriate medical standard of care and should be held liable to the plaintiff.

3. *Can governments legally dictate the kind of practice I will have as a condition of receiving my license?*

States can, and do, regulate a physician's practice by requiring physicians to treat certain patients under special arrangements dictated by the state. Only one state, however, to date has tied these arrangements to issuance of a medical license. Massachusetts does not permit licensed physicians to "balance-bill" Medicare patients.

Under federal Medicare regulations, a physician may receive payment based on a reasonable charge established by the U.S. Department of Health and Human Services. Medicare will pay 80% of that reasonable charge, and the patient must pay the rest. Under Massachusetts licensure law, however, physicians in Massachusetts are not permitted to charge Medicare patients the physician's actual cost of a treatment or service.[70] The physician is permitted to charge Medicare patients only what the Medicare schedule sets out as a fair fee. This agreement to charge no more than the Medicare schedule permits is made a condition of licensure at the time the license is granted or when it is renewed.[50]

At least one commentator has said the Massachusetts licensure requirement constitutes "license servitude" because it forces an agreement to serve particular kinds of patients at certain prices.[50] Physicians challenged the Massachusetts law in *Massachusetts Medical Society v. Dukakis,*[71] stating that the state's requirement was unconstitutional because under due process analysis a condition on a professional license must have a rational connection with the applicant's ability to practice medicine. But the court upheld the licensing requirement. The court compared physicians to lawyers, who must perform pro bono work as a condition of licensing. Thus, the court saw a relationship to the lawyer's "fitness or capacity to practice law" requirement, which is the consideration upon which lawyers are required to serve a needy section of the population without cost to the client. The court upheld the physician agreement, seeming to believe that because physicians receive a "monopoly" from the state to practice medicine, the state can impose a requirement of service to a needy segment of the population. Failure to perform this aspect of the state's license requirement would be seen as lack of capacity to practice medicine.[50]

In West Virginia, physicians make a similar kind of agreement in regard to employees of the state under a state insurance plan.[50] The physician is not permitted to charge state-insured employees more than the state's schedule of fees permits despite a particular patient's ability or willingness to pay. However, West Virginia physicians are not threatened with a licensure action if they fail to follow the state's coverage scheme. The physician may merely lose the right to treat patients in the state's plan. Similarly, other states that have imposed "balance billing" bans have not tied the ban to the physician's license. These states give the physician the option of denying treatment to patients covered by the "balance billing" law.

The Massachusetts legislation discussed above reveals that a state licensing requirement can potentially permit a state to shift a substantial portion of its health care costs to the state's physicians. It can also provide a way for a state to require its physicians to serve certain segments of the population. Thus, the physician's license becomes the state's vehicle for assuring access to care for all segments of society, as an "all or nothing" deal for physicians who want to practice. In Massachusetts, many physicians made the decision to relocate to another state.[50]

4. *With managed care assuming the responsibility for serving large segments of populations, I am concerned about being able to attract patients to my practice. Do the licensing laws guarantee me access to the managed care plans in the area so that I can be assured of having enough patients to make a living?*

"The percentage of U.S. population receiving health care through an HMO [health maintenance organization] . . . increased from 4.7% of the population in 1982 to 16.4% of the population in 1993."[9,53] Since then, HMO participation has grown to an estimated 56 million participants in 1995, or about a quarter of the national population.[92] Under managed care, an HMO or preferred provider organization (PPO) controls physician access to patients; a state's licensing laws do not guarantee that an individual physician will have access.

However, legislators have responded to the physician's dilemma by enacting "any willing provider" statutes that require managed care to accept any qualified provider who applies. At the end of 1994, approximately 24 states had enacted "any willing provider" legislation.[9,53] The statutes fall into one of four categories: 1) freedom of choice laws, which require the insurer to reimburse a non-network provider as long as the provider will accept the insurer's level of reimbursement; 2) mandatory admittance laws, which require insurers to include any provider willing to follow the terms and conditions of the

insurer; 3) due process laws, which require the insurer to follow certain procedures in creating and maintaining the plan, such as publishing participation requirements and providing an appeal process for providers; and 4) essential community provider laws, which require the insurer to contract with community providers serving medically needy and poor populations.[53]

A number of studies have said that "any willing provider" laws interfere with the insurers' plan to provide care economically because administrative costs increase and the insurer loses some ability to control care. The Federal Trade Commission has agreed and said the "any willing provider requirements may discourage competition among providers, in turn raising prices to consumers and unnecessarily restricting consumer choice in prepaid health care programs, without providing any substantial public benefit."[53] For this reason, "any willing provider" laws are being debated at the national level, and the U.S. Congress might someday be more sympathetic to insurers than state legislators have been to date.[53] For now, however, the states continue to regulate entry into the provider groups.

5. *Aren't managed care plans and third party payors "practicing medicine" without a license when making many of their coverage decisions?*

The need for cost controls in medicine has prompted federal, state, and private insurers to adopt cost-control mechanisms that either permit the insurer to dictate in advance the amount to be paid for a particular treatment or permit the insurer to monitor the course of treatment and the need for various aspects of the total treatment plan. Furthermore, since 70% to 90% percent of health care costs are controlled by doctors, ways to encourage doctors to save money are continually sought by hospitals and managed care plans.

Courts agree that only a licensed physician may practice medicine, which has been defined as diagnosing, treating, or prescribing for any physical or mental condition. Furthermore, they agree that the physician may not accept medical instructions for diagnosing and treating patients from an entity or person who is not a licensed physician. Yet, medical directives can often seem like instructions.

Mark Hall, a professor of law, has noted that

institutional or insurer directives can be either advisory or binding. The advisory directives are not problematic, for they "pose no risk of either delivering incompetent medical care or deceiving the patient about the practitioner's qualifications, the two harms protected by medical licensure."[44] General directives merely give doctors a starting point, and the doctors are free to deviate from the directives to the extent the circumstances warrant the deviation.

Binding directives, however, do not permit the physician to exercise final treatment authority. They deprive the patient of the expertise of the physician and mislead the patient about who is making the decisions. The institution or the insurer is then practicing medicine. Such treatment directives are rare, however, for almost everyone realizes the illegal effect of such directives. Therefore, instead of issuing binding controls, institutions have begun to utilize other mechanisms for controlling physician behavior. For example, in contract situations where the physician is responsible for the cost of care that exceeds the plan's limits, the physician will have little motivation to prescribe expensive treatments that will put personal finances at risk. In addition, hospitals, managed-care entities, and public and private insurers have begun to review individual physician's practices for economic efficiency in light of utilization rates and other tracking mechanisms. The threat to the physician who is labeled inefficient is that the institution or insurer may bar the physician from providing care to institutionalized patients and insureds in the plan.

Nevertheless, because any advice or determination coming from the managed care entity or insurer can affect the course of a patient's treatment, the concern remains as to whether the entity or insurer is actually practicing medicine. For example, where a pre-approval decision is mandated by the health care plan and the managed care entity decides the care is not medically indicated, then a patient for any number of reasons probably will not receive the care, despite the doctor's recommendations.[96] Thus, the patient is following the decision of the managed care entity rather than that of the physician, in obvious violation of licensing law's requirement that only licensed physicians diagnose, treat, and prescribe medication for illnesses.

6. *Third party payor directives can affect my ability to maintain my patients' trust. But could I also be held liable in a court of law for the payor's negligent decision-making? And could these negligence actions affect the status of my license?*

One of the major challenges for physicians today is preserving patient-physician trust in the managed care setting, where both patients and physicians are having to adjust to treatment limitations. As noted earlier in this chapter, one of the primary reasons for physician licensure is preservation of the patient's trust in the physician. In order to preserve that trust, physicians in managed care plans are finding that they must carefully explain treatment limitations so that patients fully understand the services offered through the managed care plan, the services offered elsewhere at the patient's own cost, and the reasons why the services offered elsewhere will not be covered by the patient's plan.[50] In other words, when acting as gatekeepers to expensive health care treatments that most patients assume they are entitled to receive, physicians run the risk of losing patient trust if patients do not fully understand that their needs must be balanced against the needs of other persons in the plan.[5,51,64]

On the other hand, physicians also are finding that they must act as patient advocates in situations where the managed care plan has denied a treatment or service that the physician believes should be provided to the patient. Thus, a second major challenge for physicians in today's managed care environment is to uphold the physician's fiduciary duty to protect the individual patient.[12,41] The role of patient advocate is consistent with the medical code of ethics' dictate to physicians to do what is best for the patient. Furthermore, since licensure is designed to eliminate quacks and charlatans so that only competent physicians are practicing medicine, the licensed physician should be charged with evaluating and advocating what is best for the patient.

The AMA's Council on Ethical and Judicial Affairs has noted that physicians are often in a situation of conflict in the managed care setting, for physicians must consider their patient's needs, the needs of all patients in the managed care plan, and possibly the physician's own financial stake in the plan.[22] To avoid conflicts, the Council made recommendations about how physicians and patients should participate in managed care plan decision-making. Some of those recommendations follow: [22]

1. Managed care guidelines for treatment restrictions or limitations should be developed at a policy level with input from the physicians in the managed care plan.
2. Patients also should participate at a policy level in decisions about restrictions on services and treatments.
3. When implementing the guidelines, physicians must disclose any treatment limitations to patients so that patients may make decisions with full information about whether to seek treatment elsewhere at their own cost. The goal here is to obtain informed consent from the patient who opts to forgo treatment from other providers in order to follow the treatment guidelines of the managed care plan.
4. Physicians must advocate directly for a patient if guidelines inappropriately restrict treatment.
5. Physicians must advocate at the policy level for patients generally if a guideline restricts treatment unfairly.
6. The managed care plan must have an effective appeals process so that patients and physicians can challenge denials.
7. Physicians should not participate in a plan that encourages care at or below minimum professional standards.
8. Physician incentives should be structured to minimize the percentage of physician income being placed at risk when making treatment decisions.

This list of recommendations highlights that managed care programs are at odds with the kind of physician autonomy envisioned in previous years by the physician's code of ethics, licensing law, and tort law. But this list also highlights the need for the physician to continue to exercise some autonomy within the managed care setting in order to avoid liability to patients who believe they have been injured as the result of managed care decision-making.

For example, the case of *Verol v. Blue Cross and Blue Shield of Michigan*[107] demonstrates that courts will place the burden of providing appropriate treatment upon the physician, even though a health care plan may deny coverage. In *Verol*, a group of physicians asserted that a pre-approval plan used by the insurer impermissibly interfered in the physician-patient relationship, because patients often opt not to have treatment where it is not covered by the insurer. The court upheld the plan and said, "[W]hether or not the proposed treatment is approved, the physician retains the right and indeed the ethical and legal obligation to provide appropriate treatment to the patient. Thus, there is no direct interference with the physician-patient relationship nor in the treatment rendered." In other words, the court stressed that the physician had the expertise to know what was appropriate and should act accordingly.

Courts will not tolerate a physician who permits a third party to interfere with the fiduciary duty owed to patients. Hence, a physician is expected to make treatment decisions based upon professional medical judgment alone. A physician can be held liable if a patient is injured as a result of a physician's decision that is impermissibly affected by the existence of pre-approval plans, clinical guidelines, financial incentives, etc. In *Wickline v. State*,[112] the physician released a patient from the hospital after a managed care decision was made that no additional hospitalization was warranted. After leaving the hospital, the patient suffered complications and later sued. The evidence in the case suggested that the physician believed that the patient should not be released from the hospital, but also felt compelled to follow the decision made by the plan's reviewers. The physician did not appeal the plan's decision or advise the patient to remain in the hospital in spite of the coverage decision. The physician was held liable.

In another case, a jury refused to hold the managed care plan liable because the physician did not exercise good judgment in managing patient treatment when faced with an adverse determination from the plan. The plaintiff in *Prien v. N.W. National Life Insurance Co. and Private Healthcare System, Inc.*,[87] was admitted to a hospital with unstable angina. The physician requested five hospital days for treatment and observation. The plan review coordinator said she could approve only two days, but the request was referred to a medical review department for determination. An additional day was authorized through medical review. As a result, the plaintiff was discharged from the hospital after three days, but two days later returned with chest pain and suffered a heart attack. The plaintiff sued the insurer and provider for releasing the plaintiff too early from the hospital.

At trial, the provider argued that the doctor did not properly evaluate the plaintiff's test results, did not communicate those results to the provider, and did not advocate a longer hospital stay. The doctor admitted that some information was not offered to the provider in support of extended hospitalization. Therefore, the jury found the provider was not negligent, for it had acted on the information provided by the doctor. Unfortunately, the plaintiff had not sued the physician, the one whom the jury obviously believed had been negligent in failing to advocate for his patient.

The cases above illustrate that a physician must continue to exercise good medical judgment in treating and managing patients even when adverse plan decisions are implicated. The physician thereby can avoid personal liability and a subsequent report to his or her licensing board of a negative outcome in the medical malpractice case.

On the other hand, managed care entities can be held liable for failing to cover a treatment recommended by the physician. This scenario is extremely likely to arise when the physician recommends a relatively new or experimental treatment for a patient and the managed care plan does not wish to cover the cost of the treatment. For example, a suit was filed in California by the family of a woman who died of breast cancer after the HMO refused to pay for a bone marrow transplant to treat the cancer.[95] The HMO argued that although it had paid for this procedure in other cases, it did not want to pay the $100,000 treatment costs in this case because the cancer had spread to the bone marrow, thus making the procedure "investigational." Nevertheless, the family won the case at trial and the jury awarded $89 million in damages for the HMO's denial of treatment that had been recommended by the doctor.

The bone marrow case illustrates that where the HMO disagrees with the physician's judgment, the HMO can be liable even when it believes a treatment to be experimental or investigational. This case also underscores the importance of including the plan's physicians in deciding which treatments generally will be covered by the managed care plan and which will be excluded as "experimental or investigational." Permitting input from the physicians only makes sense, for if the physicians in the HMO do not regard a treatment as too experimental to recommend in most cases, then the HMO should provide the coverage and avoid the repeated conflicts that occur between the physicians who recommend the treatment and the HMO that denies coverage. Agreement about what is to be covered can also help prevent lawsuits by patients who feel they have been injured by coverage decisions.

For example, at least two federal courts have examined the question of whether high-dose chemotherapy with peripheral stem cell rescue is an "experimental or investigational" treatment that a managed care provider can deny to patients. The Fourth Circuit Court of Appeals in *Wilson v. Office of Civilian Health and Medical Programs of the Uniformed Services*[114] held that the government provider's denial of payment for treatment was arbitrary and capricious because the federal regulations required only that the therapy be generally accepted, and the evidence in the case showed that the treatment is often performed with breast cancer patients.

The *Wilson* decision, however, conflicts with a Seventh Circuit decision in *Smith v. Office of Civilian Health and Medical Programs of the Uniformed Services.*[104] The *Smith* court upheld the HMO's decision to deny coverage for high-dose chemotherapy because the HMO director had found little reported scientific evidence about the procedure's effectiveness. Thus, if physicians in a managed care setting wish to perform certain treatment procedures that are appropriate in spite of relatively little scientific evidence to support the treatment, then physicians must not only advocate for individual patients but must also have input into the policy-making process of the HMO to change treatment guidelines.

Finally, an HMO also can be held liable for

negligence in its decision-making process. For example, in *Adams v. Kaiser Foundation Health Plan, Inc.*,[2] a mother had taken her child to see an HMO physician about a fever. The doctor diagnosed respiratory infection, prescribed simple treatment, and sent the family home. The child's condition worsened that night and the mother called the HMO when the child became limp and began panting. The nurse who took the call evaluated the child's condition based on the phone call with the mother and then spoke to a doctor. The nurse said she had ruled out respiratory distress, so the doctor told the nurse to have the family go to a hospital 42 miles from their home because that hospital and the HMO had negotiated discounted prices. During the trip to the recommended hospital, the family passed other hospitals. The child then went into respiratory and cardiac arrest. The parents immediately stopped at another hospital along their route, but the child had already suffered irreversible circulatory damage. The child was diagnosed with a bacterial infection.

The child's parents sued the HMO for recommending a hospital so far away when the child's condition was critical. At trial, the jury awarded a multi-million dollar verdict based on a finding that the HMO nurse did not follow HMO protocols in assessing the child's condition when the parents made the call during the night.

In summary, only a licensed physician can legally provide medical treatment to a patient. If that treatment is negligent, the physician can be held liable, particularly where the physician has let a managed care policy improperly influence the physician's medical judgment. However, if the physician exercises good medical judgment and skill in treating the patient, despite a managed care policy or decision that would be detrimental to the care the physician believes is necessary for the patient, then a court will not hold the physician liable for medical malpractice. In other words, where the patient's injury is solely the fault of the managed care plan, the physician cannot be liable, and the injured patient must seek redress from the managed care plan.

References

1. Abrams M: Alternative medicine. **Good Housekeeping.** Vol 218, March, 1994, pp 99-101

2. *Adams v Kaiser Foundation Health Plan*, No. 93 VS-7985-E (Fulton Co Ct Feb 2, 1995) (reported in **Atlanta Law Reporter 38:**201, June 1995)

3. Adler RS: Stalking the rogue physician: an analysis of the Health Care Quality Improvement Act. **Am Bus Law J 28:**683-741, 1991

4. Bandaranayake R: Maintenance of competence and/or recertification: policy considerations, in Newble D, Jolly B, Wakeford R (eds): **The Certification and Recertification of Doctors' Issues in the Assessment of Clinical Competence.** Cambridge, Engl: Cambridge University Press, 1994, pp 169-177

5. Barge J: Suits increasing for failure to spot cancer. Plaintiff's lawyers claiming cost-saving measures cost patients their lives. **ABA J 81:**16-17, 1995

6. Barnum JF: How medical fashions determine medical care. **N Engl J Med 317:**1220-1221, 1987 (Letter)

7. Baron CH: Licensure of health care professionals. The consumer's case for abolition. **Am J Law Med 9:** 335-356, 1983

8. Barzansky B, Jonas HS, Etzel SI: Educational programs in US medical schools, 1994-1995. **JAMA 274:** 716-722, 1995

9. Baxter M: Physician credentialing: new risks for patients and providers. **Md Bar J 28:**18-22, 1995

10. Birch D: Trauma doctor allegedly practiced without license. **The Dominion Post.** Oct 5, 1995, p 4B

11. Blendon RJ, Kohut A, Benson JM, et al: Health system reform. Physicians' view on the critical choices. **JAMA 272:**1546-1550, 1994

12. Boyd TH: Cost containment and the physician's fiduciary duty to the patient. **DePaul Law Rev 39:** 131-159, 1989

13. Brinkley J: U.S., industry and physicians attack medical malpractice. **New York Times.** Sept 2, 1985, p 1, sec 1

14. Carroll SL, Gaston RJ: Occupational licensing and the quality of service. An overview. **Law Human Behav 7:**139-146, 1983

15. Case S, Bowmer I: Licensure and specialty board certification in North America, in Newble D, Jolly B, Wakeford R (eds): **Certification and Recertification of Doctors: Issues in the Assessment of Clinical Competence.** Cambridge, Engl: Cambridge University Press, 1994, pp 19-27

16. Chavigny KH: Do not substitute. Physicians should teach medical students. **JAMA 268:**1190, 1992

17. Christakis NA: The similarity and frequency of proposals to reform US medical education. Constant concerns. **JAMA 274:**706-711, 1995

18. Christoffel T: Hiring on the cheap. Health care costs, the eclipse of physicians and change in licensing laws. **Public Law Forum 4:**57-79, 1984

19. Cohen HS, Mike LH: **Developments in Health Manpower Licensure. A Follow-up to the 1971 Report on Licensure and Related Health Personnel Credentialing.** Washington, DC: US Bureau of Health Services Research and Evaluation, 1973

20. Conference on Credentialing and the Public Interest: **Credentialing of Health Manpower and the Public Interest. Conference Report.** New York, NY: National Health Council, 1978

21. Cordes R: Medical boards found lax on doctor discipline. **Trial 29:**87-88, April 1993

22. Council on Ethical and Judicial Affairs, American Medical Association: Ethical issues in managed care.

JAMA 273:330-335, 1995

23. Cramblett HG: Challenges to licensing boards— 1983, in Langsley DG (ed): **Legal Aspects of Certification and Accreditation.** Evanston, Ill: American Board of Medical Specialties, 1983, pp 153-161

24. Dauphinee WD: Assessing clinical performance. Where do we stand and what might we expect? JAMA 274:741-743, 1995

25. Davis DA, Thomson MA, Oxman AD, et al: Changing physician performance. A systematic review of the effect of continuing medical education strategies. JAMA 274:700-705, 1995

26. Davis DA, Thompson MA, Oxman AD, et al: Evidence for the effectiveness of CME. A review of 50 randomized controlled trials. JAMA 268:1111-1117, 1992

27. Dawson B, Iwamoto CK, Ross LP, et al: Performance on the National Board of Medical Examiners. Part I. Examination by men and women of different race and ethnicity. JAMA 272:674-679, 1994

28. *Dent v West Virginia*, 129 US 114 (1889)

29. Derbyshire RC: How effective is medical self-regulation? Law Human Behav 7:193-202, 1983

30. Deville KA: **Medical Malpractice in Nineteenth-Century America.** New York, NY: New York University Press, 1990

31. Dolan AK: Law and the maverick health practitioner. St Louis U Law J 26:627-678, 1982

32. Dolan AK, Urban ND: The determinants of the effectiveness of medical disciplinary boards, 1960-1977. Law Human Behav 7:203-217, 1983

33. Dorsey S: Occupational licensing and minorities. Law Human Behav 7:171-181, 1983

34. Fama AJ: Reporting incompetent physicians. A comparison of requirements in three states. Law Med Health Care 11:111-112, June 1983

35. Freidson E: The reorganization of the professions by regulation. Law Human Behav 7:279-290, 1983

36. Furrow BR: The changing role of the law in promoting quality in health care. From sanctioning outlaws to managing outcomes. Houston Law Rev 26:147-190, 1989

37. Gelhorn W: The abuse of occupational licensing. U Chic Law Rev 44:6-27, 1976

38. Gelhorn W: Medical malpractice litigation (U.S.)— medical mishap compensation (N.Z.). Cornell Law Rev 73:170-212, 1988

39. *Gibson v Barryhill*, 411 US 564, 579 (1975)

40. Goldsmith J: The impact of new technology on health costs. Health Affairs 13:80-81, 1994

41. Gray P: Gagging the doctors. Time. Jan 8, 1996, p 50

42. Griffith RA: Defending physicians before boards of registration in medicine, in Gosfield AG (ed): **Health Law Handbook.** New York, NY: Clark, Boardman and Callaghan, 1994, pp 355-374

43. Gross SJ: **Of Foxes and Henhouses: Licensing and the Health Professions.** Westport, Conn: Quorum Books, 1984

44. Hall MA: Institutional control of physician behavior: legal barriers to health care cost containment. U Pa Law Rev 137:431-536, 1988

45. Health Care Quality Improvement Act of 1986, 42 USC §11101, et seq (1994)

46. Hirsch HL: Physician licensure sanctions. No longer until death do you part — an update. **Legal Aspects Medical Pract** 11:2-4, 1983

47. Hogan DB: The effectiveness of licensing. History, evidence and recommendations. **Law Human Behav** 7:117-138, 1983

48. Hogan DB: Foreword. Professional regulation— an introduction to the issue. **Law Human Behav** 7:99-101, 1983

49. Hogan DH: **The Regulation of Psychotherapists: A Study in the Philosophy and Practice of Professional Regulation.** Cambridge, Mass: Ballinger Publishing, 1979, pp 238-239

50. Holzer HM: The physician's license. An Achilles' heel? **J Legal Med** 12:201-220, 1991

51. Iglehart JK: Physicians and the growth of managed care. N Engl J Med 331:1162-1171, 1994

52. *Jaffe v State Dept of Health*, 64 A2d 330, 135 Conn 339 (1949)

53. Jiranek AL, Baker SD: Any willing provider laws. Regulating the health care provider's contractual relationship with the insurance company. **Health Lawyer** 7:1-5, Fall 1994

54. Jonas HS, Etzel SI, Barzansky B: Appendix IA. Medical schools in the United States. JAMA 272:715-719, 1994

55. Jonas HS, Etzel SI, Barzansky B: Educational programs in US medical schools. JAMA 268:1083-1090, 1992

56. Jonas HS, Etzel SI, Barzansky B: Educational programs in US medical schools. JAMA 270:1061-1068, 1993

57. Jonas HS, Etzel SI, Barzansky B: Educational programs in US medical schools, 1993-1994. JAMA 272:694-701, 1994

58. *Jones v State Board of Medicine*, 555 P2d 399 (Id 1976)

59. Jost TS: The necessary and proper role of regulation to assure the quality of health care. **Houston Law Rev** 25:525-598, 1988

60. *Kinney v Derbyshire*, 718 F2d 352, 355 (10th Cir 1988)

61. Kinney ED: Private accreditation as a substitute for direct government regulation in public health insurance programs. When is it appropriate? **Law Contemp Problems** 57:47-74, 1994

62. Koska MT: Tapping into patient bill aids quality efforts. **Hospitals** 63:32, 1989

63. Langsley DG: Medical competence and performance assessment. A new era. JAMA 266:977-980, 1991

64. Larson E: The sole of an HMO. **Time.** Vol 44, Jan 22, 1996

65. Leffler K: Economic and legal analysis of medical ethics. The case of restrictions on interprofessional association. **Law Human Behav** 7:183-192, 1983

66. Leyerle B: **The Private Regulation of American Health Care.** Armonk, NY: ME Sharpe, 1994

67. Lichter PR: Confusing licensure with education. Medicine's slippery slope. **Ophthalmology** 101:1767-1770, 1994 (Editorial)

68. Manning PR, DeBakey L: Lifelong learning tailored to individual clinical practice. JAMA 268:1135-1136, 1992

69. Marwick C: State medical boards discipline more, want role in health system reform. JAMA 271:1723-1724, 1994

70. Massachusetts General Laws Ann Ch 112, S2 (1991 and Cum Suppl 1995)

71. *Massachusetts Medical Society v Dukakis*, 637 F Suppl 684 (D Mass 1986), aff'd 815 F2d 790 (1st Cir 1987)

72. McClellan FM: **Medical Malpractice Law, Tactics and Ethics.** Philadelphia, Pa: Temple University Press, 1994

73. McGuire CH: Reflections of a maverick measurement maven. **JAMA 274:**735-740, 1995

74. McPartland PA: Mandatory continuing education. Does it really protect society from incompetent health professionals? **Risk — Issues in Health Safety** 1:329-340, 1990

75. Montague J: CME. A school for survival? **Hospitals Health Network 68:**54-56, 1994

76. Mooney BC: The patients left behind. Doctors with dubious records start fresh in other states. **Boston Globe.** Oct 5, 1994, p 1, Metro section

77. National Board of Medical Examiners: USMLE test material development and NBME discipline committees. **National Board Examiner 42:**1, Summer 1995

78. National Commission for Health Certifying Agencies: **Perspectives on Health Occupational Credentialing.** Washington, DC: US Department of Health and Human Services, 1981

79. Newble D, Jolly B, Wakeford R (eds): **Introduction: The Certification and Recertification of Doctors: Issues in the Assessment of Clinical Competence.** Cambridge, Engl: Cambridge University Press, 1994

80. Norcini JJ: Examining the examinations for licensure and certification in medicine. **JAMA 272:** 713-714, 1994

81. Norcini JJ, Davison-Saunders B: Issues in recertification in North America, in Newble D, Jolly B, Wakeford R (eds): **The Certification and Recertification of Doctors: Issues in the Assessment of Clinical Competence.** Cambridge, Engl: Cambridge University Press, 1994

82. *O'dell v Ohio State Medical Board*, 259 NE2d 169 (Ohio 1970)

83. O'Neil EH: Education as part of the health care solution. Strategies from the Pew Health Professions Commission. **JAMA 268:**1146-1148, 1992

84. Pan RJD, Ticho BS: Physician oversupply. Doing too little too late? **JAMA 274:**772, 1995 (Letter)

85. Pegalis JD, Wachsman HF: **American Law of Medical Malpractice 2d.** Deerfield, Ill: Clark, Boardman and Callaghan, 1993, §14.1-14.9

86. Physicians and Surgeons: **American Jurisprudence 2d 61:** §1, et seq (1981, Cum Suppl April 1995)

87. *Prien v NW Nat Life Ins Co and Private Health Care Sys, Inc.* No. 94 CA203SS (US Dist Ct Western Dist of Texas, Austin Div, July 1993) (reported in Hanson NP: **Health Lawyer.** Late Summer 1995, pp 12-13)

88. Quirin TM: Physician licensing and educational obsolescence. A medical-legal dilemma. **Albany Law Rev 36:**503-525, 1972

89. Rayack E: Medical licensure. Social costs and social benefits. **Law Human Behav 7:**147-156, 1983

90. Regan-Smith MG, Obenshain SS, Woodward C, et al: Rote learning in medical school. **JAMA 272:** 1380-1381, 1994

91. Review: Health system reform, physicians' views on critical choices. **Health Care Reform Lit Rev.** Vol 1, 1995

92. Rivo ML, Mays HL, Katzoff J: Managed health care. Implications for the physician workforce and medical education. **JAMA 274:**712-715, 1995

93. Rooney K, Norman J: A physician's license. The state gives and the state takes away. **Legal Aspects Medical Pract:**1-4, October 1984

94. Rose J: Professional regulation. The current controversy. **Law Human Behav 7:**103-116, 1983

95. Sanders E: Health Net settles lawsuit over refusal of treatment. **Los Angeles Daily News.** Apr 7, 1994, p B1

96. Sanders SJ: Regulating managed health care plans under current law. A radical reversion to established doctrine. **Hofstra Law Rev 20:**73-117, 1991

97. Sbarbaro JA, Caper E: A case for independent judgment: the medical society in perspective for the 1990's. **Denver U Law Rev 65:**259-266, 1988

98. Schwartz WB: In the pipeline: a wave of valuable medical technology. **Health Affairs 13:**70-79, 1994

99. Schwarz MR: Liaison committee on medical education. Past successes, future challenges. **JAMA 268:** 1091-1092, 1992

100. Seifer SD, Vranizan K, Grumbach K: Graduate medical education and physician practice location. Implications for physician workforce policy. **JAMA 274:** 685-691, 1995

101. Shryock RH: **Medical Licensing in America, 1650-1965.** Baltimore, Md: Johns Hopkins University Press, 1967

102. Skolnick AA: New data suggest needle biopsies could replace surgical biopsy for diagnosing breast cancer. **JAMA 271:**1724-1728, 1994

103. Sloan FA: **Suing for Medical Malpractice.** Chicago, Ill: University of Chicago Press, 1993

104. *Smith v Office of Civilian Health and Medical Program of the Uniformed Services*, No. 94-3744 (7th Cir, Sept 26, 1995); 64 USLW 2199 (Oct 10, 1995)

105. *Stuart v Wilson*, 211 F Suppl 700 (ND Tex 1962)

106. Todd JS: Health care reform and the medical education imperative. **JAMA 268:**1133-1134, 1992 (Editorial)

107. *Verol v Blue Cross and Blue Shield of Michigan*, 798 F Suppl 826 (ED Mich 1989)

108. Walzer RS: Impaired physicians. An overview and update of the legal issues. **J Legal Med 11:**131-198, 1990

109. Weissman JS, Epstein AM: **Falling Through the Safety Net: Insurance Status and Access to Health Care.** Baltimore, Md: Johns Hopkins University Press, 1994

110. Whitcomb ME: A cross-national comparison of generalist physician workforce data. Evidence for US supply adequacy. **JAMA 274:**692-695, 1995

111. Whitcomb ME: The role of medical schools in graduate medical education. **JAMA 272:**702-704, 1994

112. *Wickline v State*, 239 Cal Rptr 810 (Cal Ct App 1986)

113. Wilkinson D: Report questions number of W.Va. medical schools. **The Dominion Post.** Nov 17, 1995, p 4B

114. *Wilson v Office of Civilian Health and Medical Programs of the Uniformed Services*, No. 95-1016 (4th Cir, Sept 15, 1995) (**Health Law Reporter (BNA) 4:** 1671, 1995)

115. Worthington RC, Willis SE, Boyett RL: Standardized patients and licensing examinations. **Acad Med 69:** 821-822, October 1994 (Letter)

CHAPTER 21

ISSUES IN HOSPITAL PRIVILEGES AND PEER REVIEW

GRACE J. WIGAL, JD

Three important mechanisms exist for assessing physician competency: 1) the licensing process, which requires an applicant to demonstrate a minimum level of competence before a license to practice medicine is awarded; 2) the board certification process, which requires additional training and testing that verifies a higher level of competence; and 3) the peer review process conducted by the hospital medical staff, which establishes for the hospital that the physicians rendering care in the hospital setting are competent to perform the treatments and services they are providing.[134] The first two mechanisms, which were discussed in Chapter 20, do a fairly good job confirming that a practitioner possesses a certain level of knowledge and skill before the license or certification is initially awarded. But the most effective mechanism for assuring quality of care throughout a physician's lifetime of practice is probably the peer review process conducted by hospitals when deciding whether to grant or renew physician staff privileges.

Hospital peer review is effective for at least five important reasons. First, it reaches a substantial majority of practicing physicians. Second, hospital peer review satisfies almost all the attributes of an effective regulatory mechanism because the review is ongoing pursuant to procedures established by the medical staff of the hospital. Third, hospitals want to avoid liability for breach of a legal duty to conduct thorough review of all physicians who practice within the facility. Fourth, physicians ardently believe that the profession must regulate itself and are willing to participate in peer review in order to maintain control of the profession.[9(Ch.1)] Last, federal legislation now mandates thorough peer review in hospitals and in return protects hospitals in federal antitrust litigation based on peer review decisions.[43]

Each of these five reasons for asserting that hospital peer review promotes quality of care will be discussed more thoroughly below. However, recent substantial changes in both the delivery of health care services and the mechanisms for health care reimbursement are beginning to highlight that a physician's ability to control the cost of care has become a critical component of the overall assessment of whether that physician renders quality care in the hospital setting.[92] As the second part of this chapter explains, new technology permits rapid and comprehensive accumulation and assessment of utilization and outcomes data. Hospitals, managed care organizations (MCOs), insurance programs, and others can now scrutinize the quality of an individual physician's care while assessing the cost of that care. Often, peer review decisions are being made, at least in part, on the basis of cost effectiveness. Whether this increased attention to cost control results in better care is still open to debate,[28,63,101] but case law developments indicate that courts now accept economic considerations as components of the formal institutional peer review process. As a result, many physicians are learning to cope with "economic credentialing."[52] The final segment of this chapter discusses peer review in the context of MCOs and why such peer review could assure that essentially all physicians are subject to formal review of their competence to practice medicine.

Five Reasons Why Hospital Peer Review Can Be Effective

In 1972, the American Medical Association (AMA) published a peer review manual that defined peer review as "the evaluation by practicing physicians of the quality and efficiency of services ordered or performed by other practicing physicians. . . ."[9(Ch.2)] At that time, the AMA designated state or county medical societies as the appropriate bodies to review physicians in their private practices. However, assurance of the quality of health care in the hospital setting was left to the medical staff of the hospital. The AMA contemplated that the hospital medical staff would perform utilization reviews (review of hospital use, appropriateness of admissions, length of stay, services ordered, and discharge practices) and medical audits (retrospective reviews of a physician's application of knowledge in the clinical setting) to assess hospital physicians' competence.[9(Ch.2)] Although the manual's definition of peer review included a review of efficiency, no mention was made of cost effectiveness as a separate factor in the AMA's contemplated review process. Following publication of the AMA's 1972 manual, medical society peer review did not evolve as a regular and exacting regulatory process in many medical communities, and hospital peer review developed as the more effective means to continually assess physician competence. It is effective for several reasons, including the following.

1. Hospital Peer Review Applies to a Substantial Majority of Physicians

Regular hospital peer review is important because most states award the license to practice medicine for life. This means licensed physicians are relatively free of oversight if they do not practice in geographical areas with active medical societies conducting peer review of physicians in the office setting. Since many physicians would not be subject to competency review if they did not have to obtain and maintain hospital privileges, the peer review process in hospitals fulfills a beneficial regulatory purpose.

Almost all practicing physicians desire hospital privileges so that they can admit and treat their patients in the hospital when the patients become seriously ill. A physician also needs the ability to admit patients who require tests or services the physician cannot perform in his or her office. For example, the rapid advance of technology in medicine has expanded the physician's options for diagnosing and treating illness.[13] Although both patients and their doctors desire access to this state-of-the-art technology and its potentially life-saving benefits, such technology is exorbitantly expensive, and most physicians cannot afford it for a private practice. Instead, they must acquire privileges that grant permission to access and use the technology available in hospitals. Hence, few physicians practice today without exercising privileges at one or more hospitals.

Moreover, almost all hospitals have established a process for regular physician peer review to satisfy the hospital's state licensing requirements, accreditation requirements, and state and federal medical program reimbursement requirements.[20,125] In both obtaining hospital privileges and in renewing those privileges, physicians are subjected to a review process conducted by the members of the medical staff of the hospital. The staff examines the physician's qualifications and performance to determine the nature of the privileges that should be awarded. The staff then makes a recommendation to the hospital's governing board, which normally follows the recommendation.

To avoid redundant review activity, hospitals obviously seek to conduct a single form of comprehensive peer review that complies with the standards of the various accrediting teams, licensing bodies, and government insurance programs discussed below. This formal and comprehensive hospital peer review process therefore should be rigorous, applicable to all physicians in the hospital, and designed to produce meaningful data for all organizations interested in the review process. Thus, even though hospital peer review does not include a review of the physician in his or her private office practice, it does help assure that physicians are subject to competency review on a regular basis after the license to practice medicine has been awarded.

JCAHO Accreditation and Peer Review

Over 80% of the acute care hospitals in the United States are accredited by the Joint Commission on the Accreditation of Healthcare Organizations (JCAHO), a private, nonprofit organization whose primary responsibility is to regulate quality of care in hospitals.[125] Although JCAHO accreditation is voluntary in theory, it is considered quasimandatory in the industry.[69] JCAHO (formerly known as the Joint Commission on Accreditation of Hospitals, or JCAH) was organized in 1951 by the AMA and other medical associations to standardize care in hospitals. JCAHO immediately adopted standards for the hospital industry and then conducted reviews under those standards. Hospitals in substantial compliance were awarded accreditation.[115(p21)]

JCAHO's original standards focused only on structure (e.g., equipment, facilities, or personnel) and processes (e.g., treatment criteria, documentation, and decision-making processes). However, in 1992, JCAHO began a transition period to gradually phase in outcomes assessment. The transition culminated in a 1995 standards manual that no longer "articulated requirements for structures and processes as ends in themselves," but instead related "performance of essential processes to patient outcomes."[85(Foreword)] The new JCAHO standards encouraged hospitals to focus on total quality management strategies and outlined a more flexible approach to achieving quality of care. The 1995 manual contained only a third of the number of standards it contained in 1991, and the new standards focused on doing what works in an integrated system of care to achieve the best possible outcomes for patients.[29,85] Consequently, the new standards allow hospitals to be more creative and innovative in devising ways to deliver quality care in a modern facility.

Despite the recent revisions, JCAHO continues to require hospitals to conduct effective, ongoing peer review in order to receive accreditation. JCAHO's peer review standards call for "a single organized medical staff that has overall responsibility for the quality of the professional services provided by individuals with clinical privileges" and that has the responsibility of accounting to the governing body in regard to those professional services.[85(MS.1)] However, JCAHO leaves the design of the peer review process to the medical staff as long as the medical staff bylaws and rules and regulations clearly:[85(MS.3)]

- establish the framework to review the members of the medical staff;
- provide fair hearings to those receiving negative reviews and curtailed privileges; and
- provide mechanisms for corrective action where a problem in care is noted.

State Government and Peer Review

JCAHO's peer review standards have also heavily influenced how states review hospitals for compliance with state licensing requirements. Most states either have adopted JCAHO standards into their licensing regulations or have specifically adopted similar peer review standards for reviewing a hospital for licensing purposes.[29,90]

Federal Government and Peer Review

The federal government mandates peer review in hospitals in at least two ways. First, both external and internal peer review are required as a condition of participation in the Medicare and Medicaid programs.[2] For example, the Medicare conditions of participation require hospitals to assess both the credentials of an applicant before awarding privileges and the performance of the physicians who have been awarded privileges.[2] The government can deem a hospital in compliance with federal program participation requirements if JCAHO accreditation is awarded.[4,90]

However, where JCAHO accreditation is not awarded, the hospital must demonstrate that it conducts ongoing peer review in order to receive reimbursement for Medicare and Medicaid patients. Furthermore, hospitals are subject to external review by federally-funded peer review organizations that were legislatively created in 1982 to review for both cost effectiveness and quality of care in treating Medicare patients. Peer review organizations have the authority to deny reimbursement or discontinue participation when problems are found in either cost effectiveness or quality of care.[1]

The federal government utilizes a second method to encourage meaningful peer review in hospitals. The federal Health Care Quality Improvement Act (HCQIA), which is discussed in greater detail later in this chapter, protects a peer review entity by granting immunity to damage awards in antitrust litigation. The immunity, however, exists only if peer review is conducted according to the Act's guidelines that require the hospital to thoroughly screen the credentials of physicians applying for privileges, to conduct ongoing peer review of privileged physicians, to regularly query the National Practitioner Data Bank, and to promptly report to the Data Bank any adverse peer review decision.

2. Hospital Peer Review Possesses the Attributes of an Effective Regulatory Mechanism

The hospital medical staff is familiar with medical practice standards; hospital protocols; hospital resources, equipment, and services; and other important considerations in evaluating the care being rendered by a professional in the hospital environment. Therefore, the medical staff is the most appropriate entity to establish the peer review procedures and to conduct the review.

When a physician applies for staff privileges at a hospital, the hospital's medical staff bylaws stipulate the procedures to be followed in deciding whether to grant privileges. Typically, a credentials committee made up of select hospital medical staff members reviews the physician's written application and makes a recommendation to the hospital board about whether to award privileges.

If the physician is granted privileges, he or she is regularly reviewed by the peer review committee, which assesses both competency and quality of care. After conducting this periodic peer review, the peer review committee reports to the hospital board by recommending that the privileges be renewed, restricted, or suspended. This process of initial credentialing and follow-up peer review permits physicians in a hospital to self-regulate the quality of physician services rendered in that hospital setting.

Many commentators have criticized the notion that physicians can capably regulate their own profession and have argued that self-regulation amounts to "letting the fox guard the hen house."[70,71] However, the above-described process for granting and renewing hospital privileges satisfies the first five of the six attributes of an effective regulatory mechanism described by Avis Donabedian, a leader in the theory of health care assessment.[62] Donabedian asserted that a regulatory system is effective if it fulfills the following criteria:[70]

1. The system is ongoing to provide continued monitoring and reporting of data.

2. The system is regularly in place and organized so that its components are interdependent and mutually reinforcing rather than a slapped-together amalgam of random and ad hoc procedures.

3. The system monitors the outcomes of services as well as the processes.

4. The system notes when deviations from expected performance are determined, and initiates action that leads to investigation, prevention, and rehabilitation.

5. The system's formal activities express and take their quality from the shared values and objectives of the informal organization of the professionals being regulated.

6. The system meaningfully involves consumers and related professionals in the control process, as well as representatives of the professionals being regulated.

As explained below, the first five of these attributes are present when hospitals conduct meaningful peer review. Moreover, even the sixth attribute may be satisfied by the new outcomes assessment procedures being used by hospitals in their efforts to assess patient satisfaction with care and to obtain information about treatment outcomes.

Attribute 1: Hospital peer review provides continuous monitoring and reporting of data because the medical staff must regularly assess a physician's competence.

Formal peer review must be conducted every 2 years under federal HCQIA guidelines, while JCAHO requirements stipulate "ongoing" review, Medicare conditions of participation require "periodic appraisals,"[2] and the various states require differing intervals of peer review under their licensing statutes. Moreover, all physicians in the hospital setting can informally assess the competency of their colleagues on a daily basis as they observe their colleagues carrying out patient evaluation and care. Not only are these physicians ethically bound to report quality of care problems that might endanger patients, they are legally bound in many states to report evidence of incompetence. The result is an ongoing informal kind of peer review that supplements the formal and regular peer review process.

Attribute 2: The formal peer review process is continually in place and is thoughtfully organized with interdependent procedures to provide information that reinforces the total review process.

A hospital's formal peer review procedures are continually in place because they are spelled out in a document known as the hospital medical staff bylaws. The medical staff bylaws differ from the hospital's corporate bylaws, which describe the corporate operations of the hospital. The medical staff bylaws instead describe the relationship between the hospital corporation and its medical staff, delineate the duties of the medical staff, and set forth important procedures that the medical staff is to follow in carrying out its duties. By including the procedures to be used for peer review, the bylaws assure that a formal peer review process is in place at all times.

In addition to being continually in place, the medical staff bylaws usually are carefully drafted for a number of reasons. First, although the bylaws are drafted by the medical staff, neither the hospital nor the staff can unilaterally change the bylaws.[85] Courts have said bylaw provisions amount to a contract between the hospital and the medical staff,[40] and if a hospital does not follow the bylaw procedures in reviewing a physician whose privileges are denied or restricted, then the hospital is subject to suit for breach of contract.[20] For this reason, the hospital and staff should negotiate and agree upon a set of bylaw procedures that meet the needs of both the hospital and the staff in the peer review process.

The medical staff also should pay thoughtful attention to whether the procedures outlined in the bylaws are fair to all physicians subject to review. If the procedures encompass consideration of factors other than quality of care, such as economic efficiency, then the medical staff should be informed of the additional factors, should understand how those factors will be assessed, should understand the kinds of information that will be produced by review of the additional factors, and should understand the implications of that information.

The third reason the bylaws should be thoughtfully drafted concerns review by outside organizations. If the bylaws are in compliance with standards set forth by licensing and accrediting bodies, as well as the federal conditions of program compliance for Medicare, then following the bylaw procedures will help assure that the hospital's peer review process will satisfy external reviewers' expectations, as well as meet the needs of the hospital and medical staff.

In addition, thoughtful drafting and subsequent adherence to the bylaw procedures guarantees that peer review produces the kind of information that it was intended to produce: information that is meaningful to the hospital, to the collective medical staff, to individual members of the staff, and to the review process itself. The review process should be meaningful to the hospital by integrating information and pinpointing problem areas in the hospital's total services. For example, if the peer review process generates medical staff concern about the care being delivered by the obstetrics and gynecology (OB-GYN) department, the hospital then can take steps to implement new hospital procedures and guidelines to address and remedy noted weaknesses in the delivery of health care services and treatment in that particular department. The process also should show the hospital how each individual physician in the OB-GYN department is performing in the hospital setting, as well as how the individual physician is performing in relation to other physicians practicing in this and other hospital settings. Such information also can be educational and beneficial to the OB-GYN practitioner who seeks to continually improve his or her performance.

Finally, the review information can reinforce the total review process because the nature of the new information is usually important or understandable only when compared to other data gathered in present or past review processes. For example, new information about a surgeon can be compared to information gathered in past reviews to discover whether the surgeon's new operative techniques are achieving better outcomes. Such comparisons may show a trend in the physician's practice habits that should be more closely examined by the review committee, thereby triggering the need for additional review procedures and perhaps a mechanism for consultation with other members of the staff. The result is that the hospital's total review process is reinforced.

Attribute 3: The mechanism of formal peer review monitors the outcomes of treatment services as well as the process of treatment.

Physicians who are responsible for the peer review function can regularly and rather easily assess another physician's adherence to process norms. Written hospital protocols establish a range of acceptable patient treatment practices as well as a method of recording the physician's treatment. Thus, with a range of pre-defined process norms, the peer reviewers examine patient charts by looking for deviations from the norm in the physician's decision-making process.

However, the assessment of only a physician's treatment processes has some negative implications in light of quality of care. "The use of prevalent norms as a basis for judging quality may . . . encourage dogmatism and help perpetuate error."[62(p20)] Because a process review focuses on highlighting deviations from the norm, physicians may feel constrained to treat patients according to the norm, even though an alternative procedure, test, or drug might actually be preferable for the particular patient.

Courts have recognized that deviations from the normal standards of care are sometimes necessary to avoid medical malpractice. In some cases, standard procedures may be inappropriate and physicians instead are required to do what is reasonable for the patient under the circumstances.[79] Furthermore, studies have confirmed that many commonly-accepted methods of diagnosis and treatment are not grounded in scientific support[75] and therefore cannot be justified as the best way to diagnose or treat a condition. For these and other reasons, peer review procedures should be flexible enough to account for appropriate deviations in practice, and today's new peer review procedures that take into account the outcomes of treatment seem to provide that kind of flexibility.

Outcomes evaluation and its attention to the patient's opinion as well as the documentation of short- and long-term effects of treatment can provide information that process evaluation does not provide.[22,135] It gives reviewers a way to evaluate whether a physician's deviations in process actually worked for the patient. Outcomes review thereby provides the kind of flexibility that is being promoted by JCAHO as an important aspect of peer review and as a means to achieve the best result possible for the patient.

On the other hand, it is sometimes hard to tie an outcome to a specific medical decision. Furthermore, the outcome is often not known until after the patient leaves the hospital, which necessitates follow-up procedures to collect data about outcomes. For these reasons, outcomes assessment is still in its infancy, as hospitals continue to refine mechanisms to identify outcome parameters and to collect and assess outcomes data.

Attribute 4: If important deviations in either process or outcome are detected, the peer reviewers can initiate even further investigation, can require that preventative measures be taken if necessary, and can suspend privileges to carry out rehabilitation.

The heart of the effective regulatory mechanism lies in its ability to respond to and correct problems. Both JCAHO standards and the HCQIA call for the medical staff of the hospital to develop and adopt bylaws and rules and regulations to establish mechanisms for regular peer review; for corrective action, including automatic and summary suspension of privileges, if a problem with a physician's care is noted; and for fair hearings and appellate review where physicians are negatively impacted by a peer review decision.[3,85(MS.3)] The JCAHO standards are general and give the medical staff the discretion to decide both how to proceed with additional investigations and how to curtail the physician's hospital activities. The HCQIA, on the other hand, sets forth clear and specific minimum standards for review of a negative peer review decision (see subsequent section, "Effects of HCQIA"). Furthermore, both JCAHO and the HCQIA recognize the staff's need to respond to emergencies, and both give the medical staff express authority to immediately suspend privileges where warranted. Thus, the medical staff should have institutional authority to respond decisively to threats to patient safety and to suggest a plan for corrective action.

The ability of the medical staff to assess and respond to perceived problems in physician care is important in a profession where, according to the AMA, up to 10% of the members of the profession are impaired for one reason or another, including drug and alcohol addiction.[139] These statistics indicate that peer reviewers often will have to make recommendations to deny, restrict, or suspend privileges, despite the fact that the decision affects the career and livelihood of a colleague. In recognition of this dilemma, the AMA drafted and adopted the Uniform Physician Treatment Act to guide medical professionals in assisting impaired physicians to overcome problems in a manner that helps assure that they can continue working or can return to work in a timely manner.[139] A majority of states have adopted the Act, which can guide peer reviewers in making recommendations about how to proceed with physicians whose privileges will be negatively affected by a peer review decision that the physician is impaired.

However, peer review can satisfy Donabedian's fourth attribute of an effective regulatory mechanism only if physician reviewers are actually willing to take remedial steps or impose a sanction when quality of care problems are noted. In fact, some reviewers have been hesitant to act against a colleague because they feared the loss of referrals, respect, friends, and the threat of retaliation through a lawsuit brought by the disciplined physician.[72] Their fears are not without justification in light of the fact that peer review decisions have spawned more physician litigation than any other aspect of the hospital-physician relationship.[84] However, as explained in more detail later in this chapter, both the federal HCQIA and various state statutes protect participants in the peer review process as long as the reviewers are making privilege recommendations with the good faith belief that they are promoting the quality of patient care.

Attribute 5: Hospital peer review activity takes its standards from the shared values and objectives of the medical professionals working in the hospital and from the profession itself.

One problem in assessing quality of care is that variations in practice patterns are common, and little scientific evidence exists to settle a dispute over what constitutes acceptable practice in particular circumstances.[98] As a result, physicians can legitimately argue about what constitutes quality care in various environments. This disagreement can prejudice a peer review process when the physician being reviewed is utilizing a treatment regimen that the reviewers label as unorthodox.

Hospital peer reviewers, however, normally review their peers under standards and procedures that are established by consensus of the medical staff. The review procedures, which are documented in the medical staff bylaws, take into account the circumstances of the particular practice environment. Furthermore, the reviewers are members of the medical staff and are practitioners within the local community. Thus the reviewers are familiar with the hospital's and the community's resources and can define what constitutes quality in the context of a particular hospital setting. This knowledge of the practice environment should make reviewers better able to judge when practice deviations are necessary.

Furthermore, because the hospital industry now recognizes the importance of assessing quality of care by examining both process of care (whether a physician is following the protocols or guidelines for diagnosis and treatment that are established by the medical staff itself) and treatment outcomes, the medical staff of today can review a physician's practice from several different perspectives. When a physician is achieving good outcomes through non-standard treatment, the reviewers now have an improved ability to document the quality of such care. Furthermore, when reviewers can rely on both process and outcomes data, as well as their own observations, they have more information to support a negative peer review recommendation.

Attribute 6: Through outcomes surveys, consumers are now being given a more meaningful way to provide information to peer reviewers about the physician's quality of care and competency.

Although peer reviewers can observe their colleagues providing treatment to patients, and can assess treatment process and patient outcomes by studying the patient's hospital charts, patients in the past were rarely actually asked to comment upon whether they were satisfied with the quality of the physician's care. Thus, the focus of the peer review process was on technical proficiency, while the interpersonal aspect of the care provided by the physicians usually was not addressed.

Donabedian has pointed out that quality of care must be defined to include both the technical and interpersonal aspects of care.[62] He theorized that technical quality is achieved if science and technology are applied "in a manner that maximizes its benefits to health without correspondingly increasing its risks."[62] On the other hand, he admitted that the interpersonal aspect of quality care is difficult to define and assess.

Yet, hospitals in today's competitive medical market are interested in achieving not only satisfactory technical care for patients, but satisfactory interpersonal experiences as well. Because hospitals now must compete for patients, they are interested in outcomes management systems that can be used to track both the effects of medical care on patients over time and the patients' satisfaction with the care received while in the hospital.[21] Patient satisfaction, measured through surveys, today is an integral part of total system assessment.[62,97,98,136]

Hospitals are not the only entities looking at patient satisfaction. The Health Care Financing Administration (HCFA), which monitors care delivered to Medicare patients, has devised its Medicare Quality Indicator System "to include quality indicators for access, appropriateness, outcomes and patient satisfaction."[47] HCFA ultimately intends to publish some of the data for public use in its effort to provide information about physicians and hospitals. Furthermore, the Agency for Health Care Policy and Research (AHCPR) has been developing clinical guidelines to review the appropriateness of care. AHCPR has called upon panels of both physicians and consumers to develop the guidelines[75] in an effort to make the guidelines "politically as well as technically authoritative."[74] In other words, consumer input should lead to guidelines that better reflect what consumers want in health care.

This relatively new attention to consumer input and assessment of patient satisfaction is finally allowing the public to participate in regulatory and peer review processes in meaningful ways.[82] Thus, hospital peer review may in fact now be close to achieving all six of Donabedian's attributes of an effective regulatory mechanism.[56]

3. Hospitals Have a Duty to Protect Patients From Incompetent Physicians

A third reason that hospital peer review has been successful is that hospitals have a legal duty to protect patients from incompetent physicians by denying, restricting, or withdrawing hospital privileges.[87,102(p79)] When the hospital breaches its duty to carefully select a physician for privileges or to review the physician's care in the hospital, the hospital can be liable to a patient who is subsequently injured by the physician's actions or inaction in the hospital.

Since a hospital corporation does not have the legal authority to practice medicine by diagnosing or treating a patient's condition,[15] the hospital must rely upon its employee physicians and independent privileged physicians to diagnose and treat patients in the hospital. Nevertheless, courts have established that hospitals have a duty of care that runs directly from a hospital's governing board of trustees to the patients in the hospital. That duty requires a hospital to assure that only competent physicians are practicing medicine within the hospital. If the hospital is negligent in either selecting physicians or supervising them, the hospital can then be subject to liability in a suit brought by a patient who alleges injury resulting from a physician's negligent treatment provided while in the hospital. For this reason, hospitals are motivated to institute peer review mechanisms that help assure that only competent physicians are exercising privileges.

The Hospital's Duty to Patients

The hospital has a duty to exercise care when dealing with patients. The legal doctrine of *respondeat superior* makes the hospital, as the employer, liable for the civil wrongs committed by its employees acting within the scope of their employment duties.[68(p282)] Thus, a hospital is liable for the actions of all its employees from janitors to physicians. However, a hospital is not liable under this theory for the actions of independent physicians who are privileged by the hospital but technically not employed by the hospital. When a patient is injured by a physician not employed by the hospital, the patient must allege hospital liability under other legal doctrines.

Most hospital patients want to be treated by their own physicians while in the hospital, and under these circumstances the patients realize that the treating physician probably is not a hospital employee. However, if the hospital patient is not offered the opportunity to select a physician, and treatment is rendered by an "unknown" physician, the patient usually assumes that the treating physician is a hospital employee. In reality, however, patients are often treated in the hospital by independent contractor physicians who are not directly employed by the hospital. Under these circumstances, the doctrine of *respondent superior* is not applicable. Nevertheless, some courts have been willing to hold a hospital liable for physician negligence under the doctrines of "ostensible agency" and "agency by estoppel."

Under these doctrines, the hospital can be liable to the patient because non-employee physicians appear to be acting as agents of the hospital. Furthermore, these doctrines recognize that these physician "agents" of the hospital are rendering treatment in situations in which it is particularly difficult for the patient either to know that the physician is not a hospital employee or to exercise a choice about who will render that treatment.

For example, patients who enter a hospital emergency department usually assume that the physician who treats them is an employee hired to treat and admit, if necessary, those patients who must seek emergency treatment at the hospital rather than from their own physicians.[33] In addition, when a patient is referred to a hospital for specialty treatment because that treatment is available only at the hospital, the patient usually assumes that the hospital physician is employed by the hospital to render the specialty treatment.[133] In both of these scenarios, trial courts have found that when a patient has little choice about who provides treatment, and legitimately believes the treating physician is a hospital agent, then the patient has the right to recover from the hospital for any negligence on the part of the treating physician.

These cases illustrate that courts have been unwilling to impose a duty upon the patient to inquire about the relationship between the hospital and the physician.[102(p93)] For this reason, the hospital that wants to avoid liability under ostensible agency theory should inform the patient of the nature of the relationship between the hospital and the independent contractor physician.[7,104(p43)]

Attorneys representing plaintiffs in states that recognize agency theories of hospital liability should be aware that there are two slightly different legal theories for assessing ostensible agency liability.[115,145] The first theory, "pure ostensible agency," evolved from Section 429 of the Restatement of Torts (Second), which requires the plaintiff to show only that he or she had a reasonable belief that the physician was working for the hospital.[118] The second theory is based on agency by estoppel, which is explained in Section 267 of the Restatement of Torts (Second). This theory requires the plaintiff to show both a representation that the physician was a servant of the hospital and the plaintiff's actual reliance on that representation.[59] Thus, plaintiffs in jurisdictions that have adopted the theory of agency by estoppel have the more difficult job of showing reliance on a hospital representation.

Even where a physician is clearly not an employee or agent of the hospital, courts have been willing to impose liability upon a hospital for breach of its duty to exercise care in the selection of or supervision of physicians exercising privileges in the hospital. This willingness to make hospitals susceptible to liability in cases of physician malpractice stems from a general acknowledgment that the public perceives the modern hospital as a provider of medical services, relies on the hospital for high quality medical treatment, and expects the hospital to provide competent physicians as well as adequate support personnel and equipment.[104] Plaintiffs bringing lawsuits against hospitals for negligent selection or supervision of privileged physicians do so on the basis of hospital corporate negligence, a medical negligence theory grounded in two key cases.

The first case, *Johnson v. Misericordia Community Hospital*,[87] established that a hospital must perform a thorough investigation and review of a physician before granting privileges. In *Johnson*, the physician was granted privileges to perform surgery even though surgery privileges had been both denied and curtailed at other hospitals. When the plaintiff sued Misericordia Community Hospital as the result of an injury suffered during surgery, the evidence in the case revealed that the hospital had not been aware of the physician's hospital practice history. Misericordia Community Hospital was held liable for failing to establish peer review procedures that would have revealed the risk posed by granting the physician the privilege to perform surgeries in the hospital.

The second case, *Darling v. Charleston Community Memorial Hospital*,[42] established that a hospital could also be held liable for its failure to supervise a physician who has been granted privileges. In *Darling*, the plaintiff lost a leg because a cast was applied too tightly. The plaintiff was able to establish at trial that the hospital had not required the physician to stay abreast of current treatment standards, that the physician who was treating the leg was not competent to do orthopedic work, and that the hospital had not supervised the care being rendered by the physician to the plaintiff. Although the hospital argued that it had met its legal duty by carefully screening the physicians who were granted hospital privileges, the court said the hospital had the additional duty to monitor the performance of its physicians. The court said that if the hospital did not take steps to monitor the care of its privileged physicians, it thereby jeopardized the care being rendered to its patients and could be held liable in a negligence action.

Thus, hospital corporate negligence law can be used to establish liability against a hospital when that hospital has either negligently granted privileges or negligently failed to monitor physician competence after granting privileges. Use of this doctrine by plaintiffs has provided more than enough reason to prompt hospitals to institute regular and thorough review of physicians providing care in the hospital setting.

The Role of the Medical Staff in Assuring that the Hospital Meets its Duty to Patients

Because most hospitals operate as a corporation, each is run by a board of trustees that is ultimately responsible for the operations of the hospital. Because the hospital is invested with the legal duty to ascertain that only qualified doctors exercise privileges in the facility, the board also maintains the ultimate decision-making authority in privileging and supervising physicians.[102] However, the board generally lacks the expertise to either determine whether an individual physician possesses the credentials to obtain privileges or whether a currently privileged physician is competent to continue to exercise those privileges. Therefore, the board must delegate peer review to the hospital medical staff so that the staff can assess the competence of each physician and offer recommendations about whether to grant, deny, or restrict privileges.

A hospital's medical staff consists of the individual practitioners who are qualified and authorized to use the hospital to treat patients. The medical staff is typically divided into clinical departments such as dentistry, radiology, pathology, and pediatrics. Each department elects a chairperson. The medical staff also elects officers to conduct its affairs and forms staff committees with various responsibilities. The executive committee, which is composed of the elected staff officers and the chairpersons of the staff departments in the hospital, usually governs the medical staff.

A medical staff first reviews a physician when the physician applies for hospital privileges. The staff's credentials committee typically reviews the application and performs the following steps in its investigation: establishes that the applicant is properly licensed; examines the applicant's education and training; reviews the applicant's health status, ethics, and experience; reviews the applicant's history of malpractice suits, adverse licensure actions, and adverse privilege decisions; reviews his or her criminal history, if any; determines the extent to which the physician plans to use the hospital; and establishes how much professional insurance the applicant carries.[115(pp39-44)] Usually, the committee also will investigate the physician by contacting institutions where the applicant has previously exercised privileges. Furthermore, under the HCQIA, the committee must query the National Practitioner Data Bank for information about the applicant. Only after this thorough review will the credentials committee make a recommendation to the hospital board that the applicant should be privileged. Even then, the scope of the recommended privileges will be directly related to the committee's assessment of the breadth of the applicant's qualifications. For example, the committee might permit the physician to treat patients at the hospital, but might not privilege the physician to perform surgery.

Once privileges have been granted by the hospital, the medical staff also is charged with the duties of monitoring the privileged physician's competency and of closely supervising and consulting with the physician if necessary.[42,102] As explained earlier, state and federal statutory law, common law, JCAHO accreditation standards, and federal insurance programs demand such periodic review. In fact, the HCQIA requires every hospital that conducts peer review to review a physician's Data Bank file every 2 years. Such periodic review keeps the hospital informed of any changes in the physician's licensure status, medical malpractice litigation history, and privileges at other institutions.

In summary, a hospital carries out its duty to protect its patients from incompetent physicians by relying upon the hospital physicians themselves to conduct the kind of rigorous peer review contemplated by both accrediting bodies and licensing bodies charged with looking out for the public's welfare. If the hospital does not exercise care in selecting and reviewing its privileged physicians, then the hospital can be liable to a patient under the legal doctrines of hospital corporate negligence, ostensible agency, or *respondeat superior*.

4. Socialization of Physicians to the Importance of Peer Review

A sense of shared norms, values, and beliefs is an important feature of any professional community because a sense of common goals allows the profession to adapt to changes without losing sight of its underlying mission.[14(p42),91] For more than a hundred years, professionals in allopathic medicine have been socialized to and have unwaiveringly supported a mission of self-regulation. Since true self-regulation occurs only when members of the profession agree to establish standards and then assess competence based on those standards, allopathic medicine theoretically has also endorsed peer review as part of its mission.

In fact, in the mid-1800s, the AMA was organized, at least in part, to advocate the use of peer review to improve both professional status and quality of care at a time when a number of different kinds of practitioners were treating a patient population growing more and more dissatisfied with its medical care.[46,70] Later, during the early 1900s, allopathic medicine achieved true social legitimacy by making the practice of medicine more scientific. As allopathic practitioners began to gain the public's trust, they advocated that consistent quality of care could be achieved only with standardized medical school training, licensing restrictions that would screen out those without sufficient knowledge to practice medicine, and peer review that would eliminate practitioners not competent to practice.[14] Of course, such restrictions benefited the members of the profession by restricting admission. However, the public was willing to accept the notion of self-regulation, believing that with the increasingly scientific nature of the practice of medicine, only those persons trained in the profession had the expertise to regulate its members for competency. This willingness to leave review to the experts persisted through the following decades, and allopathic physicians have continued to exercise the power to set professional standards and determine whether those standards are met by individual practitioners.

Today, medical students begin to discuss the ethics and culture of self-regulation while matriculating in the various accredited medical schools across the country, and after obtaining their licenses to practice, they continue this discussion in continuing education and certification programs, as well as in the meetings of the professional organizations to which they belong. As a result, it would be hard to find a physician today who did not agree that effective regulation is possible only when the review for quality of care is performed by one with equivalent expertise—one's peers. In fact, this belief that peer review "kills two birds with one stone," in that it both works effectively and permits the profession to retain control of its destiny, explains why physicians have been willing to participate in time-consuming peer reviews and have supported state and federal legislation, such as the HCQIA, that encourages peer review.

On the other hand, physicians express misgivings about the very different kind of review now being conducted by hospitals and MCOs interested in cutting costs.[12,25] While the process of review for competence remains in the hands of medical practitioners, hospitals and MCOs have begun to scrutinize physicians for their ability to reduce the cost of care. This new focus on cost effectiveness is creating friction between physicians and the hospitals or MCOs in which they practice.[27,88,112]

Physicians have generally opposed such economic reviews because they have not been socialized to believe that the economics of their medicine is an important facet in quality of care.[71] Until recently, physicians have looked to technical competence as the benchmark for quality of care. Furthermore, physician ethical codes have historically stressed that the physician owes his or her undivided loyalty to the patient;[122] the codes did not contemplate that physicians might one day be called upon to bal-

ance the needs of one managed care patient against the needs of other patients in the managed care plan in order to preserve the limited pool of medical resources available to plan enrollees. In fact, physician ethical codes of the 20th century have stressed that the patient must have faith in the physician's technical expertise and desire to achieve the very best result for the patient, regardless of cost. Fee-for-service insurance and reimbursement mechanisms that were predominant until very recently reinforced this notion of doing everything possible for the patient. Furthermore, legal prohibitions on the corporate practice of medicine promoted physician autonomy by barring a corporation from practicing medicine through its employees. Such prohibitions were based on the fear that an incentive to profit from the employee physician's professional services might encourage the corporation to pressure the physician to provide less care to the patient.[15,128] Thus, the law attempted to protect patients by endorsing physician autonomy in making diagnostic and treatment decisions.

This historical perspective helps explain why the AMA to date has been opposed to the general idea of economic review.[108] Nevertheless, the rapidly changing medical market is demanding new attitudes toward treatment and assessment of care. Although only time will tell how the profession adapts to this challenge to professional self-regulation, it seems fairly clear that the medical profession must begin to educate its members about the importance of controlling costs in order to make health care accessible to all persons. It is equally clear that a profession socialized to self-regulation through peer review must respond to economic credentialing in a way that allows physicians to participate in setting cost parameters for treatment and in defining instances when those parameters should not be applied.[12,112]

5. Federal Legislation that Mandates Peer Review to Achieve Quality of Care

The Health Care Quality Improvement Act[3] has fostered heightened scrutiny of physician competence in the hospital setting. The HCQIA has encouraged better peer review by giving special protection to a hospital in lawsuits brought by physicians who have received adverse privilege decisions. This legislative protection exists if the hospital can show that its denial of privileges was based on quality of care concerns and that it was in compliance with other HCQIA reporting and querying requirements at the time the privilege decision was made. The HCQIA also has encouraged more meaningful peer review by creating the National Practitioner Data Bank, the first federal data bank to collect and report information about medical professionals. The Data Bank, which began its operations in 1990, has now collected a wealth of information about practitioners, and it regularly disseminates this information to peer review entities that query the system.

The HCQIA was a legislative response to a medical malpractice "crisis" that was prominently reported by the media in the early 1980s.[34] While physicians were hesitant to admit that the "crisis" was more than litigation frenzy accompanied by escalation in malpractice insurance premiums, studies revealed startling statistics that tended to show that the crisis was due to an actual increase in the occurrence of malpractice. One study claimed that about 18,000 doctors in the United States regularly committed malpractice, and that 5%-10% of the practicing physicians were impaired.[126(p1026)] Another study conducted by a team of researchers at Harvard found that about one in 27 hospitalizations resulted in disabling treatment injury, and one in four of those injuries was the result of negligence.[140(p8)] A 1984 study conducted by the Government Accounting Office also revealed that 49 of 122 practitioners disciplined by a state medical board relocated to another state and continued practicing medicine, while another 43 could not be traced and may have been practicing in undisclosed locations.[8] Thus, when read together, the studies seemed to indicate that, although most physicians were competent, those that were not competent were causing a lot of damage and getting away with it by moving from one place to another.

These alarming stories caused public outcry that came to the attention of the U.S. Congress at the same time physicians were complaining of an inability to pay for skyrocketing insurance premiums. In fact, total medical liability insurance expenditures in the U.S. rose from $60 million in 1960 to more than $7 billion in 1988.[140(p2)] Furthermore, by 1988 the average malpractice premium equaled about 6% of a practitioner's gross income.[140(p4)] Two reasons help explain why insurers had raised physician malpractice rates to this level during the late 1970s and early 1980s: 1) during this time frame the frequency of malpractice claims continued to escalate until by the late 1980s approximately 13 of every 100 doctors could expect to be sued in a given year, and 2) a substantial increase in the severity of the claims being filed occurred over that period of time (e.g., the average settlement in medical malpractice cases increased from $12,000 in 1970 to $100,000 in 1986).[140(p2)]

Congress reacted by scheduling hearings to determine how to address physician and consumer concerns. The hearings highlighted a problem with physician peer review—it was not living up to its promise of being an effective regulatory mechanism. Two important reasons were cited for ineffective peer review: 1) Physician reviewers were intimidated by the threat of litigation in cases where hospital privileges were denied or restricted. 2) No effective means existed to collect and disseminate information to hospitals, medical boards, or medical societies about incompetent physicians.

This inability to track the "rogue" physicians, who continued to practice and generate a disproportionately high number of malpractice cases, led Congress to believe that the U.S. needed a federal physician tracking and reporting mechanism. Furthermore, Congress decided that legislation was needed to encourage competent physicians in hospitals to monitor their colleagues,[61] and then to identify and report those who commit malpractice.

Congress recognized, however, that the legislation would have to offer an incentive to physicians to conduct a more stringent form of peer review, especially when the review might lead to a report being filed in a national repository for peer review information. After all, reviewing physicians might be inclined to be sympathetic and lenient when reviewing friends and colleagues. The reviewers also would have to worry about an increased potential for backlash and litigation based on negative reviews. The final legislation, the HCQIA, was drafted to address these concerns by including a *quid pro quo* for improved peer review—entities that followed the legislation's mandates to conduct periodic review, and to report peer review findings, would enjoy limited immunity in lawsuits brought by physicians who were adversely affected. Although some state peer review statutes already had granted such immunity in cases based on state law claims,[2,31] the state statutes had been unable to protect peer reviewers in cases alleging violations of federal antitrust law.[125] Thus, the HCQIA gave heightened protection to peer review entities because, in addition to providing immunity to state law claims, the Act granted immunity in cases raising *federal* antitrust issues as well.

The HCQIA created the National Practitioner Data Bank, which serves as a national repository for information about physicians that can be queried by licensing bodies, by hospitals making privileging decisions, and by professional societies making certification decisions. Congress specifically stated in the first section of the Act that the legislation and the Data Bank were intended to address "(1) the increasing occurrence of medical malpractice claims, (2) the need to 'restrict the ability of incompetent physicians to move from State to State,'(3) the threat to peer reviewers of liability for their peer review recommendations, and (4) the 'overriding national need to provide incentive and protection for physicians engaging in effective professional peer review.'"[115]

Congress believed that the improved access to information about physicians and the security provided to peer reviewers by the immunity provisions would lead to the following benefits for consumers and hospitals: 1) better decisions about who would be granted hospital privileges; 2) a concomitant improvement in the quality of hospital care; and 3) an ultimate reduction in the number of malpractice claims being filed against hospitals.

In addition, Congress hoped that consumers could be better protected from incompetent physicians who were not subject to regular hospital peer review because the following legislative requirements of the Act would make it eas-

ier to identify those physicians as well:

1. The Act required insurance carriers to report all claims paid on behalf of a physician in a medical malpractice action.

2. The Act required medical societies or any other professional body conducting peer review to report adverse membership decisions made on the basis of competence.

3. The Act required state medical boards to report all negative actions taken against a physician's license, and also encouraged the boards to query the Data Bank on a regular basis to discover new information about licensed physicians practicing in the state or applying for a license to practice in the state.

Specific Provisions of the HCQIA

The Act is written broadly to protect any "professional review body" engaged in peer review activity.[3] Thus, hospitals, MCOs, professional societies, and other organizations conducting peer review can claim immunity as long as the "professional review body" can show compliance with the Act's querying and reporting requirements. This immunity applies to every person participating as a member of the review body. It also applies to persons who provide information to the review body, unless the information proves to be false and the informant knew the information was false.[2]

The Act protects adverse "professional review actions" taken in regard to physicians (including dentists practicing in hospitals), but only if the review action was based on concerns about competency or professional conduct.[3,115] Thus, review actions applying to other health professionals, such as laboratory technicians, are not covered by the Act, and review actions taken for reasons unrelated to competency and professional conduct are not protected by the Act. For example, a review action taken for purely economic reasons would not be protected.

The immunity provisions protect against liability for damages in suits based on both state and federal laws. Immunity, however, is not complete. First of all, the immunity provisions cannot be asserted in suits brought by patients. The Act was never intended to insulate reviewers from liability to patients injured by a negligent physician. Instead, the Act is designed to protect peer review entities from liability in cases brought by disgruntled physicians who seek damages that stem from allegedly unwarranted peer review decisions. Nevertheless, HCQIA immunity is limited even in the physicians' suits, because the Act does not insulate a defendant reviewer from claims that seek injunctive relief, that are brought by an attorney general of a state or federal government, or that are brought under federal civil rights provisions.[115]

Despite these limitations and exceptions, the HCQIA's immunity provisions are important because they supplement the various states' immunity statutes[37] and provide immunity in the dreaded federal antitrust actions that often result in treble damage awards for successful complaining physicians.[38,84]

A peer review entity that wants to assert an HCQIA immunity defense can do so only if the review body can show that it provided the plaintiff physician a fair opportunity to participate in the peer review decision-making process (see "Effects of the HCQIA" in this chapter). In addition, the peer review body must be able to show that it has met the Act's reporting and querying requirements, as explained below.

Reporting Requirements. The HCQIA requires a Data Bank report to be filed in four instances: 1) when a malpractice payment is made on behalf of a health care practitioner; 2) when a state board takes an adverse licensure action; 3) when a health care entity takes an adverse professional review action lasting longer than 30 days; and 4) when a professional society takes an adverse action that is based on a review of competence or professional conduct and that affects membership in the society.[3,115]

In regard to the malpractice payment, the Act requires an entity making a payment in the name of *any health care practitioner* (including practitioners other than physicians) to report the payment to the Data Bank. This reporting requirement applies to insurers as well as hospitals and other organizations providing health care services and conducting peer review. The report, which must be made even if the payment is made to settle a nuisance suit prior to litigation, must include the name of the practitioner, the amount of payment, names of orga-

nizations with which the practitioner is associated, and a description of the facts that led to the malpractice payment.[3]

Furthermore, a health care entity that takes a professional review action adversely affecting a physician's clinical privileges for longer than 30 days must report the action to the state medical board.[3] This reporting requirement, which applies only to adverse decisions made in regard to physicians, also stipulates that a health care entity must report to the state board any case of voluntary surrender of clinical privileges if the physician surrendering privileges is under review and trying to avoid an investigation. Because professional medical societies are included in the definition of health care entities that must report, such societies must report any decision made on the basis of competence that adversely affects a physician's membership in the society.

In summary, a peer review body can assert that it has met HCQIA reporting requirements, and therefore may be immune to suit, if it also can show timely reporting of medical malpractice payments to the Data Bank and reported adverse privilege decisions to the state medical board. Under the HCQIA, the medical board then assumes the duty of reporting information about hospital privileges to the Data Bank.

This medical board duty to report to the Data Bank is an important aspect of the HCQIA's framework. It was hoped that if medical boards were the reporting conduit for adverse hospital privileges decisions, the boards would keep more detailed and updated files on individual physicians. Furthermore, an adverse privilege decision would be likely to prompt the board to review a physician's licensure file for other evidence that might indicate a need for the board to investigate the physician's competence to practice medicine.

Congress also hoped that the HCQIA provisions requiring the medical boards to report all adverse licensure actions to the Data Bank would ultimately result in a federal bank of information that would allow the various states to more readily identify those physicians who might try to move from one state to another to practice medicine after being subjected to licensure restrictions or revocation. Thus, the HCQIA requires state boards filing an adverse licensure report to include the reasons for the licensure action, as well as any other information available in regard to the circumstances of an adverse action.[3,115]

Querying Requirements. Congress's goal of improved information dissemination could not be achieved without requiring health care entities to ask for the Data Bank's information. Because most physicians exercise hospital privileges, Congress focused on hospitals and made them responsible for requesting Data Bank information each time a licensed health care practitioner applies for hospital privileges.[3] Furthermore, the hospital must query the Data Bank every 2 years to obtain updated information about all practitioners who are exercising privileges in the hospital.[3]

This querying process is expensive for hospitals, which must pay a flat fee for each query. However, the expense of querying may actually save a hospital money in the long run. When a physician sues the hospital as a result of an adverse privilege decision, the HCQIA protects the hospital if it can show that it properly queried the Data Bank and then relied on the Data Bank's information in rendering the adverse privilege decision. HCQIA immunity applies even though the Data Bank information may have been false or incomplete, as long as the hospital was not aware of the problem with the information and therefore relied in good faith on the Data Bank data. Thus, a hospital that invests money in querying the Data Bank may actually save litigation expenses at a later date.

Furthermore, querying might assist the hospital in escaping liability for damages in cases of physician malpractice and negligent credentialing. If the hospital can show that it relied on the Data Bank information in making its decision to grant privileges to the physician, and the Data Bank information revealed nothing that would put the hospital on notice of a problem with the physician, then the hospital might be able to prove to a jury that it breached no duty to the patient in credentialing the physician.

Confidentiality Provisions. The public is not entitled to query the Data Bank for information.[3,106] Data Bank information is available only to medical boards, hospitals, and other health care entities making privilege decisions or conducting regular peer review activity. These entities are strictly prohibited from subsequently releasing Data Bank information to the public, and the information also is not subject to subpoena in civil and criminal actions.

An exception to these confidentiality provisions exists, however, in a negligence case brought against both a hospital and physician. When a plaintiff's attorney can show that the hospital failed to request information from the Data Bank as required by the HCQIA, the Data Bank information can be released to the attorney to show what the hospital would have known had it properly queried the Data Bank. The Data Bank report, however, may be used only in that litigation.[3,115]

Effects of the HCQIA

Due-Process Standards. The HCQIA has helped define due process in privilege decisions. Because loss of privileges is so detrimental to a physician's ability to successfully practice medicine, the Act recognizes that a physician is entitled to minimum due process procedures before the privileges can be restricted, denied, or revoked. The Act states that peer review entities do not have to strictly comply with its list of minimum due process procedures, but the entities must provide similarly "adequate notice and hearing procedures." Inevitably, after passage of the Act, hospitals modeled their notice and hearing procedures on the Act's requirements, but in so doing have found the procedures are sometimes onerous.[49] Recognizing this to be true, courts applying the HCQIA have generally stated that the review body's failure to meet all the Act's due process requirements does not by itself constitute a due process problem sufficient to nullify the Act's protections. However, courts have required hospitals claiming HCQIA immunity to show that deviations from the Act's due-process requirements continue to provide adequate notice and hearing procedures under the circumstances of the case.[49]

Under the Act a peer review entity must:[3,49]

1. give the physician notice that a review action might be taken against the physician;

2. give the physician the reasons for the action;

3. inform the physician of the right to request a hearing and have legal counsel present at the hearing;

4. inform the physician of the time frame in which the hearing request must be made;

5. provide the physician a summary of the physician's rights in the hearing;

6. give the physician notice of the time, place and date of the hearing;

7. give the physician a list of the witnesses before the hearing;

8. inform the physician that the right to the hearing will be forfeited if he or she does not appear; and

9. conduct the hearing before a mutually acceptable arbiter, a noncompeting hearing officer appointed by the hospital, or a panel of noncompetitors appointed by the hospital.

The Act also stipulates that after the hearing, the physician has the right to receive a written recommendation from the arbiter, officer, or panel, and the right to receive from the hospital a final written decision that delineates the reasons for the decision.

Improved Dissemination of Information. Peer review entities are querying the Data Bank in record numbers. During its first year of operation in 1990-91, the Data Bank received almost 40,000 queries about practitioners, but 4 years later it was getting almost 600,000 queries annually.[36] While hospitals are required to query the Data Bank about both new and renewal applications for privileges, the hospitals' share of requests rose only about 19% during the first 4 years of Data Bank operation. The increase in queries was driven mostly by MCOs voluntarily seeking information about physicians.[36] Thus, the Data Bank has become an important source of information to many kinds of health care entities concerned about physician competence.

Improved Participation in Peer Review. Realizing that much more information is now available to health care entities seeking information about individual physicians,[36] applicant physicians have become more willing to provide thorough and accurate information to credentials and peer review bodies. In other words, physicians want to be the first to disclose and explain information that will be available through other sources.[48,115(p79)]

Furthermore, physicians have reason to more willingly serve as peer reviewers. Recent court decisions verify that courts are properly granting summary judgment to defendant reviewers in suits based on peer review actions when the defendants can show they have met HCQIA immunity requirements.[38,43,49,111,115(p80)]

Finally, the Data Bank is producing valuable aggregated data. It is true that many physicians continue to object to the reporting requirements, in part because a physician must report all payments made to settle a claim, including a payment made to settle a nuisance suit.[6,130] Thus, many physicians feel that a Data Bank report about an individual physician can be misleading about competency.[64] However, the Data Bank's cumulative information is now being used to study patterns in licensure actions, privilege decisions, and medical malpractice litigation that can eventually assist reviewers in interpreting an individual's Data Bank report. For example, one study revealed that small, seemingly unimportant malpractice claims are indicative of a physician who is more likely to become embroiled in much more serious malpractice litigation in subsequent years.[142]

Possible Negative Effects. The HCQIA's reporting provisions have had at least two unintended negative effects. First, the reporting provisions probably have affected a physician's willingness to settle a malpractice case.[143] Any payment made on behalf of a physician to satisfy a judgment or to settle a malpractice case is reportable to the Data Bank. However, physicians are highly successful defendants in medical malpractice cases in that they win in approximately 80% of the cases brought against them.[115(p81)] For this reason, rather than settle the case and make a Data Bank report about the settlement, many physicians opt to litigate the case and possibly escape both liability and the Data Bank report. Thus, the HCQIA may be a hindrance in some settlement negotiations.

The HCQIA also may be prompting hospital peer reviewers to suggest 30-day suspensions of clinical privileges rather than more long-term solutions to quality of care concerns.[65] The HCQIA does not require a peer review entity to report an adverse privilege decision that is in effect for only 30 days or less. Thus, peer reviewers may be inclined to recommend a sanction that is not reportable to the Data Bank rather than one that is reportable and more likely to be litigated or challenged.[61,115]

ECONOMIC CREDENTIALING, PEER REVIEW, AND QUALITY OF CARE

This chapter has stressed that hospital peer review emerged as the most effective tool of professional self-regulation during the latter half of this century because hospital peer review was a regularly-ongoing process to identify and correct deficiencies in quality of care. In fact, as explained above, both state and federal statutory law evolved to encourage meaningful peer review by protecting peer reviewers who made negative privilege decisions based upon concerns about a physician's ability to render appropriate and adequate care.[3,137]

But in today's cost-conscious medical market, hospital peer review has begun to encompass more than the hospital medical staff's examination of quality of care. Hospital managers now are reviewing a physician's ability to render high-quality care in an environment that urges the physician to reduce costs and increase efficiency. Thus, a majority of hospitals now either perform or wish to perform what might be called "hybrid" peer review that looks at both competency and ability to contain costs.[19,134]

This focus on the economics of care has resulted in physician fear that quality of care concerns may begin to take a back seat to economic screening in some institutions. In fact, one recent publication stated that what doctors fear most in today's health care marketplace is their steady erosion of control over the practice of medicine, including their lack of control over peer review decisions being made on the basis of economic considerations.[12] Such fears are justified if a hospital's administration wants to examine only a physician's economic practice patterns in order to decide whether to grant or renew privileges, a practice known as "pure economic credentialing." Under pure economic credentialing, physicians are selected for participation and are retained only on the basis of an ability to practice medicine within certain cost guidelines. Of course, pure economic credentialing does not encourage the physician to make decisions based on what is best for the patient; the physician's medical decisions are more likely to be based on the cost of the care. Pure economic credentialing is understandably opposed by the AMA, and it has not yet been endorsed by courts or adopted by hospitals.[105]

Many hospitals, however, are presently using or making plans to use a form of hybrid economic credentialing. In the 1980s, economic problems forced nearly 700 hospitals in the United States to close.[40] Furthermore, many remaining hospitals experienced a rapid decline in the number of inpatient admissions during the early 1990s. In fact, in urban settings, some hospitals saw up to a 60% drop in the number of beds filled on a daily basis.[41] Several developments contributed to this drop in utilization and the resulting economic woes for hospitals.

The first major development to affect the hospital market occurred when the federal government in 1983 adopted a prospective system of Medicare reimbursement based upon diagnosis-related groups (DRGs).[4] Under the DRG system, a hospital could bill a fixed flat fee for each Medicare patient, with the fee being determined by the patient's diagnosis rather than by the costs actually incurred by the hospital. The DRG system was adopted in response to soaring Medicare costs under the pre-existing fee for service system of reimbursement, which encouraged physicians and patients to overutilize Medicare benefits. The DRG prospective reimbursement system was designed to encourage a hospital to treat Medicare patients within the government's reimbursement ceilings. Under the DRG scheme, a hospital that does not treat a patient within the imposed diagnostic "cost ceiling" is not permitted, under program guidelines, to bill either Medicare or the patient for the cost of care beyond the imposed cost cap. Over time, the DRG system proved to be successful in making hospitals attentive to costs and utilization of program assets, but the DRG reimbursement system also has been the impetus for major changes in hospital-physician relationships.[122]

The DRG system was bound to affect hospital-physician relationships because 70%-90% of hospital costs are controlled by the physicians[73] who diagnose and treat patients in the hospital setting.[93] Hospital management consequently had an incentive to pressure physicians into reducing the risk to the hospital of incurring costs beyond the DRG ceilings. More specifically, management began to encourage individual physicians to place patients in high reimbursement rate DRGs that provide more money for hospital treatment costs, to conservatively utilize hospital resources during the patient's hospital stay, and to discharge patients as early as possible.[5(p395)] Thus, under DRG prospective reimbursement mechanisms, hospital management actually had to encourage a reduction in the number of inpatient days in the hospital (one reason for the reduction in inpatient days that ultimately led to a financial crisis for some hospitals having trouble filling existing beds)! Furthermore, hospital administrators could no longer be satisfied with reviewing privileged physicians only for competency and quality of care; management needed to review each doctor for his or her ability to keep patient treatment costs below reimbursement rates.

The second major development to affect the hospital market occurred when state governments followed the federal government's lead by implementing similar controls over health care expenditures. Some states adopted DRG-type prospective reimbursement schemes, but an even greater number began using MCOs for delivery of health care to state enrollees (both employees and indigent persons receiving care under Medicaid programs). The MCOs usually were set up to both insure and provide health care services to each enrollee for a capitated cost established on a yearly basis. Such plans placed emphasis on outpatient rather than inpatient hospital treatments, which ultimately affected both the number of hospital admissions and length of stay of the patient while in the hospital. Even where fee-for-service plans were retained for state employees, some states legislatively capped reimbursement for physicians and hospitals electing to service state insurance program enrollees.[73] The caps, along with the drop in government enrollees' inpatient admissions and lengths of stay, forced many hospitals to both close departments and floors and attempt to increase the number of private-pay patients entering the hospital.

However, hospitals found little help when turning to the private sector. At the same time government insurers were trying to rein in hospital costs, private insurers were reacting to employers' complaints about the rising costs of employee health insurance benefits.[73] Private insurers also sought out MCO plans (e.g., health maintenance organizations (HMOs) or preferred provider organizations (PPOs)) to meet the private sector's demand for cost reduction, and MCOs proved to be very good at getting people out of the hospital quickly or keeping them out entirely. Furthermore, hospitals discovered that most MCOs utilized in the private sector also required hospitals to accept fixed, capitated payments for insureds who had to enter the hospital. In fact, a 1994 hospital study predicted that by 1996, approximately 92% of hospital contracts with MCO insurers would be capitated arrangements. This private sector focus on cost savings through capitation assured the emergence of economic credentialing as a component of the total hospital peer review process.

Today, very few patients enter the hospital under fee-for-service or self-pay terms. Thus, hospital management's best interests now lie in attracting and keeping competent physicians on staff who can adapt their practice habits to provide high-quality care with the kind of economic efficiency demanded by prospective reimbursement schemes that are capitated. The new approach to credentialing and peer review, which looks at both clinical and financial measures of quality, permits hospital boards to satisfy both the board's fiduciary duty to the hospital to keep the hospital financially stable and the hospital's duty to patients to provide high-quality care. This need in the 1990s for hybrid economic credentialing has prompted hospitals to begin educating physicians about two things: 1) the hospital's need to contain costs; and 2) the cost effectiveness of the individual physician's practice patterns. With recent advances in computer hardware and software capabilities,[21] hospitals can provide individual assessments of cost effectiveness by gathering and analyzing data that is then organized in sophisticated physician practice profiles. Such profiles can compare each physician's cost efficiency to that of other physicians in the hospital, as well as to that of other physicians in regional and national data bases.[92] To determine economic efficiency, a hospital can collect data to reflect many variables, including the kind of patients admitted by the physicians (e.g., Medicare, Medicaid, or private payer), patient length of stay and charges per admission by DRG or other reimbursement scheme, utilization review denials from the insurers, bad debt, malpractice settlements and awards, and physician market share.[131,134]

In addition to the financial data, hospitals can use medical guidelines, utilization review information, credentials information, and routine practice data to create over time a more complete picture of each physician's practice and competency during a defined time period.[21] Furthermore, outcomes data can be collected by procedures that permit patients to provide information about health outcomes and satisfaction with care.[135] Thus, outcomes data can provide an important piece of the total picture of competency.[56]

Hospitals' two-pronged strategy of first educating physicians about institutional cost concerns, and then assisting physicians in identifying their own impact upon the hospital's financial well-being, seems to be working to hospitals' advantage. Physicians are reporting that they have begun weighing the costs of alternative treatments. For example, one physician reported that he now orders oral medications rather than intravenous medications.[131] Others report that they sometimes take a "wait and see" approach before ordering expensive tests,[131] while others now realize that a pill costing $100 is cost effective if it keeps a patient out of the hospital for a day.[12] Thus, physicians seem to have accepted a certain degree of economic review[92] as a valid component of their total peer review process.

One commentator has noted that development of clinical practice guidelines, outcomes measures, and provider profiles has had many advantages for hospitals in addition to helping physicians understand the need to become cost effective. For instance: a hospital will have a better understanding of how it is delivering health care; accumulated data will assist the hospital in identifying and highlighting variations in physician practices; the data will provide a way to fairly and objectively identify nonconforming physicians and to request explanations for the nonconformities; and the data will provide new benchmarks for judging total physician performance.[21] Furthermore, physician profiles can be shared with other hospitals making credentialing decisions.

Case law also recognizes a hospital's need to take cost considerations into account when deciding who to appoint or reappoint to a medical staff. Courts have emphasized that hospitals must act for the public good, and lowering cost is a worthy societal purpose.[45] Furthermore, courts have recognized that economic survival of the institution may dictate that physicians be screened for their ability to contain costs.[21] Some courts have gone so far as to state that an ability to contain costs might be symptomatic of quality.[54,96]

Even when a hospital decides to close the staff or award an exclusive contract to a physician group in order to save money, courts have recognized that benefits to the public could justify the hospital's actions.[32,58,76,117] For example, if the hospital OB-GYN staff delivers 200 babies per year, and almost 200 doctors exercising privileges perform the deliveries, then the hospital cannot assess a doctor's performance. But if the OB-GYN staff is limited to 20 physicians who perform all the deliveries, then regular peer review and assessment will be meaningful.[92] Limiting the size of the staff improves quality of care by guaranteeing that the staff is experienced and continues to improve through beneficial peer review.[39,73] Thus, hospitals making economic decisions that can be justified in quality of care terms are highly likely to prevail in physician suits alleging purely illegal, economic motives in the hospitals' privilege decisions.[72]

Finally, the new hybrid credentialing process helps promote one of the elements of the effective regulatory mechanism outlined in the first part of this chapter: continual monitoring of performance accompanied by immediate follow-up. With hybrid credentialing, hospitals continually monitor a number of screens that can pinpoint deviations in practice patterns. Thus, the screens remove some of the subjectivity from the review process and provide immediate, hard data about performance. The data is also collected in a manner that can be easily reviewed and quickly made available to individual physicians so that both the hospital and physician can immediately begin discussing and addressing noted problems.

Despite these noted benefits of hybrid credentialing, physicians generally oppose economic credentialing because it jeopardizes physician autonomy and threatens traditional medical staff peer review. Peer review has historically been conducted only by medical experts—the physicians.[92] Physicians correctly point out that economic review is against public policy if it leads hospital administrators to devalue the medical staff's review of professional competence and to favor computer data that can be reviewed by administrators without medical staff involvement. Physicians fear that too much focus on computer data will elevate cost concerns above concerns about quality of care and patient safety.[141] Physicians also argue that economic credentialing policies are beneficial and in the public interest only to the extent that they support a plan to improve the total quality of care rendered by physicians in the hospital setting;[40] if economic credentialing is in place merely to improve the hospital's profit, it is an unconscionable means of professional review.

Case law supports physicians in regard to this latter position, because no appellate court has yet upheld a hospital's privilege decision that was clearly based on economic factors alone.[73] While one trial court in Florida upheld a hospital's decision to deny privileges to a surgeon merely because he headed a department in another hospital and might therefore have an economic conflict of interest, the surgeon did not appeal the decision and the hospital eventually granted privileges.[123] The decision has no value as precedent for several reasons: it was never tested in an appellate court, it does not reflect existing law, and it was based on a state statute that seemed to give the hospital a right to make an economic decision.

To physicians' relief, pure economic credentialing has not yet been adopted by any hospital, in part because decisions based on economics alone foreclose a hospital from asserting statutory peer review immunity. State and federal immunity statutes are designed to protect only those peer review decisions that are based on quality of care. The HCQIA protects peer review entities in federal antitrust litigation only if the decision was made with the "reasonable belief that the action was in the furtherance of quality health care,"[3] while most state peer review immunity statutes protect decisions

made in "good faith" that the decision promotes quality of care in the hospital.[115(p68)] For this reason, most hospitals have and will turn to a hybrid form of credentialing, where both quality and cost can be considered when making credentialing decisions.

Hospitals will also favor hybrid credentialing because pure economic credentialing may result in hospital liability under antitrust law; privilege decisions based on economics alone may equate to an illegal and anticompetitive restraint of trade that is compensable to the damaged physician.[40] A discussion of antitrust law is beyond the scope of this chapter, but to avoid this legal quagmire, hospitals and medical staffs should consult an attorney to assist in drafting bylaw peer review provisions that do not violate antitrust rules, that give medical staff members adequate notice of how economic considerations will factor into a peer review decision, and that protect the hospital by seeking a patient mix that does not unduly risk financial instability resulting from nonreimbursable costs.[99]

The main reason that hospitals will avoid pure economic credentialing, however, is that it could trigger a loss of the public's trust.[112] In today's competitive market, a hospital could not survive a reputation of ignoring quality of care issues when selecting physicians. It probably also could not survive the rash of malpractice lawsuits based on negligent credentialing theories.

MANAGED CARE AND PEER REVIEW

This chapter has stressed that the hospital credentialing and peer review process has for many years promoted quality of care by exercising significant influence over physicians' practice of medicine in the hospital setting. But, when President Clinton's effort to nationalize medicine ultimately led to a revolution in health care financing and delivery in the mid-1990s, the hospital's role in regulating quality of care began to diminish for at least three reasons.

First, a substantial number of Americans are enrolled in MCOs. The MCOs emerged in the private sector to deliver health care services with the express purpose of cutting the cost of those services (e.g. HMOs, PPOs, preferred provider arrangements (PPAs), exclusive provider organizations (EPOs), and other hybrid MCOs).[102(p152)] Although MCOs had already been in existence for many years, the 1994 national health care debate highlighted the need to cut the cost of health care to employers so that they could assure that all working Americans were covered by adequate heath care plans. In the wake of the national debate about cost and coverage, managed care enrollment skyrocketed. In 1992, approximately 37 million Americans were enrolled in HMOs, but by 1995 that number had risen to more than 46 million.[132] One study projected that the enrollment would reach 65 million by the beginning of 1997.[129] This phenomenal growth in managed care enrollment set the stage for increased physician participation in managed care—the second reason the hospitals' role in regulating quality of care has begun to diminish.

Just as hospital privileges in past years were a necessary component of a physician's ability to obtain and keep patients, the ability to access patients in the MCOs has become essential to the physician who is practicing in an area deeply penetrated by MCO models of health care delivery. For example, about 45% of the population of California is enrolled in a managed care plan.[95] One California doctor explained the impact on his practice: although he had no capitated patients in 1990, approximately 50% of the patients he now serves are in capitated health care arrangements.[100] As for the rest of the country, one projection is that 40%-60% of the U.S. population will be enrolled in managed care plans by the year 2000.[26] Thus, because most physicians are now or will soon be participating in MCOs,[51,61] the physician selection and review processes used by the MCOs could become just as important to the assurance of high-quality physician care as the hospital peer review process has been in the recent past.[105]

A third reason the hospital's role in regulating the quality of medical care has diminished is that patients are now spending less time in hospitals.[121] Both private insurers and MCOs have promoted less-expensive outpatient treatment options and have pushed for decreases in length of stay for patients who must be admitted to the hospital. For this reason, much of the physician care that used to be provided in the hospital setting is now being rendered either in the rapidly proliferating outpatient centers or in the physician's private office. Thus, physicians simply have less need to see patients in the hospital setting.

Both the medical profession and the public have recognized the importance of hospital peer review. The HCQIA is evidence of an agreement between consumers, legislators, and practitioners to regulate quality by reviewing physicians in their hospital practices. But the changes explained above point out that both patients and doctors are spending less time in hospitals. This trend de-emphasizes the importance of the hospital in patient treatment and highlights the need to establish credentialing and peer review mechanisms to monitor physicians who are practicing in managed care systems. Although federal regulations require each MCO to have a quality assurance program to review physicians,[23] there is no clear responsibility for credentialing and peer review in today's managed care systems.[16] The challenge now is for MCOs to decide how to assume their obvious duty to help in the regulation of physician competence. Certainly, only competent providers should be given access to the organizations, and such providers should be regularly reviewed.

However, this need to monitor access has spawned tension between MCOs and physicians, who argue that they are unfairly being excluded from MCO participation, that they are being reviewed by MCOs on the basis of their cost efficiency rather than their ability to render quality care, and that MCOs are interfering in the patient-physician relationship. These and other issues are discussed below.

MCO Access Issues

To maintain their cost effectiveness, MCOs generally seek out those physicians who can render care in a cost-efficient manner. Other factors considered by the MCO are geographic location, historical utilization, credentials, and range of services,[86] all of which are criteria often examined by hospitals when determining who should receive privileges under hybrid economic credentialing guidelines. But many doctors are being excluded from MCO participation, as is evidenced by MCO enrollees' primary complaint about today's plans: lack of access to desired physicians.[81]

In fact, physicians have accused MCOs of unfair exclusion and have mounted campaigns in various parts of the country for legislative enactments that allow them to maintain access to their patient base. Such statutes, generally known as "any willing provider" laws, have been directed at limiting an MCO's ability to dictate which physicians the MCO enrollees are permitted to see. "Any willing provider" laws have been described as falling into one of four categories:[86]

1. those that require the MCO to reimburse a physician as long as the physician agrees to accept the MCO level of reimbursement;

2. those that require the MCO to: a) admit any physician who agrees to abide by the MCO's contract provisions, including cost of service schedules,[11] and b) adopt a provision guaranteeing patients the right to choose their physicians;

3. those that require the MCO to provide due process to physicians by giving notice about how to join and by setting up an appeal process for physicians terminated from MCO participation; and

4. those that require the MCO to contract with physicians who provide essential services to certain segments of the community, particularly the poor population.

By 1995, at least four states had adopted "any willing provider" laws that applied to most classes of health care providers[77,80] and many more had adopted laws that applied only to pharmacy services.[86] In addition, the U.S. Congress was considering such legislation.[13,58,86]

Congress's willingness to consider "any willing provider" legislation may be contradictory, however, of its stated purposes in enacting the HCQIA. The HCQIA was aimed at improving the hospital physician selection and peer review process in order to assure that only competent physicians would be awarded privileges. "Any willing provider" legislation, on the other hand, can take away an MCO's discretion in selecting physicians to participate, and therefore can represent a step backward for the MCO that is attempting to select only high-quality physicians in order to maintain or improve the qual-

ity of patient care in the MCO.[89]

"Any willing provider" laws that do not take into account a screen for cost effectiveness can also represent a step backward in the war against health care costs by denying an MCO its ability to use cost effectiveness as one of a number of factors in choosing participating physicians. In fact, several studies have indicated that "any willing provider" statutes can increase the cost of health care by increasing administrative costs, increasing costs associated with patient litigation, and reducing the MCO's ability to negotiate successfully for lower provider costs.[86] For these reasons, legislators need to carefully consider how to permit the MCO to choose those providers who can provide good and affordable care. In other words, an MCO's right to exclude physicians on the basis of cost and quality must be balanced against a physician's right to be involved in the MCO if the physician can meet the MCO conditions of participation.[27]

Ultimately, participating physicians must become more knowledgeable about the *business* of medicine, become more involved with MCO credentialing and peer review processes, and participate in MCO decision-making with regard to physician contracts and patient coverage issues. Hospital peer review has been successful because physicians were regulating physicians. Physicians now must take the initiative to solve new kinds of physician credentialing problems arising in the MCO setting.[12,18]

Quality-of-Care Issues

Although the objective of hospital credentialing and peer review traditionally has been improved quality of care, hospitals now must also review for efficiency in order to continually assess the financial stability of the hospital institution. Similarly, an MCO must also review physicians to assess each doctor's costs related to patient care. One commentator used the following example to explain why some measure of economic credentialing is vital to the financial well-being of the MCO.[142]

Assume that one physician has 100 patients for whom the treatment costs total $2,000. Assume a second physician also has 100 patients, but the treatment costs total $3,000. The first physician's cost per patient is $20, while the second's cost per patient is $30. Where the MCO has contracted to treat each patient for $25, the first physician is making the organization money, while the second physician is losing money with each patient treated.[143] This is information that is crucial to the MCO.

Nevertheless, this example also illustrates the potential danger of economic credentialing: the two physicians' economic credentials rather than their medical credentials might become the deciding factor in whether they can continue to participate in the MCO. Under pure economic credentialing, the position of the second doctor probably would be terminated. However, additional data from peer, utilization, and outcome reviews might reveal that the second doctor is treating more seriously ill patients. Furthermore, the data might reveal that the second doctor has better patient outcomes with the seriously ill patients because he uses treatments that are slightly more expensive, but that are also are more effective. In fact, the more expensive treatment might lead to higher rates of cure that ultimately will keep the patients out of the system. Thus, the second doctor's higher costs might be justified from a quality of care standpoint, and physician number two should not be terminated on the basis of an economic screen alone.

This example illustrates why physicians must become more involved with MCO peer review and development of treatment policies. As one commentator has noted, "it simply is not possible to have persons other than physicians develop rationing guidelines for physicians to implement."[112] Physicians should be included in the process of writing the organization's treatment guidelines,[22,88] implementing those guidelines, and then reviewing physician performance under those guidelines.[119] MCO physician peer review could help assure that quality is not abandoned to preserve financial stability,[66] while at the same time assuring that MCO physicians continue to be educated about ways to save costs and preserve financial stability.[109] Furthermore, physician participation in review could encourage MCOs to establish procedures that assure due process fairness in termination proceedings and thereby also reduce conflict between physicians and MCOs.[30,88]

MCO Tort Liability Issues

How to effectively conduct physician peer review is a critical emerging issue for MCOs because courts have begun to find MCOs liable in cases of physician malpractice.[146] Just as courts have utilized theories of *respondeat superior*, ostensible agency, and hospital corporate negligence to find hospitals either vicariously or directly liable to a patient injured while in the hospital, courts are now finding MCO liability where the facts of the case justify application of one of these three theories.

For example, many HMOs contract directly with a physician and exercise the kind of control over the physician that is typical in an employer/employee relationship. When an employer/employee relationship exists, the MCO can be held liable for the physician's negligence under the doctrine of respondeat superior. This legal doctrine holds the MCO responsible for the employee physician's negligent acts that are within the scope of employment.[16,17] Even where the MCO contracts with a physician to perform services as an independent contractor, as is usually the case in a PPO, the MCO can be liable under the doctrine of ostensible agency. A court may apply this theory to find MCO liability when the physician appears to be an agent of the MCO, the MCO enrollee patient is not free to choose a physician not on the MCO's list of providers, and the MCO indicates that the plan's physicians are agents of the MCO. For example, the plaintiff in *Decker v. Saini*[44] successfully argued that the HMO was liable under ostensible agency principles because of representations made in the HMO literature distributed to enrollees.

The facts of the *Decker* case indicated that the HMO published literature asserting that its primary care physicians provided the "best care" available. The plaintiff enrollee's primary care physician referred the plaintiff to a non-member doctor who did not diagnose the plaintiff's cancer. In finding that the HMO could be liable under the ostensible agency theory, the court noted that the patient viewed the primary care physician as an HMO agent, the HMO represented that the primary care physician was its agent, and the plaintiff relied on the primary care physician, in part because the HMO represented that the physician offered the best care available. Based on these facts, the court said the HMO could be liable under ostensible agency theory.

The *Decker* court went on to point out that HMOs should be liable for the negligence of their physician providers, because HMOs would have no incentive to associate with and keep the best physicians if the HMO could not be held liable for associating with less than competent physicians. Furthermore, the court said that allowing the HMO to escape liability for the negligence of the nonplan physician to whom the case was referred would simply encourage the HMO to use specialty physicians outside the plan. Other courts have agreed with the *Decker* court's reasoning and found that when a managed care case raises questions about whether the negligent physician was an ostensible agent of the MCO, the case should be sent to the jury to determine whether the MCO should be held liable.[16,17,24,103]

Finally, at least two courts have said that, just as a hospital has certain nondelegable duties that run directly to the hospital's patients, an MCO has a nondelegable duty to select and retain only competent physicians and a duty to enforce policies to ensure quality of care.[103,116] In other words, these courts believe an MCO can be liable for its own acts of negligence in selecting, retaining, and supervising independent contractor physicians that are practicing within the MCO system.

The ERISA Pre-emption Issue

The Employee Retirement Income Security Act of 1974 (ERISA)[57] was "designed to promote the interests of employees and their beneficiaries by regulating the creation and administration of employee benefit plans."[114] In fact, because the U.S. Congress sought to achieve nationally uniform administration of employee benefit plans,[120,124] Congress wrote the Act to include a pre-emption provision. ERISA regulates employee benefit plans that "relate to" medical care, accidents, disability, or death, and the ERISA pre-emption provision applies to all state laws except those that regulate insurance. Thus, ERISA pre-emption principles will apply to a judicial claim brought under state law if the

court finds the claim "relates to" an ERISA employee benefit plan.

For this reason, many MCO defendants in medical malpractice cases remove a plaintiff's MCO negligent selection or retention claim to federal court and then assert an ERISA pre-emption defense to bar the plaintiff's claim against the MCO. The success of this defensive strategy depends upon which court is hearing the case because the federal circuit courts are split on whether ERISA pre-empts such claims.

Some circuits that have been responsive to a pre-emption argument have stressed continued concern about cost containment and the need to protect emerging systems that purport to deliver medical care at reduced costs.[16,17] These courts have permitted a pre-emption defense by finding that the process of credentialing MCO physicians is an administrative function of the plaintiff's medical plan, and the claim therefore is "related to" the plan.[50,60,110] In other words, these courts would say a malpractice claim against an MCO is really an attack on the benefit plan itself, and ERISA was designed to control such attacks.[127]

Other courts have distinguished negligence claims brought on the basis of ostensible agency and have not found pre-emption.[53] These courts have found that the claim against the MCO is actually based on a professional malpractice claim against the physician, so the claim against the MCO does not "relate to" the benefit plan itself.[55] One court seemed to go farther by suggesting that peer review and other assessments of quality of physician care are activities that go beyond simple plan administration. Thus, negligent credentialing and supervision cases brought as corporate negligence cases also are not "related to" ERISA.[94]

This split of authority has led to inequitable results in malpractice cases. In fact, courts in jurisdictions that recognize ERISA pre-emption have noted that plaintiffs in these jurisdictions may have no legal remedy against the MCO when ERISA pre-empts the claim, even though both injury and negligence are obvious.[16,17,35] It is now up to Congress or the Supreme Court to revisit ERISA and address this unforeseen problem associated with a statutory scheme designed to protect beneficiaries of employee health plans.[16,17,127]

Physician-Patient Issues

As fee-for-service care has declined, MCOs have turned to capitation or salary mechanisms for paying physicians. Salaried physicians are common in HMOs, which usually attempt to contract with physicians who give all their time to the HMO. Physicians in salary arrangements are typically referred a certain number of patients, and the physician obviously has an incentive to limit the number of patients for whom he or she is responsible.[112]

Preferred provider groups, however, are usually made up of physicians who have contracted with an MCO to give only a part of their time for a fixed, capitated cost per MCO patient served.[112] Such physicians have an incentive to increase the number of patients they serve and possibly to rely more upon services provided outside their offices such as hospital diagnostic tests and referrals.

To encourage salaried physicians to treat patients within HMO cost guidelines, and to discourage capitated physicians from overusing outside services or making too many referrals to expensive specialists, some MCOs have created a system of financial rewards and penalties that affects how much money the physician receives from the MCO. Where the physician treats patients within MCO cost parameters, the physician is financially rewarded, but the physician is also financially at risk for patients whose treatment costs exceed the guidelines or capitated cost figure. Often, patients are not aware of these financial arrangements that are likely to interfere in the fiduciary patient-physician relationship.

Furthermore, some MCOs have contractual "gag clauses" that bar doctors from telling patients that their MCO plan creates financial incentives[67,83,143] or that alternative or more advanced treatments than those provided by the MCO might be helpful to the patient. Physicians have strongly objected to such clauses because they further interfere with the patient-physician relationship.[64]

In response to both physician and consumer complaints, many state legislatures have considered "patient fairness acts" that would limit physician incentive plans and MCOs' ability to "fire" doctors who give patients information about alternative treatments or limitations in the MCO health care plan.[10,80] In addition, the U.S. Congress has stepped in to assure that Medicare and Medicaid patients do in fact receive such critical information.

The Omnibus Budget Reconciliation Act of 1990 (OBRA 90) addressed incentive plans that apply to physicians who treat Medicare or Medicaid patients. OBRA 90 bars specific payments made directly or indirectly to doctors to induce them to reduce or limit medically necessary services.[138(p3)] Furthermore, if the incentive plan places the physicians at substantial financial risk for services ordered or arranged, but not furnished directly, then the MCO must provide stop-loss protection and conduct patient surveys to assess the access to and satisfaction with services.[78,138]

The Health Care Financing Administration issued final regulations in 1996 that will implement these OBRA 90 provisions and govern the manner in which MCOs may make incentive payments to providers.[138] The final regulations, which became effective in January 1997, require MCOs to make survey results, as well as information about plan incentive arrangements, available to Medicare and Medicaid plan enrollees upon request.[78] Thus, OBRA 90 and its accompanying regulations seek to address problems that affect patients' ability to make informed decisions about their health care and to accurately assess the quality of care provided by the MCO.

Final Notes on MCO Peer Review

As managed care has mushroomed in the health care market, physicians have found that they must be credentialed by a number of MCO providers, each of which has the goal of finding qualified and competent physicians who can practice medicine within the MCO cost guidelines. Centralized or integrated credentialing services have been proposed to reduce redundant efforts in screening physicians and to provide comprehensive information that would meet the informational needs of the various MCO providers.[144] In fact, state-wide associations representing physicians, hospitals, and MCOs in California seem to have taken a step toward endorsing integrated credentialing by adopting a standardized credentialing application that ultimately could be used by an integrated credentialing center.[144] However, centralized credentialing will not be feasible until concerns about loss of control over confidential information can be appeased, and until the proponents of centralized credentialing know whether such services can be organized to provide the kind of thorough and professional peer review activity that is protected by federal and state statutes.

In the meantime, one way for MCOs to lessen consumer dissatisfaction with their limited choice in physician providers is to ensure that all physicians within the MCO are qualified and competent. Meaningful peer review conducted when selecting and reviewing MCO physicians would not only assure the MCO that its physicians were less likely to spawn costly malpractice suits, but would also help build the public's trust in the MCO's ability to deliver high-quality care.[89] Because so many Americans now must participate in an MCO plan for their health care services, it is time for state and federal regulators to support legislation that fosters meaningful peer review at the MCO level. When both hospitals and MCOs are reviewing providers, the consuming public will again be able to believe that most physicians who are delivering health care treatments and services are being watched by the experts—their peers.

Furthermore, in the MCO environment, full-risk capitation agreements may provide an answer for many physicians disillusioned by their loss of autonomy. This shift of risk from the insurer to the physician provider allows the insurer to stop trying to contain costs by managing physician treatment decisions. Physicians who have assumed the full risk of capitation also can gain from the arrangement, because they can keep the money that they save through more efficient delivery of health care.[107] Realizing that capitation might be an answer to their problems, many physicians are now advocating that they can replace the MCOs altogether, and in so doing can reduce administrative costs, improve peer review, and take more control over how care is delivered.[12,88,105,107,113] Moreover, recent federal legislation removed many legal barriers for physicians who want to organize into a network that provides health care services by contracting directly with employers and other payers.[113]

Finally, changes in how health care is delivered to the public obviously will continue to occur in the years to come as physicians and insurers seek arrangements that meet their various needs. The trump card that physicians can continue to exercise through this process of change is the fact that only a physician can be licensed to practice medicine and only a licensed practitioner has the expertise to assess the quality of care provided to patients by other physicians. Thus, physicians can continue to assert the need for professional autonomy in deciding what constitutes quality care, who will be permitted to deliver that care, and who will control the process of making treatment decisions.

REFERENCES

1. 42 CFR §Parts 462-476 (1996)
2. 42 CFR §Part 482 (1996)
3. 42 USC §11111 et seq (1994) (Health Care Quality Improvement Act)
4. 42 USC §1395 (1994)
5. Abraham KS, Weiler PC: Enterprise medical liability and the evolution of the American health care system. **Harvard Law Rev 108:**381-436, 1994
6. Access, quality, cost: Practitioner Data Bank — Doc loses bid to delete his name. **Am Health Line 3:**189, Jan 6, 1995
7. *Adamski v Tacoma General Hospital*, 579 P2d 970 (Wash 1978)
8. Adler RS: Stalking the rogue physician: an analysis of the Health Care Quality Improvement Act. **Am Bus Law J 28:**683-741, 1991
9. American Medical Association: **Peer Review Manual**. Chicago, Ill: American Medical Association, 1972
10. Amos DS: Medical balancing act. Doctors weigh patient needs against insurers' rules. **St Louis Post-Dispatch.** Apr 1, 1996, p 10 (1996 WL 2760284)
11. Arkansas Acts, 1995, ' 505, amended by 1995 Arkansas Acts 1193
12. Azevedo D: Taking back health care — doctors must work together. **Med Econ 73:**156-167, June 24, 1996 (1996 WL 9421553)
13. Baxter MJ: Physician credentialing: new risks for patients and providers. **Md Bar J 28:**18-22, Jan-Feb 1995
14. Begun JW, Lippincott RC: **Strategic Adaptation in the Health Professions. Meeting the Challenges of Change.** San Francisco, Calif: Jossey-Bass Publishers, 1993
15. Bell JA, Jewell CM: The corporate practice of medicine prohibition: past, present, and future. Healthcare Mergers and Acquisitions. **ABA: Forum on**

Health Law. 1995

16. Benesch K: Emerging theories of liability for negligent credentialing in HMOs, integrated delivery and managed care systems. **Health Lawyer 9:**14-19, Fall 1996

17. Benesch K: Managed care liability: an expansion of familiar theories. **Health Lawyer 9:**8-14, 1996

18. Blendon RJ, Kohut A, Benson JM, et al: Health system reform: Physicians' views on the critical choices. **JAMA 272:**1546-1550, 1994

19. Blum JD: Economic credentialing. A new twist in hospital appraisal processes. **J Legal Med 12:** 427-475, 1991

20. Blum JD: The evolution of physician credentialing into managed care selective contracting. **Am J Law Med 22:**173-203, 1996

21. Blum JD: Hospitals, new medical practice guidelines, CQI, and potential liability outcomes. **St Louis U Law J 36:**913-945, 1992

22. Boehm FH: An unethical ploy. **The Tennessean.** Mar 19, 1996, p 7A (1996 WL 4942559)

23. Bouey PS: Peer review in the managed care setting. **PLI/Comm 471:**279, 1988

24. *Boyd v Albert Einstein Medical Center*, 547 A2d 1229 (Pa Super 1988)

25. Boyd TH: Cost containment and the physician's fiduciary duty to the patient. **DePaul Law Rev 39:** 131-159, 1989

26. Brook RH, Kamberg CJ, McGlynn EA: Health system reform and quality. **JAMA 276:**476-480, 1996

27. Brown LC, Anderson JM: Walking the provider panel selection tightrope. **Inside Health Law 1:**3-5, Jan 1996

28. Burge J: Suits increasing for failure to spot cancer. Plaintiffs claiming cost-saving measures cost patients their lives. **ABA J 81:**16-17, 1995

29. Butler KA: Health care quality revolution: legal landmines for hospitals and the rise of the critical pathway. **Albany Law Rev 58:**843-870, 1994/1995

30. Cappasso T: Doctors move to limit HMOs' meddling with patients. **The State Journal-Register.** Jan 24, 1996, p 1 (1996 WL 5786978)

31. *Cardwell v Rockford Memorial Hospital,* 555 NE2d 6 (Ill 1990)

32. *Centeno v Rosville Community Hospital,* 167 Cal Rptr 183 (1979)

33. *Clark v Southview Hospital and Family Health Center,* 68 Ohio St 3d 435 (1994)

34. Colantonio MA: The Health Care Quality Improvement Act of 1986 and its impact on hospital law. **WVa Law Rev 91:**91-124, 1989

35. *Corcoran v United Healthcare, Inc,* 965 F2d 1321 (5th Cir 1992)

36. Crain Communications Inc: Hospitals warming to use of Physician Data Bank in hiring. **Modern Healthcare.** Jan 16, 1995 (1995 WL 2495025)

37. Creech CD: The medical review committee privilege. A jurisdictional survey. **NC Law Rev 67:** 179-231, 1988

38. Cross LL: Is HCQIA protecting peer review from antitrust claims? **Health Span 10:**11-13, June 1993

39. Crowley LT: The growing use of exclusive contracts by hospitals. **NY Law J 213:**73, April 18, 1995

40. Dallet B: Economic credentialing: your money or your life! **Health Matrix 4:**325-363, 1994

41. Dantzker D: Maintaining viability of health care

institutions as we move into a managed care environment. **The Second John E. Jones Symposium on Health Policy.** April 18, 1996

42. *Darling v Charleston Community Memorial Hospital,* 211 NE2d 253 (Ill 1965)

43. Darricades J: Medical peer review: how is it protected by the Health Care Quality Improvement Act of 1986? **J Cont Law 18:**263-283, 1992

44. *Decker v Saini,* 14 Employee Benefits Cases 1556, 1991 WL 277590 (Mich Cir Ct, Sept 17, 1991)

45. *Desai v St Barnabas Medical Center,* 510 A2d 662 (NJ 1986)

46. Deville KA: **Medical Malpractice in Nineteenth-Century America.** New York, NY: New York University Press, 1990.

47. Diamond JT, Weil DA: Clinical practice guidelines: quality, utilization, and the changing standard of care. **Health Lawyer 7:**9-12, Fall 1994

48. Dinnell, D: Hospital and consumer groups debate merits of Data Bank. **Wichita Bus J.** Mar 24, 1995, Section B

49. Donovan RE: The health care quality improvement act in the courts: fast-acting cure for physician peer review headaches? **J Health Hosp Law 28:**5, 257-268, 312, 1996

50. *Dukes v United States Health Care Systems of Pennsylvania, Inc,* 848 F Supp 39 (ED P 1994)

51. Eaton L: Aetna to buy U.S. Healthcare in big move to managed care. **New York Times.** Apr 2, 1996, pp A1, C8

52. Economic credentialing economics widely used in reviewing doctors. **Modern Health Care,** Nov 16, 1992 (1992 WL 7801950)

53. *Edelen v Osterman,* DC DC, No. 96-1655, 10/31/96. **Health Law Reporter (BNA) 5:**1695, 1996

54. *Edelman v John F Kennedy Memorial Hospital,* No. C-2104-80 (NJ Sup Ct 1982), *cert denied,* 475 A2d 585 (1984)

55. *Elesser v Hospital of Philadelphia College of Osteopathic Medicine,* 802 F Suppl 1286 (1992)

56. Ellwood PM Jr, Lundberg GD: Managed care: a work in progress. **JAMA 276:**1083-1086, 1996

57. Employee Retirement Income Security Act of 1974, Pub L No. 93-406, 88 Stat 829, 29 USC §§1001-1461 (1994)

58. Feinstein RA: Economic credentialing and exclusive contracts. **Health Lawyer 9:**4-11, Fall 1996

59. Ferraro DA: Apparent agency: estoppel/detrimental reliance/proximate cause — an evolution from case law to statute. **J Health Hosp Law 29:**38-42, 1996

60. *Frappier Estate v Wishnov,* Fla Dist Ct App 4th Dist, No-95-0669, 5/8/96. **Health Law Reporter (BNA) 5:** 858, 1996

61. Freudenheim M: Managed care empires in the making. Companies build networks to stay ahead of a hard-charging field. **New York Times.** Apr 2, 1996, pp C1, C8

62. Furrow B, et al: **Liability and Quality Issues in Health Care.** St Paul, Minn: West Publishing, 1991

63. Furrow BR: The changing role of the law in promoting quality in health care: from sanctioning outlaws to managing outcomes. **Houston Law Rev 26:** 147-190, 1989

64. Gale AH: When bad things happen to good doctors. **Mo Med 89:**720-726, 1992

65. Gavzer B: Why some doctors may be hazardous to

your health. **Parade Magazine.** Apr 14, 1996, pp 4-6

66. Glassheim J: Health care reform already with us. Fresno physician hopes quality care is not sacrificed because of costs. **The Fresno Bee.** May 21, 1995, p B7 (1995 WL 7412686)

67. Gray P: Gagging the doctors. **Time.** Jan 8, 1996, p 50

68. Green R, Reibstein R: **Employer's Guide to Workplace Torts.** Washington, DC: Bureau of National Affairs, 1992

69. Griffith RL, Parker JM: With malice towards none. The metamorphosis of statutory and common law protections for physicians and hospitals in negligent credentialing litigation. **Texas Tech Law Rev 22:** 157-209, 1991

70. Gross SJ: **Of Foxes and Henhouses. Licensing and the Health Professions.** Westport, Conn: Quorum Books, 1984

71. Hagen LA: Physician credentialing: Economic criteria compete with the Hippocratic oath. **Gonzaga Law Rev 31:**427- 474, 1995/1996

72. Haines S: Hospital peer review systems. An overview. **Health Matrix 2:**30-32, Winter 1984/1985

73. Hall M: Institutional control of physician behavior: legal barriers to health care cost containment. **U Pa Law Rev 137:**431-536, 1988

74. Havighurst CC: Practice guidelines as legal standards governing physician liability. **Law Contemp Prob 54:** 87-117, 1991

75. Havighurst CC: Practice guidelines for medical care: the policy rationale. **St Louis U Law J 34:**777-819, 1990

76. *Hay v Scripps Memorial Hospital-La Jolla*, 228 Cal Rptr 413 (Cal App 4 Dist 1986)

77. Health Care Law - HMO Regulation—Arkansas requires HMOs to accept any provider willing to join their networks. **Harv Law Rev 109:**2122, 1996

78. Health Maintenance Organizations, Competitive Medical Plans, and Health Care Prepayment Plans, 42 CFR §Part 417 (1996)

79. *Helling v Carey*, 519 P2d 981 (Wash 1974)

80. Hellinger FJ: The expanding scope of state legislation. **JAMA 276:**1065-1070, 1996

81. HMO gives members direct access. **The Herald-Sun** (Durham, NC). June 18, 1996

82. Hospital, patient input key to quality reforms. **Hospitals.** Oct 20, 1989, pp 77-78

83. Iglehart JK: Physicians and the growth of managed health care. **N Engl J Med 331:**1167-1171, 1994

84. Jaffee C: The Health Care Quality Improvement Act: antitrust liability in peer review. **Tort and Insurance Law J 24:**571, Spring 1989

85. JCAHO: **Accreditation Manual for Hospitals.** Chicago, Ill: Joint Commission on Accreditation of Hospitals, 1995

86. Jiranek AL, Baker D: Any willing provider laws: regulating the health care provider's contractual relationship with the insurance company. **Health Lawyer 7:**1-6, Winter 1994-1995

87. *Johnson v Misericordia Community Hospital*, 294 NW2d 501 (Wisc App 1980)

88. Johnson J, Kent C, Prager LO: Fairness, not force: doctors urged to guide managed care changes. **Am Med News.** Dec 25, 1995, p 3 (1995 WL 10600214)

89. Jordan KA: Managed competition and limited choice of providers: countering negative perceptions through a responsibility to select quality network physicians. **Ariz State Law J 27:**875-952, 1995

90. Jost TS: The Joint Commission on accreditation of Hospitals: private regulation of health care and the public interest. **Boston Coll Law Rev 24:**835-923, 1983

91. Jost TS: The necessary and proper role of regulation to assure the quality of health care. **Houston Law Rev 25:**525-598, 1988

92. Kadzielski MA, Fenton H, Lang DA: The Hospital medical staff: what is its future? **Whittier Law Rev 16:**987-1004, 1995

93. Kadzielski MA, Meinhardt RA, McCabe TA: Peer review potpourri: new developments in credentialing and privileging. **Whittier Law Rev 15:**51-73, 1994

94. *Kearney v US Healthcare, Inc*, No. 94-2625 (ED Pa Aug 3, 1994)

95. Kertesz L: Over HMO's high margins and lower payments, they are negotiating full-risk contracts. **Modern Healthcare.** Feb 5, 1996, p 24 (1996 WL 7525591)

96. *Knapp v Palos Community Hospital*, 465 NE2d 554 (Ill App Ct 1984)

97. Koska MT: Hospital CEOs divided on use of economic credentialing. **Hospitals 65 (6):**42-48, 1991

98. Koska MT: Outcome management stresses patient input. **Hospitals 63 (21):**32, 1989

99. Lang DA: **Managing Medical Staff Change Through Bylaws and Other Strategies.** Chicago, Ill : American Hospital Publisher, 1995

100. Larson E: The soul of an HMO. **Time.** Jan 22, 1996, pp 44-52

101. Leyerle B: **The Private Regulation of American Health Care.** Armonk, NY: ME Sharpe, 1994

102. MacKelvie CF, Mauro MH: **The Trustee's Guide to Board Duties, Liabilities, and Responsibilities.** Chicago, Ill: Probus Publishing, 1993

103. *McClellan v Health Maintenance Organization of Pennsylvania*, 604 A 2d 1053 (Pa Super 1992)

104. McClellan FM: **Medical Malpractice—Law, Tactics, and Ethics.** Philadelphia, Pa: Temple University Press, 1994

105. Mellas LA: Adopting the judicial approach to medical malpractice claims against physicians to reflect Medicare cost containment measures. **U Colo Law Rev 62:**287-319, 1991

106. Miller FH: Illuminating patient choice—releasing physician-specific data to the public. **Loyola Consumer Law Rep 8:**125-135, 1996

107. Miller FH: The promise and problems of capitation. **Am J Law Med 22:**167-172, 1996

108. Moore JD Jr: AMA proposals aim to bolster doc standing. **Modern Healthcare.** 1995, p 32 (1995 WL 2495962)

109. Morreim EH: Economic disclosures and economic advocacy. New duties in the medical standard of care. **J Legal Med 12:**275-329, 1991

110. *Nealy v US Healthcare HMO*, 844 F Suppl 966 (SD NY 1994)

111. Ogden BP: Peer review and the HCQIA's civil damages immunity. **Health Lawyer 7:**8-9, Spring 1994

112. Orentlicher D: Paying physicians more to do less: financial incentives to limit care. **U Richmond Law Rev 30:**155-197, 1996

113. Pear R: Doctors may get leeway to rival large companies. Shift in antitrust rules. Change would ease way for physicians to join forces in health market-

place. **New York Times.** Apr 8. 1996. pp A1, A10

114. *Pilot Life Ins Co v De-deaux,* 41 US 41, 44 (1987)

115. Pollard MJ, Wigal GJ: **Hospital Staff Privileges: What Every Health Care Practitioner and Lawyer Needs to Know.** Chicago, Ill: Health Administration Press, 1996

116. *Raglin v HMO Illinois, Inc,* 595 NE2d 153 (Ill App 1 Dist 1992)

117. *Redding v St Francis Medical Center,* 255 Cal Rptr 806 (Cal App 2 Dist 1989)

118. **Restatement of Torts, Second.** St. Paul, Minn: American Law Institute, 1979

119. Rinella L: The use of medical practice guidelines in medical malpractice litigation — should practice guidelines define the standard of care? **UMKC Law Rev 64:**337-355, 1995

120. Rinn C: ERISA and managed care: the impact of Travelers. **Health Lawyer 8:**19-21, Early Spring 1996

121. Robinson JC: Decline in hospital utilization and cost inflation under managed care in California. **JAMA 276:**1060-1064, 1996

122. Rodwin MA: Strains in the fiduciary metaphor: divided physician loyalties and obligations in a changing health care system. **Am J Law Med 21:** 241-257, 1995

123. *Rosenblum v Tallahassee Memorial Regional Center,* No. 91-589 (Cir Ct Leon County, Fla, filed June 22, 1992)

124. Roth RL: Recent developments concerning the effect of ERISA pre-emption on tort claims against employers, insurers, health plan administrators, managed care entities, and utilization review agents. **Health Lawyer 8:**3-7, Early Spring 1996

125. Rypma J: The physician cartel—potential hospital federal antitrust liability in class-based denial of staff privileges to clinical psychologists. **Drake Law Rev 39:**509, 1989/1990

126. Scibetta PL: Restructuring hospital-physician relations. Patient care quality depends on the health of the hospital peer review. **U Pitt Law Rev 51:** 1025-1059, 1990

127. Sculnick DH: HMO liability and ERISA preemption for medical malpractice. **Health Lawyer 8:**8-12, Early Spring 1996

128. Serbaroli FJ: Corporate practice of medicine: a clear and present danger. **Health Lawyer 7:**6-7, Spring 1994

129. Showstack J, Lurie N, Leatherman S, et al: Health of the public: the private-sector challenge. **JAMA 276:** 1071-1074, 1996

130. Slobodzian JA: Judge says physicians on list can't sue to clear their name. **The Philadelphia Inquirer.** Jan 5, 1995 (1995 WL 5738007)

131. Slomski AJ: Hospitals wield a heavy club against high-cost doctors. **Med Econ 68:**57-69, Oct 7, 1991

132. **Statistical Abstract of the United States.** Washington, DC: US Dept. Of Commerce, Bureau of Census, 1995

133. *Sztorc v Northwest Hospital,* 496 NE2d 1200 (Ill App Ct 1986)

134. Taber JC, King JP: Caught in the crossfire: economic credentialing in the health care war. **Detroit Coll Law Rev 4:**1179-1214, 1994

135. Tarlov AR, Ware JE Jr, Greenfield S, et al: The Medical Outcomes Study. An application of methods for monitoring the results of medical care. **JAMA 262:** 925-930, 1989

136. VanderVeer JB Jr: Pleasing patients: It's the little things that count. **Med Economics.** June 24, 1996, pp 177-180

137. WVa Code §30-3C-2 (1986 Replacement Volume)

138. Wachler AB, Avery PA: Physician incentive plan regulations: implications for managed care organizations and providers. **Health Lawyer 8:**1-5, Late Spring 1996

139. Walzer RS: Impaired physicians: An overview and update of the legal issues. **J Legal Med 11:**131-198, 1990

140. Weiler PC: **Medical Malpractice on Trial.** Cambridge, Mass: Harvard University Press, 1991

141. Weinmann R: Economic snooping on doctors could imperil patients. **The Plain Dealer.** Jan 22, 1996, p 9B (1996 WL 353237)

142. Weinmann RL: Medical red-lining? **The Commercial Appeal.** Jan 28, 1996, p B4 (1996 WL 3201803)

143. Wertkin MG: The relationship between physicians' malpractice claims history and later claims. **JAMA 273:**1487-1489, 1995

144. Willett DE: Centralized credentialing. **Health Lawyer 9:**12-13, Fall 1996

145. Wilson CT, Dellinger AM (eds): Staff membership and clinical privileges. **Healthcare Facilities Law. Critical Issues for Hospitals, HMOs, and Extended Care Facilities.** Boston, Mass: Little, Brown, and Co, 1991, pp 3-64

146. Woods D: Changing health care system brings new legal risks. **Am Med News 14:**38-46, Dec 11, 1995 (1995 WL 10600190)

CHAPTER 22

THE IMPORTANCE OF THE MEDICAL RECORD

CONRAD J. PESYNA, BS

The medical record serves several purposes, including: providing a basis for planning patient care and for continuity in evaluating the patient's condition and treatment; furnishing documentary evidence of the course of the patient's medical evaluation, treatment, and change in condition during a hospital stay or an ambulatory care or emergency visit; documenting communication between the responsible practitioner and any other health care professional contributing to the patient's care; assisting in protecting the legal interests of the patient, the hospital, and the responsible practitioner; and providing data for continuing education, research, and administrative use.

Complete and accurate medical records are indispensable for the proper care of patients and are the focal point of communication among health care providers. The content of the medical record must be sufficiently detailed and organized to enable the practitioner to provide continuing care to the patient, to determine what the patient's condition was at a specific time, and to review the diagnostic and therapeutic procedures performed and the patient's response to treatment. Also, this information helps a consultant to render an opinion or another practitioner to assume the care of the patient at any time.

The well-executed record is more important now than ever before. As care becomes more complex and large numbers of professionals become involved in the treatment of each patient, a complete and consistent record gains in value. It is the prime communication medium for planning and orchestrating patient care. A well-kept record is also vital to practitioners who may care for that patient years in the future and, perhaps, miles from the original treatment center. The computer-based longitudinal medical record will facilitate this ongoing treatment.

The medical record is a legal document. Although the medical record is protected by the laws of confidentiality, scores of people both inside and outside of the hospital may properly gain access to it. Every medical record is also, under certain circumstances, legally discoverable (open to examination) and admissible as evidence in court cases. "As time passes, memories dim and conflicting arguments are voiced; juries tend to believe the record."[1] Photocopies may be released upon request and receipt of a properly signed authorization.

Experts agree that in malpractice cases, the content and quality of the medical record are pivotal. "It is invariably the most important factor in the case. All else, including the practitioner's credentials, personality and reputation, pale in comparison."[1] Incomplete, sloppy, contradictory documentation can make even the best care seem negligent. The current litigation crisis, in which multimillion dollar claims are not uncommon, mandates that this document be well maintained for the defense of clinical decision-making.

The medical record also aids in the retrieval of pertinent information required for utilization review and quality assurance activities. Monitoring systems that assess the quality of care provided to patients are dependent upon the information contained in medical records. Evaluators extract clinical data from the medical record, compare elements of treatment with predesignated standards of care, and determine whether deviations from these standards were justified. These analyses often identify patient management problems and suggest solutions that may ultimately improve the quality of patient care. Medical records often are used to help identify problems with patient treatment before the problems prompt lawsuits or external reviews.

Risk management issues are a growing concern with regard to the medical record. The Joint Commission on Accreditation of Healthcare Organizations (JCAHO) now requires risk management programs as a condition of accreditation. Professional review organizations have expanded their review mechanisms to focus on quality of care. Some states require the reporting of incidents.

The medical record is crucial to health care finance. The record is the instrument that ensures adequate reimbursement. Prospective payment systems have made the medical record the basis of payment for many patients' hospital stays, and this has resulted in more responsibility and increased levels of complexity of work for medical record departments. Soaring costs have stimulated third-party payors to scrutinize records thoroughly for documentation justifying admission, services provided, length of stay, and quality of care before they will certify payment of bills. The advent of managed care also demands a well-organized record.

The medical record is utilized in planning and cost-containment activities. Rising health care costs increase the need for accurate, reliable medical information to help planners evaluate the cost-effectiveness of the health care delivery system. As the economic environment leads to changes in the structure of health care delivery (e.g., health maintenance organizations (HMOs) and multi-hospital systems), clinical information also will be called upon to support some of the administrative functions of health care providers such as investing, acquisition, finance, and marketing. Data will be used to review trends and project future case mixes, profitability, and market share in an effort to maintain a competitive edge.

Among the other activities in which medical records are used are credentialing, privileging, education, research, discharge planning, support of patient claims for personal injury and workers' compensation, and the generation of case-mix and management-related data. It is the medical record that must provide the objective information needed to support the reappointment decisions of the medical staff and the performance appraisals of other clinical disciplines.

CONTENTS AND RULES

Included in the medical record are various demographic data including the patient's name, address, date of birth, next of kin, and a unique number that identifies the patient in the system. The medical history obtained from the patient, with the chief complaint, details of the present illness, and, when appropriate, the assessment of the patient's emotional, behavioral, and social status, is also described. In addition, it contains relevant past, social, and family histories, as well as an inventory of body systems. For children and adolescents, an evaluation of development and consideration of educational status and needs is included, as appropriate. The results of the physical examination are recorded, as well as the results of laboratory tests, diagnoses, and changes over time.

To ensure that the maximum possible information about a patient is available to the professional staff providing care, the unit record system is used. It may not be feasible to combine all inpatient, ambulatory care, and emergency records of an individual patient into a single unit record. If it is not, a system is established to routinely assemble all record components when a patient is admitted to the hospital or appears for a prescheduled ambulatory care appointment. An alternative requires placing in the ambulatory care record, or combined ambulatory care/emergency record file, copies of pertinent portions of each inpatient medical record, such as the discharge report, the operative note, and the pertinent laboratory reports.

No standard nationally-recognized format exists for the organization of a medical record. Each health care facility determines its own forms, format, and filing arrangement according to the institution's needs. All forms included in the medical record must be approved by the institution's medical records committee. Nothing may be removed or deleted from a medical record. No irrelevant or facetious notations should be made, nor may the record be edited or marked in any way.

The quality of the medical record depends in part on the timeliness, completeness, meaningfulness, authentication, and legibility of the informational content. If the medical record lacks detail, is inaccurate, or is incomplete, the patient, the hospital, and/or the physician may be affected. The indexed data will reflect these inadequacies, and financial reimbursement and research will be handicapped.

Medical records contain valuable and confidential information and are to be safeguarded by everyone who uses them. Hospital medical records are to be kept in the Medical Record Department or at the site of patient care services. Medical records of inpatients must be returned to the Medical Record Department on the day of discharge. Medical records requested by clinics should be returned within predetermined timeframes after the visit. Access to medical records of all patients shall be afforded to all staff physicians and dentists in good standing, and to other persons as authorized by the hospital administrator for bona fide study and research, consistent with preserving confidentiality of personal information concerning the patient. Medical records may be borrowed only by authorized borrowers, who must adhere strictly to established guidelines for request and return of records. Persons with records checked out to them must always make them immediately available for patient care. Medical records may be used

outside the Medical Record Department for specific occasions, such as conferences and meetings. A physician or physician group practice must apply similar restrictive measures as a means of preserving patient confidentiality.

All medical records are the property of the hospital or a physician and/or physician group practice and should not be removed from the respective facility without permission from a hospital administrator or the primary physician at an office site, even if a subpoena has been served.

The length of time medical records should be retained will vary depending on the purposes for which the record is being kept. In formulating a record retention policy, a health care institution must be guided by its own clinical, scientific, and audit needs, and the possibility of future patient litigation. In some jurisdictions, a health care institution is not required by law to preserve its records for any given length of time. The appropriate period of retention may be affected by the statute of limitations for bringing a legal action for an injury or breach of contract. In most states, the period of the applicable statute of limitations is less than 10 years. Under the "discovery rule," however, the statute of limitations does not begin to run until the patient could reasonably discover the existence of the injury, which may be several years after a failure to diagnose or properly treat. Also, the statute of limitations may be longer for a minor, although many states require that an action for personal injuries sustained by a minor be filed within a few years after he/she attains maturity.

Inasmuch as a hospital or other health care institution is seldom requested to produce medical records older than 10 years for clinical, scientific, legal, or audit purposes, it is ordinarily sufficient to retain the medical records 10 years after the most recent patient care activity in the absence of legal considerations. Accordingly, it is recommended that complete patient medical records in health care institutions usually be retained, either in the original or reproduced form, for 10 years after the most recent patient care activity. After 10 years, such records may be destroyed unless destruction is specifically prohibited by statute, ordinance, regulation, or law, provided that the institution:

1. Retains basic information such as dates of hospital admission and discharge, names of responsible physicians, records of diagnoses and operations, operative reports, pathology reports, and discharge summaries for all records destroyed.
2. Retains complete medical records of minors for the period of minority plus the applicable limitations period prescribed by statute in the state in which the health care institution is located.
3. Retains complete medical records of patients under mental disability in like manner as those of patients under minority.
4. Retains complete patient medical records for longer periods when requested in writing by one of the following:
   a) an attending or consulting physician;
   b) the patient or someone acting legally in his/her behalf; or
   c) legal counsel for a party having an interest affected by the medical records of the patient.

It is unnecessary for a health care institution to preserve medical records that duplicate other official records that will be kept permanently. Thus, keeping records for the sole purpose of proving birth or age, residence, citizenship, or family relationship is not necessary.

MEDICAL RECORDS DEPARTMENT ACTIVITIES

Coding

Coding is done by analysts responsible for coding inpatient, ambulatory surgery, outpatient, and emergency department records. Coding analysts apply all pertinent diagnosis and procedure codes using the "International Classification of Diseases-Ninth Revision-Clinical Modification" and "Current Procedural Terminology" codes. Each analyst reviews staff notes, ancillary reports, and dictated reports to determine the diagnoses and procedures appropriate for coding and Diagnostic Related Group (DRG) assignment. In order to ensure accurate coding, as well as optimization of reimburse-ment, coding analysts may utilize the Medical Transcription Dictation, Clinical Laboratory, Clinical Pathology, Billing and Receivables, and Patient Management systems.

Coding analysts interact with physicians and other hospital employees (e.g., those from the catheterization laboratory and radiology) for clarification of coding issues. The ambulatory surgery and outpatient cases may also be abstracted into the computerized medical records system to establish a comprehensive data base. Codes are then entered into a medical record abstracting system and grouped into the appropriate DRG. Some prospective payment accounts have an attestation attached for physician signature prior to billing.

Cancer Registry

A cancer registry is part of the American College of Surgeons Accredited Cancer Program that must follow state law and involves reporting all malignancies to the state's Department of Health and Human Services. The cancer registrars identify, abstract, code, and keypunch data about patients diagnosed and/or treated for cancer. Each patient is followed annually to document progress of disease or treatment. All reportable cancer diagnoses are maintained in a registry database to enhance reporting capabilities at the state and federal level. In addition, comparison and statistical reports help to facilitate research.

Trauma Registry

The trauma registry is required for a Level I trauma center as mandated by the American College of Surgeons. The trauma registrars identify, abstract, code, and keypunch medical and financial data about patients admitted with blunt or penetrating trauma. The registry usually coordinates all requests for comparison data and patient identification information needed for research when a hospital trauma registry system is used in conjunction with the hospital mainframe computer. The registrars are responsible for reporting all head injuries to the state Head Injury Foundation.

CONFIDENTIALITY

The American public is more worried about privacy now than ever before. According to a recent Louis Harris poll conducted for Equifax, Inc., a record 83% of the public is concerned about threats to their privacy—particularly their medical records.[1]

The current legal obligation to maintain confidentiality of health information derives from a patchwork of state licensure laws and regulations, specific statutes and regulations about medical record confidentiality, Medicare's Conditions of Participation, standards of the JCAHO, and various court decisions. However, information that may be protected in one state may not have protection in another state. An independent national medical privacy board should be created to hold hearings, issue regulations, and enforce standards.

All medical information contained within the health care system should be designated as sensitive, and penalties should be imposed for unauthorized disclosures. However, patients should have the right to inspect their medical records and have a procedure for correcting or updating them.

The following principles are included in the American Health Information Management Association (AHIMA) Fair Health Information Practices Act of 1994:[2]

- Health care information concerning a patient must be collected only to the extent necessary and only for a lawful purpose.
- The patient has the right to know what health care information is maintained, by whom, and for what purpose the information is to be used.
- All persons maintaining health care information must prepare formal, written statements of their fair information practices and give each patient a copy and explanation of their practices.
- Patients have the right to access their health care information and the right to a copy after payment of a reasonable charge. They also have the right to have information amended or corrected on request.
- Any person maintaining, using, or disseminating health care information shall implement reasonable safeguards for the security of information, as well as its storage, processing, and transmission.

ELECTRONIC MEDICAL RECORD SYSTEMS

Since the first attempts to create electronic patient records in the 1960s, there has been a difference of opinion concerning their value. Some people believed that computerization would be useful, while others believed that it would not be useful or practical, and that it would not gain user acceptance.

A few electronic medical record systems began to be installed in the early 1960s. But development of the electronic patient record has been slow for four reasons: 1) speech technologies, database technologies, communications, multimedia technologies, and most of all, the appropriate software packages have not been fully developed; 2) the case for fully functional electronic patient record systems has not been made to the point where the average caregiver clearly sees that the capabilities and benefits more than justify the costs; 3) more legislation and standards development are needed; and 4) the legal environment in every state is ill-prepared for the creation of paperless patient record systems.[7]

However, today market forces (such as integrated delivery systems and health information networks) are influencing the adoption of automation and the creation of, or at least parts of, electronic medical records. In addition, new hardware and software can reduce the administrative costs inherent in paper and other forms of records, can more efficiently manage the ever greater amount of information related to caring for an aging population, and can help practitioners provide better care.

To develop electronic patient record systems, providers must purchase hardware, software, and services such as integration and consulting, and educate themselves and their staffs about new work processes. Since there is no standardized product, every hospital, clinic, or provider's office must consider its own needs and develop a customized system. In addition, because of constant improvement in hardware and software, these systems must be periodically upgraded.

In 1991, the Institute of Medicine released an influential report, "The Computer-Based Patient Record: An Essential Technology for Health Care."[8] This report led to the creation of the Computer-Based Patient Record Institute, an advocacy group that is supported by corporations in the health care, insurance, and data-processing industries. Last year's proposals for health care reform and bills currently before Congress include provisions for the establishment of a national health care data network. Such a network would contain records on every medical encounter in the United States. These measures at the federal level reflect the effectiveness of efforts to promote the computer-based patient record.

It is now suggested that the computerized medical record must fulfill the following objectives:[5]

- support patient care and improve the quality of care;
- enhance the productivity of health care professionals and reduce the administrative costs associated with health care delivery and financing;
- support clinical and health services research;
- accommodate future developments in health care technology, policy, management, and finance;
- ensure patient data confidentiality at all times.

Providers who intend to automate their medical records face a number of important legal issues that they must resolve to ensure they maintain their accreditation and protect themselves from liability. Federal and state statutes, regulations, and accreditation standards specify the form of medical records, how long the facility must maintain them, and confidentiality requirements. Complying with these requirements is essential for licensure and certification. Further, having medical records in a legal format so that they are admissible as evidence in a trial, such as malpractice litigation, is an essential part of a good risk management program. But the law has not caught up with the technology, and

providers wishing to automate their medical records face a bewildering array of often conflicting laws and regulations.

Before automating, one must determine whether the state and the licensing authority even permit the use of electronic media for storing medical records, since the law varies from state to state. If they do, one must determine government requirements and private accreditation standards for what medical records must contain to ensure that records are complete and that the appropriate portions are automated. One must also determine government requirements and private accreditation standards for storage media. Some states permit automation but require that providers retain certain parts of a medical record in another format, such as paper or microfilm. One must determine whether computerized medical records produce admissible evidence in the local jurisdiction because records will do little good if they cannot be used in court for the benefit of patients and staff. The Federal Rules of Evidence and the laws of many states provide for the admission of medical records into evidence in court, either under the business record exception to the hearsay rule or under a special variation of the business record exception specifically covering medical records. Even if a state statute or administrative regulation provides for the use of electronic medical records and their admissibility in court, the state may nonetheless require long-term storage in paper or some other form, such as microfilm. One must also review the medical staff bylaws to determine whether the medical staff should revise them to allow for electronic medical records.

One must determine whether state and licensing authorities permit authentication of medical records by computer entry because state laws concerning authentication of medical records vary widely. Some state and licensing authorities do not address how providers must authenticate entries in medical records. Others simply require providers to complete and maintain medical records in accordance with recognized professional standards. However, others are very specific as to how a provider must authenticate an entry. All permit handwritten signatures, many permit initials, and some permit stamped signatures, often specifying conditions upon the use of such stamps. Others prohibit stamped signatures. Some permit authentication by computer key, and others have introduced legislation to do so.[5]

Once the government and the licensing authorities change their requirements to authorize electronic medical records in all jurisdictions, developing a legally sufficient system will be fairly easy. Because the federal government intends to mandate the use of electronic medical records, such authorization appears likely to be forthcoming.

The greatest concern about electronic patient records is the problem of confidentiality. Even before the introduction of the computer, confidentiality deteriorated as care provided by large groups became more common. The number of people authorized to read medical records has increased dramatically in the past two decades because of the growing reliance on insurance to pay medical bills and the growth of oversight activities. In the current health care environment, a widening audience of outside observers now watches the performance of doctors, nurses, and patients. Anticipation of the availability of computerized patient records appears to be generating even more extensive claims of a need to know. The authors of the IOM report stated that the number of parties with a potential need to know was so large that they would not even attempt to provide a complete list. The authors nevertheless listed many parties not directly involved in patient care. Obviously, medical information, as well as the wide array of other data in electronic records, is considered valuable by many commercial enterprises (including HMOs and various kinds of health care networks, insurers, pharmaceutical firms, medical-equipment firms, and research enterprises), as well as by employers, detectives and information brokers, political campaign managers, and others. Parties with a desire to know the contents of medical records use various strategies, some of them illegal or of borderline legality, to obtain information from those who have access to the records on the basis of a need to know. However, computerized records, particularly if embedded in large networks designed to collect comprehensive lifelong data, in which large numbers of people are given access to data, can rapidly accelerate this trend. Even security measures, such as passwords and encryption, may have limited efficacy.

Currently, there is a patchwork of state laws, all with different standards, and no national guidelines for keeping medical records secure. This issue was discussed by health security officers at "The Conference on Health Information Security" in September 1996 in Chicago, Illinois. This complicates release of information across state lines. For example, a patient is treated in State A, but his/her insurance company is headquartered in State B. The State A hospital must send the records to State B for the claim, but State B has less stringent standards for privacy than State A. Is the hospital in State A responsible if the information is improperly disclosed under State B's less stringent standards? Does the disclosure in State B make it a tort in State A? These are the type of questions health security officers must deal with under the current system.[3]

Legislation at the federal and state levels needs to be established and standardized in order to accomplish two goals: 1) to protect privacy, the individual patient's right to keep confidential information created or maintained as part of the health treatment and payment process; and 2) to insure security, the integrity of data and assurance that it cannot be manipulated from its original form. It would be ideal to have federal legislation to establish national standards.[2] The AHIMA has worked with the Federal Information Privacy Commission and others to come up with model legislation to govern the collection, use, and disclosure of electronic health care records, and includes:[6]

- Disclosure provisions that would prohibit anyone except the patient from disclosing health care information without authorization.

- A patient's valid authorization that would identify the patient and describe the health care information to be disclosed and the person to whom it was disclosed. This authorization would also include the purpose of disclosure and a time limit on patient authorization.

- A record of disclosure that would include the name, address, and institutional affiliation of the person to whom the health care information was disclosed, the date and purpose of disclosure, and a description of the information disclosed.

One proposed solution for the lack of security is to pass a pre-emptive federal law, which would allow the federal government to promulgate and enact standards pertaining to electronic medical records. A first step has already been taken with the passage of The Health Insurance Portability and Accountability Act of 1996.[4] Under this act, security regulations will be set by the U.S. Secretary of Health and Human Services, who will determine the minimum standard for health care organizations from state to state.[3]

Regardless of the status of the local jurisdiction's laws authorizing such systems, providers and their attorneys will want to carefully review the legal requirements for medical information to develop systems in such a way as to meet their individual requirements. Even if pertinent statutes, regulations, and accreditation standards in the local jurisdiction permit the use of electronic medical records, the medical staff should make the decision to adopt them and specify the rules for using them in a given facility[5] in a manner that will fill the institution's needs without subjecting the facility to unnecessary liability.

Much work remains to develop improved electronic record keeping and the legal environment in which it can function. The computerized record ideally would be a multipurpose document with a standardized format and nomenclature. However, there are a multiplicity of problems with standardized formats and record keeping. Also, the suitability of a single record for many purposes (e.g., business, clinical, research, and public health) is questionable. Concerned parties need to be proactive and submit their views about the development of laws and rules concerning electronic records to federal and state governments and to licensing authorities so that they adopt statutes and regulations that meet providers' and patients' needs and do not put unnecessary impediments in the way of adopting a cost-effective electronic medical records system. However, recent advances in hardware and software make the electronic record feasible, useful, and an inevitable development in modern medicine.

References

1. Fox LA, Imbiorski W: **The Record That Defends Its Friend.** 4th ed. Chicago, Ill: Care Communications, 1989
2. HR 4077, 103rd Congr, 2d Sess (1994)
3. Pisiewski K: Toward an electronic patient record. **Med Rec Inst 5:**August/September 1996
4. Pub L No. 104-191, 110 Stat 1936 (August 21, 1996)
5. Tomes JP: **Compliance Guide to Electronic Health Records: A Practical Reference To Legislation, Codes, Regulations and Industry Standards.** New York, NY: Faulkner & Gray, 1994
6. Waegamann CP: Toward an electronic patient record. **Med Rec Inst 4:**May, 1996
7. Waegemann CP: Toward an electronic patient record. **Updates Standards Devel 3:**12, 1995
8. Woodward B: Sounding board. The computer-based patient record and confidentiality. **N Engl J Med 333:** 1419-1422, 1995

CHAPTER 23

Managed Care Organizations

Daniel R. Sullivan, MD, JD, and Perry Oxley, JD

The cost of health care in the United States has risen over the past two decades at a startling pace. Health care costs rose 10.4%, more than double the rate of inflation, during the 1980s, and costs are expected to double in the next decade to $2.1 trillion.[36] The extraordinary increase of health care cost is attributable to the increased cost of individual services compounded by an increased frequency of encounters by patients.[6] In response to rising health care costs, managed care was developed. Managed care plans "are health care financing and delivery arrangements designed to reduce the cost per service and the volume of services utilized through organized relationships with health care providers."[6] Managed care plans are a response to the traditional indemnity plans of unrestricted choice of provider and unrestricted fees paid for individual services. Under traditional indemnity plans, there are no incentives for patients to choose efficient providers or for physicians to control the number of services rendered.[35] In fact, indemnity plans provide financial benefits for increased services. Managed care uses "financial incentives and management controls to influence the behavior of patients and providers."[6]

Managed care plans usually have certain distinct elements. These elements include credentialing, patient incentives, provider reimbursement incentives, utilization management, quality assurance and primary care gatekeepers. Credentialing is arranging "with selected providers to furnish comprehensive services to members."[6] Patient incentives are inducements for persons covered under the plan to use health care providers participating in the plan, while provider reimbursement incentives are enticements for providers participating in a plan to be cost-efficient.[51] Utilization management is a series of procedures used to contain the number of services and type of services rendered.[6] Quality assurance involves programs that assure appropriate care even though incentives are placed on the provider and the patient to reduce cost and volume.[6] A managed care plan uses primary care physicians in a "central role in the delivery of care, often serving as a 'gatekeeper' regulating utilization of specialty, ancillary and hospital services."[6]

Managed Care Entities
Health Maintenance Organizations

"HMOs [health maintenance organizations] are state licensed entities that offer a comprehensive set of health benefits to members on a prepaid basis."[6] An HMO provides a health plan to enrollees with comprehensive health care services,[28] and by doing so incurs the financial risks associated with overuse of health care services.[24] With the exception of emergency care, enrollees of an HMO are required to receive their health care services from HMO-approved providers in order to have coverage.[24]

In order to contain health care costs, HMOs employ physician-incentive payment plans that are different from those for physicians taking part in fee-for-service delivery models.[6] They also engage in utilization management activities including pre-admission review, admission review, concurrent review, estimated length of stay, diagnosis validation, outpatient procedure certification, code rebundling, discharge planning, and case management.[6] Evaluations conducted prior to hospital admissions are called pre-admission reviews. Evaluations conducted within 24 hours of an emergency admission or a non-scheduled obstetrical inpatient admission are called admission reviews. Evaluations conducted during an inpatient stay are referred to as concurrent review.[6] These reviews assess medical necessity and length of stay.

HMOs may control costs by using the admission diagnosis acquired from admissions information to estimate the covered person's length of stay (estimated length of stay), which should not be exceeded without review or approval, or if the hospital is reimbursed based on diagnosis, by inspecting the diagnosis for accuracy ("diagnosis validation").[6] An HMO may also review the health care services recommended for a covered person before the procedure occurs to determine medical necessity ("outpatient procedure certification").[6] Further, HMOs may require hospitals to bill for an entire procedure, referred to as "code rebundling," instead of individual sub-parts to avoid improperly inflated payments.[6] HMOs attempt to keep hospital stays to an appropriate length by prearranging for care by "discharge planning."[6] Finally, HMOs may establish procedures for cases likely to require extensive hospitalization or intensive therapy, termed "case management," to assure that the most appropriate level of services is provided on an efficient basis.[6]

There are five basic models of an HMO,

which are distinguished by the relationship of the HMO with its affiliated physicians. The first model is the "staff model," which occurs when "the HMO employs the physicians who render services at HMO owned or controlled facilities."[24] Under the staff model, the HMO is the primary provider of medical services. The second type of model is the group model, which occurs when an HMO contracts with a multispecialty physician group to deliver services to HMO covered persons.[23] Physicians are not employed by the HMO, but are employed directly by the group practice. The third model is the Independent Practice Association (IPA), which "is made up of individual practitioners, all of whom have their own private practices but contract for the provision of health care services to HMO enrollees."[24] The fourth model is the "direct contract model," in which an "HMO contracts directly with individual physicians or practices to provide physician services to its members."[6] The fifth model is a Network Model, in which HMOs have a variation of provider methods. These arrangements may include staff, group, IPA, and direct contracts.[6]

HMOs typically are regulated by states and may be federally qualified.[6] Under state regulatory acts, HMOs usually are required to have a license, and the state insurance commission and health department typically are involved. Among the items regulated by a state HMO act are "premium rating requirements, governing body and organizational requirements, comprehensive health benefits which must be provided, protection against insolvency, minimum capitalization, net worth and surplus requirements, grievance procedures, quality assurance requirements, and reporting requirements."[6] HMOs are regulated as health insurance companies and must have reserves and assets.[28] Federal qualification is not a requirement for operation under state law, and not all HMOs are federally qualified. HMOs that are federally qualified ". . . have certain marketing advantages through a federal mandate which requires employers to offer HMO coverage."[6]

Preferred Provider Organizations

A "preferred provider organization" (PPO) is

an entity that contracts with a provider panel of physicians to deliver medical services to persons covered under the PPO plan.[28] Participating providers ". . . agree to abide by utilization management procedures and agree to accept predetermined reimbursement (usually discounted fees)."[6] The PPO gives covered persons incentives to use it by making out-of-pocket costs greater when the covered person obtains care outside the PPO provider panel.[6] PPOs are not regulated directly by any federal statute. However, many state statutes do regulate financial and operating aspects of PPOs.[26] Further, if risks are associated with a PPO, the PPO may be subject to regulations which pertain to a health insurance company or HMO.[28]

The three generally recognized PPO plans are "gatekeeper," "open panel," and "exclusive provider organization."[24] In a gatekeeper PPO, each enrollee must choose a primary care provider from the provider panel of physicians. This physician is responsible for providing the majority of health care services to the enrollee and must authorize specialists and other provider referrals.[24] Under this plan, the enrollees must pay all or much of the fee if they receive care without the primary care provider's approval.[24] The open panel PPO allows enrollees to choose their health care providers without having all services approved by a designated primary care physician.[24] An open panel PPO provides financial incentives for covered persons to use the PPO network. Such incentives include lower deductibles and co-insurance payments.[24] The exclusive provider organization PPO is similar to the open panel PPO in that there is no primary care provider to approve medical services, but it differs in that enrollees must pay the entire bill for services outside the PPO network.[24] The advantage over an open panel is that the enrolled must use the PPO network.

Point of Service Plans

A "point of service" plan contains elements of both an HMO and a PPO.[6] Unlike most forms of PPOs, an enrolled person must select the primary care physician to act as a gatekeeper for specialty and hospital services in a point of service plan.[6] Under the point of service plan, ". . . the covered person has the option, at the time of service, to use out-of-network providers, but at a reduced level of benefits."[6]

Integrated Delivery System

An integrated delivery system (IDS) "is a single organization which provides hospital, physician and other health care services to patients."[28] The three critical components of an IDS are insurance, hospitals, and physicians.[25] The insurance component, a term used loosely, includes the type of insurance entity the parties have chosen (e.g., HMO, PPO, and point of service) plus management functions such as marketing the network and overseeing the distribution of receipts within the network.[25] The hospital component consists of all institutional facilities in the network.[26] Nursing homes, outpatient facilities, and freestanding emergency centers may be incorporated in the network.[25] These institutions may operate under single or joint ownership, a partnership, or as independently-owned facilities that affiliate by contract.[25] Physicians are the largest component, and due to their numbers often become members of single integrated group practices that align themselves in order to contract in an IDS. Alignment may take place via contract or partnership, or by an insurer or hospital that acquires a number of physician practices.[25] These contractual networks of individual practicing physicians resemble an IPA.[26] A hospital or insurer may employ physicians, contract with them, or make them equity partners. For example, a "management services organization" takes place when an insurer acquires all of the physical assets of a physician practice and then independently contracts the services of the physicians.[25]

Once each component has aligned horizontally, there are a multitude of ways the components may integrate vertically to form an IDS. However, there are three main models of classification that generally characterize vertical integration. The first model may be called a "totem-pole" institution and is the most tightly integrated.[25] These institutions are characterized by top to bottom "ownership or control of all three components of a fully-integrated delivery system."[25] "In the simplest manifestation, this would be an ordinary staff-model HMO that owns its own hospital, employs its own physicians, and markets its own insurance."[25] The second model may be called the "three-legged stool." Under this model, the three components are separately managed entities that are affiliated together by some commonality of ownership or contract.[25] A holding company ". . . might tie the three together, or one of the three components—usually the insurer or the hospital—might be the dominant party."[25] The third model occurs when the three components are linked more loosely. Under the third model, the components of an IDS may be "linked in a loose, contractual network with no common ownership."[25] Another utilization of the third model occurs when only a portion of the network is composed of a looser contractual network. For example, "a hospital-based PPO might own the insuring entity and contract with doctors, or a staff model HMO might employ its doctors and contract with hospitals."[25] The final version of the third model occurs where "the hospital and physician stand on approximately equal footing, commensurate with a partnership arrangement."[25]

An organization often linked to an IDS is a Physician Hospital Organization (PHO), which is "a venture between a hospital and its medical staff, or multiple hospitals and medical staffs, used to contract, typically on a risk basis, with managed care plans."[6] A PHO may become a part of an IDS network by integrating physicians and hospitals into joint ventures in the same manner that an IPA horizontally integrates physicians.[6] The PHO entity is responsible for contracting with a managed care plan, for providing covered services in exchange for capitation or percentage of premium, and for reimbursing the providers rendering services.[6]

The regulatory control of IDS organizations varies with the many possible models, and a complete discussion is beyond the scope of this chapter. Generally, an IDS with little integration is affected by regulatory issues "ranging from antitrust to statutory restrictions on physician referrals."[27] As the integration of management becomes more extensive and asset ownership becomes more diverse, many of the same concerns manifest themselves. Finally, as the IDS becomes fully integrated in "the financing and delivery of health care, the system faces regulation similar to that of an insurance company or health maintenance organization."[27]

HEALTH CARE FINANCE

Managed care entities sometimes utilize a payment method called "capitation" in order to achieve their financial goal of holding down the cost of health care. In capitation, a "physician or medical group receives a fixed monthly payment for each member that elects to receive medical care from the physician or medical group."[6] Capitation may be accomplished by ordinary capitation, global capitation, and intermediary entity capitation. In ordinary capitation, a fixed amount is paid to a physician or physician group for expected professional services to patients. Global capitation is a fixed amount paid to a physician or physician group for expected professional services and other services to patients. The services include but are not limited to specialty services, ancillary services, and inpatient services.[6] In an intermediary entity capitation, the fixed payment or percentage of premium collected by the payor flows directly to an intermediary entity, which contracts with individual providers.[6]

Capitation affects the allocation of risk associated with providing health care by fully or partially shifting accountability from one entity to another entity. For example, a payor makes a capitation to a physician group for professional services to be provided to patients. Upon receipt of the payment, the physician group assumes the risk that the cost of services to patients may rise above the fixed monthly payment, which would cause it to lose money. The different types of capitation illustrate the shifting of risk between different entities. For example, intermediary entity capitation shifts the risk of loss to the intermediate entity, who is forced to control the costs of providing health care in order to be profitable.

Within a managed care entity, physicians may receive reimbursement for professional services rendered through several different methods. These methods include salary, capitation, discounted fee-for-service, discounted fee-for-service with withholds, and incentive plans for withholds. Physicians who receive a salary are employed by the payor, which includes HMOs, insurers, and self-insured employers or intermediary entities, and are paid a fixed sum for their services. As mentioned in the preceding paragraph, physicians also may be paid directly by capitation under ordinary or global capitation. Under the discounted fee-for-service payment method, physicians are paid for each service rendered at a reduced rate which is established by negotiation with the payor or intermediary entity.

A variant of the fee-for-service payment is the fee-for-service payment with withholds. Under this method, "a percentage of each fee-for-service payment is withheld in an incentive fund."[6] Targeted budgets that also include costs for certain health care services not rendered directly by the physician are set for physicians to meet. If the targets are met, the amount withheld is returned. However, some or all of the withheld amount may be retained by the payor if the targeted budget is not met.[6]

Hospital reimbursement methods include discounted charges, per case charges, per diem rates, capitation, and percentage of premiums. Under the discounted charges method, hospitals are paid at a rate that is discounted from their published charges. The discount levels may be tied to volume. An agreement between a payor and a hospital may provide for charge reductions at certain predetermined volume levels. Hospitals may be compensated by per diem rates, which are fixed daily payments to provide all or different categories of services. Under the per case charges method, prospective payments based on the diagnosis of the patient at the time of admission are made to the hospital. As with physicians, hospital capitation occurs when "the hospital (that has agreed to admit covered persons) receives a fixed monthly payment for each covered person who selects a primary care physician. . . ."[6] Finally, under the percentage of premium method, a fixed monthly payment, based on a percentage of premium collected by the payor, is made for each individual covered by the payor.

MEDICARE AND MEDICAID MANAGED CARE CONTRACTING

Concepts of managed care are increasingly being used in Medicaid and Medicare contracting. The term "Medicaid managed care" is interpreted by the Medicaid Bureau within the Health Care Financing Administration (HCFA) as encompassing: "(1) full capitation programs; (2) partial capitation programs; (3) primary care case management programs; and (4) programs offered by health insuring organizations."[30] Full capitation programs are arrangements in which a managed care entity with whom the state Medicaid agency has contracted is at risk for a comprehensive range of Medicaid services.[49] Partial capitation programs are entered into with a prepaid health plan in which the contracts provide, at their own risk, two or fewer established categories of services.[30] A Primary Care Case Management program takes place when "Medicaid clients either select or are assigned to a primary care physician who has the responsibility to serve as the case manager for the client, referring the persons when necessary, and continuing to monitor the care. In Primary Care Case Management, the physician is playing a gatekeeper role, and he or she is compensated for both the gatekeeper role and any services they provide."[30] The last type is the "health insuring organization," which refers to entities similar to IPA model HMOs that arranged for services and became operational prior to January 1, 1986.[30]

The Medicare program has two parts. Part A is a mandatory insurance program covering inpatient hospital services and post-hospital care of individuals eligible for social security retirement and disability benefits.[45] Part B ". . . is a voluntary program of supplemental medical insurance covering generally eighty percent of the 'reasonable charge' for physician services and certain other medical and health services, which services include outpatient hospital services, x-rays, laboratory test, medical supplies, and durable medical equipment."[39,46] Through the HCFA, the Secretary of Health and Human Services administers Part B with fiscal carriers who determine whether a claimed service or item is medically necessary. Further, the carriers establish "reasonable charges" for covered services by utilizing criteria prescribed by statute and by the Secretary.[47]

The Secretary may enter into contracts with eligible HMOs or competitive medical plans (CMPs).[48] The two types of authorized Medicare contracting with eligible HMOs are "risk-sharing" and "reasonable cost reimbursement" contracts. In a risk-sharing contract, "the Secretary pays the HMO/CMP monthly in advance an amount determined under the terms of section 1876 on a capitation basis depending upon the number of its enrollees."[39] "Under reasonable cost reimbursement contracts, the Secretary pays the reasonable costs incurred by HMO/CMP as actually incurred."[39]

LIABILITY ISSUES

As managed care has become more widespread, liability for negligent health care has expanded from physicians to managed care entities. First, a managed care entity may be vicariously liable for negligent health care on the basis of respondeat superior or ostensible agency. Second, corporate negligence based upon negligent selection and negligent control of the physician may be used to hold a managed care entity liable for negligent health care. Finally, a managed care entity may be liable under a corporate negligence theory based upon the corporation's independent acts of negligence, such as management of utilization control systems, or directly liable under a breach of contract theory. For those plans subject to the Employee Retirement Income Security Act (ERISA) of 1974,[19] the ERISA pre-exemption has a definite effect on the liability of a managed care entity.

A managed care entity may be found vicariously liable for the negligent health care of its health care providers under several theories. Under the doctrine of respondeat superior, an employer may be found vicariously liable for the acts of an employee within the scope of his employment.[2,3] A staff model HMO may be found liable for negligence of physicians under the doctrine of respondeat superior because it employs its own physicians.

The doctrine of respondeat superior usually does not apply to physicians under an independent contract because the physicians are not supervised or controlled by the managed care entity.[19] Those entities that independently contract with physicians, instead of employing them, may be liable for provider negligence, however, under the theory of ostensible agency. A managed care entity is subject to liability under the theory of ostensible agency if services

rendered by the health care provider are accepted in reasonable belief that the services are being rendered by the managed care entity.[37]

In *Boyd v. Albert Einstein Medical Center*,[7] the court determined that an HMO could be vicariously liable for an independent contracting physician's malpractice under an ostensible agency theory. In making this determination, the court found that two factors are relevant in a finding of ostensible agency: "(1) whether the patient looks to the institution, rather than the individual physician for care, and (2) whether the HMO holds out the physician as its employee."[7] The court reasoned that an HMO could lead an enrollee to perceive the HMO as his or her health care provider and the doctors as its agents, through marketing materials, credentialing activities, and referral practices.[7]

The representations made to HMO subscribers may be determinative in deciding whether an agency relationship exists between an HMO and a health care provider. In *Raglin v. HMO Illinois, Inc.*,[38] an HMO published a statement on its subscriber certificate which stated that the HMO could not make medical judgments and that it could not furnish medical care. Further, the plaintiff failed to show reliance on the HMO's representations. In *Raglin*, the court held that the agency relationship did not exist under the facts of the case.

Further, in order to establish liability on the theory of ostensible agency, a plaintiff must demonstrate a reliance on representations by a managed care entity that the physicians were its agents or employees. In *Chase v. Independent Practice Association, Inc.*,[9] the plaintiff testified that she did not know certain health care providers were members of an IPA and that she was not told the health care providers were not employed by the HMO. The court held that the plaintiff's testimony did not establish the requisite reliance.[9]

Direct liability of managed care entities generally arises under a corporate negligence theory. Many states accept the doctrine of corporate negligence as a viable theory to hold hospitals liable for their selection of staff physicians.[37] Courts have extended the theory to managed care entities, which may be liable "for their failure to adequately investigate their medical care providers' credentials or competence."[31,37] In

Harrell v. Total Health Care, Inc.,[26] the court, utilizing corporate negligence, found that "an HMO may be liable for negligently selecting contracting physicians."[26] In *Harrell*, the court found that an HMO limited its members' choice of physicians to those it selected, who were unqualified or incompetent.[26] The court concluded that the HMO owed a duty to adequately check the credentials of its physicians and to investigate the physician's background in the community.[26] Most PPO plans differ from the HMO identified in *Harrell* because PPO plans usually give members greater freedom of choice in selecting providers. Accordingly, under the *Harrell* rationale, courts may determine that PPOs do not owe the same standard that HMOs owe to their members.

A managed care entity may be liable for its independent acts of negligence under a corporate negligence theory, and this category focuses primarily on utilization review. Generally, utilization review "refers to external evaluations of medical care that are based on established clinical criteria and are conducted by third-party payors, purchasers or health care organizers to evaluate the appropriateness of medical care."[5] Utilization review may be carried out by the payor's physicians, payor's nurses, payors, purchasers' health care organizers, or outside health management. Appropriate care is determined on the basis of correct setting of the care and correct level of care.

Because patients may purchase uncovered services, utilization review is constructed for the sole purpose of determining the medical justification for a service. However, if medical treatment is not covered, many patients will decline the treatment based on financial constraints. Additionally, if care is not covered, a treating physician may decide not to provide the care in a managed care plan. "If a patient suffers a bad result, the payor may be sued on the theory that a defect in the utilization review process resulted in the patient failing to receive necessary or appropriate medical care."[15] Almost all third party payors have internal appeals mechanisms for patients that are denied coverage. Physicians must be cautious that denial of payment does not absolve the physician of the responsibility to actively pursue the standard of care and to be an advocate of payment for indicated care.

Wickline v. State of California[53] was the first case to find that liability can be imposed on third-party payors for their negligent implementation. The court stated that: "Third party payors of health care services can be held legally accountable when medically inappropriate decisions result from defects in the design or implementation of cost containment mechanisms as, for example, when appeals made on a patient's behalf for medical or hospital care are arbitrarily ignored or unreasonably disregarded or overridden. However, the physician who complies without protest with the limitations imposed by a third party payor, when his medical judgment dictates otherwise, cannot avoid his ultimate responsibility for his patient's care."[53] Almost all third party payors have internal appeals mechanisms for patients who are denied coverage. Physicians must be cautious that denial of payment does not absolve the physician of the responsibility to actively pursue the standard of care and to be an advocate of payment for indirect care.

In *Wickline*, the court dealt with the imposition of liability for utilization review under the Medi-Cal program. In *Wilson v. Blue Cross of Southern California*,[54] the court extended the *Wickline* decision beyond the context of Medi-Cal patients to include those insured under a private insurance policy. Courts have attributed liability to third party payors for failure to inform a patient of the right to appeal.[41] Further, when a utilization review physician fails to conduct an independent review, courts have found the denial of benefits to be arbitrary and capricious.[40]

Another possible theory of direct liability is breach of contract. Under the breach of contract theory, a managed care entity breaches its health care services contract by failing to provide the qualified medical providers pursuant to the contract.[33] The factual basis for breach of contract claims is the quality of the coverage provided and not the failure to provide coverage, which is an important distinction for purposes of ERISA pre-emption analysis.[13]

Despite the most egregious factual scenario, ERISA may pre-empt a patient action that is based on state law. This important federal law is deregulatory in nature, limiting state regulation of employment-related health plans. In order for

ERISA to apply, there must be a private employer-sponsored health care coverage plan.[13] Further, ERISA generally "applies to HMOs to the extent HMO coverage is purchased through a health benefits program sponsored by a private employer."[13] Accordingly, ERISA does not apply to governmental or church entity sponsored plans[20] or to group insurance, unless the employer contributes to the program for the employees.[21]

ERISA sets forth that it "shall supersede any and all state laws insofar as they may now or hereafter relate to any employee benefit plan."[22] In *Shaw v. Delta Air Lines, Inc.*,[42] the Court found that a state law "relates to" an employee benefit plan ". . . if it has a connection with or reference to such a plan."[42] Accordingly, ERISA may pre-empt a state law that has no express link to an employee benefit plan. The reach of ERISA's pre-emption has been limited where the state law connection to an employee benefit plan is "too tenuous, remote or peripheral a manner to warrant a finding that the law 'relates to' the plan."[42] In order to determine whether or not a state theory of liability relates to an employee benefit plan, it becomes important to examine typical state actions in light of a claims factual basis.

The first group of state actions are those involving liability of employee benefit plans, which are based on the quality of care received. Courts generally have found that ERISA pre-empts state actions for direct or vicarious liability against the HMO in cases involving the quality of care. In *Dukes v. United States Health Care Systems of Pennsylvania, Inc.*,[18] the United States Health Care Systems of Pennsylvania (USHC), an HMO, was sued on behalf of Darryl Dukes, a deceased patient, on claims of direct liability under the theory that the HMO was negligent and had vicarious liability under the theory that the malpracticing physician was an ostensible agent of the HMO. The court found that the "plaintiff's allegations of ostensible agency 'relate to' Mr. Dukes' benefit plan because the allegations focus on how USHC described to Mr. Dukes its plan benefits and its relationship with its care-providers."[18] Further, the court found that the "malpractice claim against an HMO 'relates to' a benefit plan because the claim is based on the circumstances of medical treatment provided pursuant to the plan."[18]

Some cases have found that claims for direct liability were pre-empted by ERISA while claims for vicarious liability were not pre-empted. In *Jackson v. Roseman*,[29] the court found a medical malpractice action against an HMO for its physician under the theory that vicarious liability was not pre-empted by ERISA. The court reasoned that actions based on vicarious liability do "not involve a direct claim to recover benefits, enforce rights under the plan, or clarify future benefits, as contemplated under 29 U.S.C.s 1132(a),"[29] which it found necessary for ERISA pre-emption. The court found instead that the focal point of a negligence claim was whether "negligent care of individual providers caused him injury."[29] Further, the court stated that issues of agency alone are insufficient to implicate the policy concerns of ERISA pre-emption.[29] Some courts have found that neither direct liability nor vicarious liability was pre-empted.[33]

Another category of possible ERISA pre-emptions are those based on coverage decisions. In *Corcoran v. United Healthcare, Inc.*,[16] the court found that a state claim of malpractice against a utilization review organization is pre-empted by ERISA if the plan is subject to ERISA.[15] In *Kuhl v. Lincoln Nat'l Health Plan*,[32] the defendant, the Lincoln National Health Plan (LNHP), refused to pre-certify a heart procedure, and by the time that the LNHP certified the procedure and the surgery, the surgical team was not available. The plaintiff died awaiting a transplant, and his estate brought suit for medical malpractice, intentional infliction of emotional distress, tortuous interference with contract, and breach of contract. In *Kuhl*, the court held that the plaintiffs' state law claims were pre-empted by ERISA because they arose from LHNP's administration of plan benefits.[32]

EMERGING TECHNOLOGIES AND THE INVESTIGATIONAL EXCLUSION

Medical technology is constantly expanding while managed care entities are geared to maintain costs and decrease the volume of services rendered. These two forces interact when managed care entities attempt to limit the amount of services rendered by using investigational exclusions. In order to contain costs, managed care entities exclude medical procedures that are not yet proven to work.[1] In order for a claim to be denied on investigational grounds, an investigational exclusion must exist in the plan.[1]

If a health plan denies health care services that should be covered under the plan, liability may exist. A person denied medical services may bring a suit under a contract or tort theory. Under a contract theory, a provider may be liable for breach of contract if the contract called for the services to be delivered and they were not delivered. The determination of whether the particular service should have been delivered under an agreement is fundamental, and the answer lies within the interpretation of the contractual language of a specific plan. Generally, courts set minimum requirements that a health care plan's investigational exclusion contain: "(i) sound criteria for making the decisions and (ii) a description of the decision making process; these must be (iii) not ambiguous, and (iv) sufficient to put the subscriber on notice of what is not covered."[1] Further, a structure for patients to appeal decisions concerning care should be in place to allow patients a form of recourse for improper decisions within the health care plan.[1]

Liability also exists under a tort theory for both negligent administration of benefits and misleading advertising. If a patient is denied medical services that should have been delivered under the plan, the court may find the plan liable for delaying review, conducting an incomplete review, conduction of an out-of-date review, or review for cost containment as opposed to quality of care.[1] In addition, an action may be made against the plan for misleading advertising, which occurs when a plan subscriber relies to his or her detriment on claims made by the plan.[1] Misleading advertising may occur when health services are not available or are inadequate as a result of an investigational exclusion, which may result in a claim of fraud.

ANTITRUST

Antitrust law attempts to promote competition by prohibiting certain agreements among potential competitors and other practices that have the effect of limiting the number of competitors, artificially inflating prices, or otherwise interfering with the operation of a free market. As the types of managed care entities expand, antitrust issues become more and more prevalent. At the outset, readers should note that antitrust is an extensive field, and this section will cover only the most important areas of antitrust law relating to health plan and network formation. The two primary categories of antitrust issues in managed care are "horizontal" (combining of entities providing similar types of services) and "non-horizontal" (combining of entities providing different types of services).

Antitrust laws fall under three statutory enactments. First, under the Sherman Act,[43] Section 1 prohibits restraining trade by contract, combination, and conspiracy, which all require a collective movement between two or more individuals or entities;[14] Section 2 prohibits monopolization and attempts or conspiracies to monopolize.[44] Second, under the Clayton Act,[10] Section 3 prohibits exclusive dealing arrangements, which may substantially lessen competition;[11] Section 7 bans mergers, joint ventures, consolidations, or acquisitions of stocks or assets that are predisposed to create a monopoly or substantially lessen competition.[12] The Department of Justice ". . . may bring federal or civil action under the Sherman and Clayton Acts in federal district courts, or private parties may bring suit."[28] Third, under the Federal Trade Commission (FTC) Act,[23] unfair methods of competition and unfair or deceptive acts or practices are prohibited. "The FTC Act is enforced in administrative proceedings subject to federal judicial review."[23]

The first horizontal antitrust issue concerns hospital mergers. Hospitals may avoid antitrust liability by falling within the "safety zone" established by the FTC and Department of Justice. The safety zone takes effect if "one of the hospitals (1) has an average of fewer than 100 licensed beds over the three most recent years, and (2) has an average daily inpatient census of fewer than 40 patients over the three most recent years."[51] If the hospital merger falls outside the "safety zone," the FTC and Department of Justice will apply a five-step test in the Horizontal Merger Guidelines. The analysis includes

"(1) assessment of the merger's effect on concentration; (2) determining the likely adverse effects of the merger on competition based on concentration and qualitative factors; (3) assessment of entry barriers; (4) assessment of efficiencies; and (5) determining whether either firm is a failing company and whether the failing-firm defense applies."[50] The FTC and Department of Justice apply the five step test with particular emphasis on whether: "... (1) the merger would not increase the likelihood of the exercise of market power either because of the existence post-merger of strong competitors or because the merging hospitals provide sufficiently different services; (2) the merger would allow the hospitals to realize significant cost savings that could not otherwise be realized; or (3) the merger would eliminate a hospital that likely would fail with its assets exiting the market."[51] Further, a safety zone has been created to take advantage of existing new equipment where neither of the merging hospitals could support the equipment.[51]

The second horizontal antitrust issue concerns physician practice mergers. With respect to antitrust laws, the primary concern of physician mergers is between competing physicians and not integration of specialists. With physician practice mergers, the *1992 Horizontal Merger Guidelines*[50] can be applied as they are to hospitals.

The third horizontal antitrust issue concerns the formation of partially integrated provider networks, such as IPAs and PPOs. An analysis of antitrust law begins with determining if the alleged violation is a "naked" price-fixing agreement, which is per se unlawful because the agreement can significantly harm competition and is without redeeming value. In the alternative, an alleged antitrust violation may be "ancillary" to the pricing agreement.[34] An alleged antitrust violation is ancillary "if it is reasonably necessary for the arrangement to achieve its designed procompetitive effect...."[34]

Agreements relating to partially integrated provider networks may escape antitrust liability by falling within a "safety zone" if they meet specific criteria. The FTC and Department of Justice will not challenge an alleged violation, absent extraordinary circumstance, if an exclusive physician network joint venture comprises

less than 20% of the physicians in each physician specialty community who practice in the relevant geographic market and have active hospital staff privileges.[52] For a non-exclusive physician network, the safety zone expands to 30% or less of the physicians in each physician specialty. Although the FTC and Department of Justice address physician networks specifically, the same "analysis would apply equally to networks of other competing providers, including hospitals."[34] Even if an alleged violation falls outside the safety zone, "it will be viewed under a rule of reason analysis and not as per se illegal either if physicians in the joint venture share substantial financial risk or if the combining of the physicians into a joint venture enables them to offer a new product producing substantial efficiencies."[51]

If an alleged antitrust violation escapes per se liability, it is viewed under the rule of reason, which requires an examination of the purpose, operation, and effect of the trade restraint to conclude as to whether the purpose or result of the agreement significantly harms competition, or if redeeming economic benefits of the arrangement exist.[28] In order to determine if the agreement has anticompetitive effects, the courts examine whether the network has significant market power, which is determined by the network's market share and the presence of entry barriers prohibiting similar networks from competing.[34]

Antitrust laws also affect nonhorizontal formations of managed care entities, such as health care purchasers, networks, or health plans contracting to form exclusive contracts with health care providers, individual providers, or individual networks. Specifically, one problem present in "exclusive contracts" is a "requirements contract," in which "a purchaser will buy all its requirements of a particular good or services from a single source."[34] Another problem is an agreement not to compete, which occurs when "a seller agrees to sell its services to a single purchaser and not to its competitors."[34]

Usually, courts test exclusive contracts between a health care purchaser and a provider under the rule of reason, which requires identifying and balancing the competitive and anticompetitive effects of the contract.[34] In *Capital Imaging Associates, P.C., v. Mohawk Valley Med-*

ical Associates, Inc.,[8] the court explained the analytical framework of exclusive contracts and antitrust law. First, the plaintiff must prove "that the challenged action has had an actual adverse effect on competition as a whole in the relevant market. . . ."[8] If the plaintiff meets the burden of proof, the defendant must "offer evidence of the pro-competitive 'redeeming virtues' of their combination."[8] If the defendant is successful in presenting the necessary proof, the plaintiff must prove that "any legitimate collaborative objectives proffered by defendant could have been achieved by less restrictive alternatives."[8]

With respect to "exclusive contracts," the theories of antitrust violations depend upon having a high degree of foreclosure, which could lead to competitors leaving the market due to decreased business, the erection of barriers to competition, and ultimately the health care purchaser exercising market power. Accordingly, the courts usually identify competitive and anti-competitive factors in order to determine the degree of foreclosure.[34] In order of importance, the first factor is the health care purchaser's market share which, as a general guideline, is considered safe if 10% or less and is a cause for concern if over 35%. The second factor is the contract duration. The third "factor is whether the contract is really exclusive"[34] because some contracts that state they are exclusive are not and others that do not state they are exclusive may be exclusive. The fourth factor concerns the motivation for the exclusive contract which, if motivated by the purchaser, shows the purchaser's beliefs that the contract is competitive. The fifth factor is whether or not other exclusive contracts exist in the market. The final factor is whether increased barriers to entering the market have resulted from the contract.

The second type of exclusive contracts that are affected by antitrust laws are those that contain covenants not to compete. Such contracts are scrutinized under the framework announced in *Capital Imaging Associates, P.C.*[8] The antitrust theory used for these actions is that covenants not to compete "may become an entry barrier preventing competitors of the purchaser from being able to obtain an 'input' essential for it to compete effectively with the purchaser that has the . . . [exclusive contract]."[34] Accordingly, "if the market for private health-care financing in which consumers purchase is competitive, or if actual and potential competitors in that market can obtain the health-care services they need to compete, then the exclusive should create little antitrust risk."[34] Thus, the primary factor in cases concerning covenants not to compete is the percentage of the market for providers the covenant covers.[52]

ETHICS AND MANAGED CARE

Cost containment is essential to managed care, and physician financial incentives to contain costs are an important element in containing costs. Often, physician financial incentives present doctors with critical ethical decisions which are unique to managed care entities. Two general areas of concern are conflicts with the allocation of care among patients and conflicts between physician financial gain and the best care for patients. These conflicts of interest will be discussed in light of newly released guidelines issued by the American Medical Association (AMA) Council on Ethics and Judicial Affairs.[17]

The first guideline established by the AMA is that physicians must not allow the health care system to interfere with the delivery of patient care and that "physicians must continue to place the interests of the patient first."[17] The principle of placing the patient's care before any other factor runs throughout the guidelines published by the AMA.

Managed care entities utilize cost containment methods to eliminate inefficiencies and to limit the "availability of tests or procedures that offer only small or uncertain benefits or that provide a likely benefit but at a great expense."[17] Decisions concerning who will receive care and who will not often create ethical conflicts. The AMA guidelines provide principles for dealing with the problems associated with allocation decisions. The AMA states that "any broad allocation guidelines that restrict care and choices . . . should be established at a policy making level so that individual physicians are not asked to engage in ad hoc bedside rationing."[17] Further, under the AMA guidelines, physicians should have an active role in constructing allocation guidelines by contributing "their expertise to any allocation process and . . .

[advocating] for guidelines that are sensitive to differences among patients."[17] In order to accomplish the above, the guidelines state that managed care plans need to develop structures to facilitate physician input into allocation guidelines and, further, that allocation guidelines should be reviewed on a regular basis.[17]

Even if the AMA guidelines are used to develop allocation guidelines, physicians must advocate any care they believe will materially benefit their patients without regard to allocation guidelines or gatekeeper directives.[17] Additionally, the guidelines state that "adequate appellate mechanisms for both patients and physicians should be in place to address disputes regarding medically necessary care," and, under appropriate circumstances, physicians have a responsibility to initiate appeals for patients.[17]

Under the requirements of informed consent, managed care entities must fully disclose all material information to patients, and full disclosure "requires that managed care plans inform potential subscribers of limitations or restrictions on the benefits package when they are considering entering the plan."[17] For physicians, "full disclosure includes informing patients of all their treatment options, even those that may not be covered under the terms of the managed care plan."[17] The AMA guidelines further state that "physicians should not participate in any plan that encourages or requires care at or below minimum professional standards."[17]

The second area of ethical concern considered by the AMA guidelines is conflict between physician financial gain and the best care for patients. Managed care entities use fee withholds, capitation payments, and other financial incentives to motivate physicians to contain costs, and, accordingly, the AMA concluded that "financial incentives are permissible only if they promote the cost effective delivery of health care and not the withholding of medically necessary care."[17] In order to accomplish this result, the AMA established three criteria for incentive plans. First, the guidelines state that all "incentives to limit care must be disclosed fully to patients by plan administrators on enrollment and at least annually thereafter."[17] Second, they recommend that limits be placed on the amount of fee withholds and other incentives and that the calculation of incentives should be

based on the efficiency of a group of physicians instead of the performance of one physician.[17] Finally, they state that "health plans or other groups should develop financial incentives based on quality of care."[17]

In conclusion, it should be noted that the AMA guidelines include patient responsibilities. The guidelines state that patients have a responsibility to be aware of the extent of their health care benefits, to exercise autonomy by participating in the formation of benefit packages, and to be careful in the selection of their health care coverage.[17]

REFERENCES

1. Ader M: **Managing Emerging Technologies.** Washington, DC: Managed Care Law Institute, National Health Lawyers Association, 1993, pp 1-28
2. American Law Institute Restatement (Second) of Agency §219 (1958), American Law Institute, St Paul, Minnesota
3. American Law Institute Restatement (Second) of Torts §69 (1984), American Law Institute, St Paul, Minnesota
4. American Law Institute Restatement (Second) of Torts §439 (1977), American Law Institute, St Paul, Minnesota
5. Bales JF III, Demarco LA: **Selected Topics in Medical Malpractice Litigation.** New York, NY: Practicing Law Institute, 1993
6. Boochever SS: **Overview.** Washington, DC: Managed Care Law Institute, National Health Lawyers Association, 1993, pp 1-18
7. *Boyd v Albert Einstein Medical Center*, 547 A2d 1229 (Pa Super Ct)
8. *Capital Imaging Associates, PC, v Mohawk Valley Medical Associates, Inc*, 996 F2d 537 (2d Cir), *cert denied*, 510 US 946 (1993)
9. *Chase v Independent Practice Association, Inc*, 583 NE2d 251 (Mass App Ct 1991)
10. Clayton Act §1, 15 USC §12-27 (1994)
11. Clayton Act §3, 15 USC §14 (1994)
12. Clayton Act §7, 15 USC §18 (1994)
13. Conrad RJ Jr, Seiter PD: Health plan liability in the age of managed care. **Def Couns J 62:**191-200, 1995
14. *Copperweld Corp v Independence Tube Corp*, 467 US 752 (1984)
15. Corcoran ME: **Liability.** Washington, DC: Managed Care Law Institute, National Health Lawyers Association, 1993, pp 1-34
16. *Corcoran v United Healthcare, Inc*, 965 F2d 1321 (5th Cir 1992), *cert denied*, 506 US 1033 (1992)
17. Council on Ethical and Judicial Affairs, American Medical Association: Ethical issues in managed care. **JAMA 273:**330-335, 1995
18. *Dukes v United States Health Care Systems of Pennsylvania, Inc*, 848 F Supp 39 (ED Pa 1994)
19. Employment Retirement Income Security Act, 29 USC §1001-1461 (1994)
20. Employment Retirement Income Security Act,

29 USC §1003 (1994)

21. Employment Retirement Income Security Act, 29 USC §1002 (1) (1994)

22. Employment Retirement Income Security Act, 29 USC §1144 (a) (1994)

23. Federal Trade Commission Act §1, 15 U USC §45 (1994)

24. Freiburg JP: The ABCs of MCOs: an overview of managed care organizations. **Ill Bar J 81:**584-589, 1993

25. Hall MA: Managed competition and integrated health care delivery systems. **Wake Forest Law Rev 29:**1, 1994

26. *Harrell v. Total Health Care, Inc,* 78 SW2d 58 (M 989)

27. Hitcher CH, et al: Integrated delivery systems: a survey of organizational models. **Wake Forest Law Rev 29:** 273, 1994

28. Jackson RL, Levy KW: **Innovations in Managed Care.** New York NY: Practicing Law Institute, 1994

29. *Jackson v Roseman,* 878 F Supp 820 (D Md 1995)

30. Joffe MS: Medicaid and managed care, in Gosfield AG (ed): **Health Law Handbook.** Deerfield, Ill: Clark, Boardman, and Callaghan, 1994, pp 177-195

31. *Johnson v Misericordia Community Hosp,* 301 NW2d 156 (Wis 1981)

32. *Kuhl v. Lincoln National Health Plan,* 999 F2s 298 (8th Cir 1993), *cert denied,* 510 US 1045 (1994)

33. *McClellan v. Health Maintenance Org of Pennsylvania,* 604 A2d 1053 (Pa Super Ct 1992)

34. Miles JJ: **Managed Care, Managed Competition, and Antitrust.** Washington, DC: Managed Care Law Institute, National Health Lawyers Association, 1993, pp 1-47

35. Morreim EH: Cost containment and the standard of medical care. **Calif Law Rev 75:**1719-1763, 1987

36. Note: Universal access to health care. **Harv Law Rev 108:**1323-1340, 1995

37. Prise HL: The proper extension of tort liability principles in the managed care industry. **Temple Law Rev 64:**977, 1991

38. *Raglin v HMO Illinois, Inc,* 595 NE2d 153 (III App Ct 1992)

39. *Roen v Sullivan,* 764 F Supp 555 (D Minn 1991)

40. *Salley v Dupont,* 966 F2d 1011 (5th Cir 1992)

41. *Sarchett v Blue Shield of California,* 43 Cal3d 1 (1987)

42. *Shaw v Delta Air Lines, Inc,* 463 US 85 (1983)

43. Sherman Act §1, 15 USC §1-7 (1994)

44. Sherman Act §2, 15 USC §2 (1994)

45. Social Security Act §1811, 42 USC §1395c-i (1994)

46. Social Security Act §1831, 42 USC §1395j-w (1994)

47. Social Security Act §1842, 42 USC §1395u(a) and (c) (1994)

48. Social Security Act §1876, 42 USC §1395mm (1994)

49. Social Security Act §1903(m)(1), 42 USC §1396b (1994)

50. US Department of Justice and Federal Trade Commission: **1992 Horizontal Merger Guidelines.** Washington, DC: US Government Printing Office. 57 (No. 176) **Federal Register** 41552 (Sept 10, 1992)

51. US Department of Justice and Federal Trade Commission: **Statements of Antitrust Enforcement Policy in the Health Care Arena. 4 Trade Reg Rep** (CCH), Chicago, Ill, pp 13, 152 (1994)

52. *US Healthcare, Inc, v Healthsource, Inc,* 986 F2d 589 (1st Cir 1993)

53. *Wickline v State of California,* 239 Cal Rptr 810 (Cal Ct App 1986), *review dismissed,* 741 P2d 613 (Cal 1987)

54. *Wilson v Blue Cross of Southern California,* 35 Cal Rptr 377 (1990)

CHAPTER 24

Health Insurance, Medicare, and Medicaid

Sandra A. Price, JD

Health Insurance

Health insurance is purchased by persons desiring to protect themselves from catastrophic financial losses in the event they need major health care services. Employers often provide health insurance as a benefit of employment. In either circumstance, health insurance is a contract between the patient and the insurance company. The patient pays a premium, generally on a monthly basis, and the insurance company agrees to accept the patient's risk of illness (i.e., financial cost of illness) and spread this risk out over a group of patients.

Providers' Rights and Responsibilities

Health care providers are not parties to this contract, and therefore do not have rights or responsibilities to either party in connection with the insurance contract. However, providers can voluntarily assume some of the parties' responsibilities if they desire or if they are not careful. For example, clauses in the health insurance contract often require the patient to notify the insurance company and obtain approval before the patient can "purchase" or receive services. Because health care providers are third parties, they do not have a duty to obtain permission from the insurance company before proceeding to provide the service. However, if providers tell patients that the provider will obtain permission for a procedure, they have voluntarily agreed to take on the patient's obligation under the contract. Once a provider offers this service, patients may come to rely on the provider doing the same in the future. This practice can become expensive for physicians if their staff provides these services for all patients.

There is currently a lawsuit in the West Virginia circuit courts[18] that is attempting to redefine the nature of the relationship between health care providers and insurance companies. In this case, a patient entered the hospital and the insurance company did not pay the subsequent bills for hospital or physician services. When the physician's practice attempted to collect payment from the patient's estate, the patient's estate filed suit against the physician's practice plan. The complaint alleged that the practice plan knew the insurance company had denied a precertification request to pay the charges and had failed to inform the decedent of all matters relevant to her care and treatment while under the physician's supervision. Thus, either: 1) the defendant (practice plan) breached its duty to inform the patient of the denial; or 2) the defendant breached its contract with the patient to inform the patient of the denial. Obtaining precertification has not been a duty or responsibility of a health care provider. The above-referenced case alleges that the physicians created a duty for themselves by providing assistance in obtaining precertification in the past.[18]

Confidentiality and Consent to Disclose

Since health care providers generally are not parties to the health insurance contract, they cannot release confidential patient information to the insurance company without the patient's permission. Physicians or their office staff should always have their patients' consent in writing prior to release of confidential patient information to third party payors. If confidential patient information is released to a health insurance company without written consent of the patient, the provider could be sued for breach of privacy. If the patient refuses to consent, the patient can and should be held personally responsible for the cost of the service.

The release of patient information is even more complex when insurance companies hire an independent company to process claims. Providers should notify patients and get consent before releasing health care information to a claims processing company.

Some types of medical records are more sensitive, and thus better protected, than others. Often both state and federal law specifically prohibit and/or restrict the right of the provider to release patient information to third parties for treatment of psychiatric problems, alcohol and/or drug abuse, venereal disease including HIV (human immunodeficiency virus) status, and prenatal care for minors. For example, Federal Confidentiality Rules (42 CFR Part 2) state that patient records which identify, diagnose, or contain prognosis or treatment records for drug and/or alcohol abuse rehabilitation are confidential and may only be disclosed under certain circumstances.[2]

To disclose information to an insurance company, the patient should sign a written consent for the disclosure and the consent should include: 1) the name of the provider permitted to disclose; 2) the name of the individual/organization to whom disclosure is made; 3) the name of the patient; 4) the purpose of disclosure; 5) how much/what information is to be disclosed; 6) the signature of the patient or legal guardian; 7) a statement that the consent is revocable at any time except to the extent that the provider already acted in reliance thereupon; and 8) a date, event, or condition upon which consent will expire if not revoked beforehand. Before consent is obtained, the provider cannot even disclose that the person is/was a patient at his/her office or facility. A typical consent clause reads:

> I am responsible for paying for services provided to me and agree that any insurance benefits for my account be paid directly to provider. I certify that all information supplied by me in applying for payment by any third party is true and accurate. I authorize release of my medical bills to the person whose insurance is paying all or part of my account. I further authorize my provider to release my medical records and any other information relating to my care, specifically including information relating to psychiatric or substance abuse treatment and/or HIV status to any person or company who may need them for my continuing care and/or for purposes of paying all or part of my account.

This consent clause informs patients about the release of information and obtains the patient's consent to release such information.

In addition to the above consent, each disclosure made must be accompanied by the following written statement:

> This information has been disclosed to you from records protected by Federal confidentiality rules (42 CFR Part 2). The Federal rules prohibit you from making any further disclosure of this information unless further disclosure is expressly permitted by the written consent of the person to whom it pertains or as otherwise permitted by 42 CFR Part 2. A general authorization for this release of medical or other information is NOT sufficient for this purpose. The Federal rules restrict any use of the information to criminally investigate or prosecute any alcohol or drug abuse patient.[9]

Health care facilities generally create a rubber stamp with this statement and stamp each page of confidential information before it is released to a third party.

It is thus imperative that physicians know and understand state and federal requirements before releasing medical records to third party payors.

Restrictions on Disclosure for Minor Patients

Although state law varies, many states also restrict parents' access to medical records of minor patients (under the age of 18) for specific treatments. For example, in West Virginia a physician can treat a minor patient without parental consent or knowledge for the following conditions: 1) addiction to controlled substances;[27] 2) addiction to alcohol;[26] 3) venereal disease (including HIV);[24] 4) birth control;[25] and 5) prenatal care.[25] Alabama allows a patient to consent to medical, dental, health or mental health services if the patient is 14 years or older, or graduated from high school, or is married or divorced, or is pregnant, or has a child. In addition, any minor can consent to treatment of pregnancy, venereal disease, drug dependency, alcohol toxicity, or any reportable diseases.[10] In Idaho, minors 14 years or older are allowed to consent to the diagnosis and treatment of any infectious, contagious, or communicable disease.[17] California allows minors to consent to medical or dental care if the patient is 15 years or older, living alone, and managing his/her own finances. Patients 12 years or older are allowed to consent to mental health counseling and treatment (but excludes convulsive therapy and psychosurgery) if they are mature enough to participate intelligently in the care and are either a danger to themselves or others or an alleged victim of incest or child abuse; they can also consent for diagnosis and treatment of infectious, contagious, or communicable diseases, or medical care and/or counseling relating to drug- or alcohol-related problems (excluding methadone).[11]

Many states that allow minor patients to consent to specific treatments also add that in those circumstances parents are not liable for the cost of the medical care provided. In addition, billing the parent's insurance carrier could be construed as notifying the parent because the insured (parent) generally receives an explanation of benefit form from the insurance company which tells the patient's name, date of service, provider name, and amount of payment (if any). The parent would then have knowledge that health care was provided to the minor child. Therefore, providers should either arrange for direct payment from the minor patient or obtain the minor's consent to bill their parent's insurance company before proceeding.

MEDICARE AND MEDICAID

The Medicare/Medicaid system of reimbursement is an extremely complex subject. For specific information physicians should consult either a provider reimbursement manual, a Medicare/Medicaid reimbursement specialist, or a book written by such a specialist. A physician should also consult a Medicaid specialist in his/her state to learn the particulars about the local program.

General Information

The Medicare program[4] consists of three parts and was enacted by the federal government in 1965 to help pay for health care for a select group of individuals. This group includes: individuals over 65 years of age who qualify for Social Security or railroad retirement benefits; individuals receiving Social Security payments because of a disability (after a waiting period); and persons with end-stage renal disease. Part A is generally known as hospital insurance; Part B covers outpatient services, physician services, durable medical equipment, comprehensive rehabilitation facilities, and diagnostic tests; and Part C covers miscellaneous provisions of the program.

Federal law 42 USC 1395 *et seq* created the Medicare program, fraud and abuse language, and prohibits self-referral and kickbacks; the False Claims Act[1] deals with providers that filed false claims for Medicare and Medicaid dollars; and 42 USC 1301 and 1320a-7a provide criminal sanctions for self-referral and other prohibited actions in the Medicare program.

Medicaid[7] is a joint state-federal program that provides medical assistance to approximately 36 million low-income adults and children.[12] It was enacted in 1965 at the same time as Medicare, but as a separate program. All states chose to participate in the program. States submit plans for approval, and, once approved, receive varying amounts of federal matching funds. According to 42 USC 1396d, the federal government pays between 50% and 83% of a state's Medicaid expenditures depending upon the state's average per capita income. The federal government pays 55% of a state's Medicaid expenditures if the state has a per capita income equal to the national average; if the state's per capita income is higher than average, it receives fewer federal dollars, and if the per capita income is lower than average, it receives more federal dollars.[7]

Federal law 42 USC 1396 *et seq* created the Medicaid program and allows each state to create a Medicaid plan and submit it for approval. Because each state has broad discretion in formulating its Medicaid plan, Medicaid programs differ from state to state. The law requires all states to provide medical assistance to certain groups of patients (i.e., people who receive Aid to Families with Dependent Children, Supplemental Security Income, and certain low-income pregnant women and children who do not receive welfare payments). States can elect to cover additional people. States also have flexibility in determining what services will be covered: some states offer a wide range of benefits such as inpatient, outpatient, and physician services, long-term nursing home care, dental expenses, eyeglasses, and preventive services.

The Health Care Financing Administration (HCFA) of the United States Department of Health and Human Services was created in 1977 to administer both the Medicare and the Medicaid programs.

In 1995, Medicare and Medicaid spending accounted for 31% of all U.S. health care expenses.[19] Medicare enables medical insurance to be available to approximately 40 million Americans.[21] The Congressional Budget Office estimated that Medicare paid $32.8 billion to physicians in fiscal year 1995.[16]

Coverage

Several coverage issues should be addressed when a physician is trying to decide whether a patient is covered by Medicare. The threshold questions are whether the patient is a Medicare beneficiary, and, if so, is this particular service a covered benefit under the Medicare program? No payment is made for: personal comfort items; routine physical checkups, eyeglasses or eye examination; orthopedic shoes; custodial care; cosmetic surgery; care, treatment, filling, removal, or replacement of teeth or supporting structures; flat foot, subluxations of the foot, or routine foot care; or if the provider is an immediate relative of the Medicare beneficiary.[5]

If the patient and service are covered, there are other requirements for payment. The physician must personally examine the patient or visualize some aspect of the patient's condition (e.g., interpret a laboratory test or an x-ray film) before the physician can bill for a procedure. Also, for coverage to apply, the service must be: 1) medically "reasonable and necessary," 2) of a quality which meets professionally recognized standards of care, and 3) supported by evidence showing the medical necessity and quality.[3] Such evidence consists of medical records which must be maintained for at least 5 years and which must contain, at a minimum, information that would allow a review agency to determine the procedure was medically necessary, was actually performed, and was performed competently.

In *Enaw v. Dowling*,[13] Dr. Augustin Enaw, a provider in New York's Medicaid program, was ordered to make restitution of $318,583 plus interest and was banned from participation in Medicaid for 5 years. The charges against Dr. Enaw were based on demonstrated record-keeping deficiencies which included insufficient information and/or inadequate documentation to justify the tests ordered or medication prescribed.[13]

Medicare Reimbursement

In the past, physician services were reimbursed at a rate related to charges; since 1993, the payment system is called a Resource-Based Relative Value Scale (RBRVS). Many factors go into determining what fee a physician will receive for any given service provided to the patient. According to 42 USC 1395w-4(b)(1), payment amounts for a service shall be equal to the product of the relative value for the service multiplied by the conversion factor for the year multiplied by the geographic adjustment factor. (Additionally, special rules apply to fees for radiology, anesthesiology services, and electrocardiogram interpretations.) Three factors go into setting a relative value for each physician service. These components are: a work component that reflects physician "time and intensity" in providing the service, a practice expense component that reflects practice overhead costs other than malpractice, and malpractice expenses associated with the service. Relative values must be reviewed by the Secretary of Health and Human Services at least every 5 years. Currently, there are three separate conversion factors. The conversion factor for surgery is $39.45, for primary care is $36.38, and for nonsurgical procedures is $34.62.[15] Conversion factors are updated annually. Finally, the Secretary establishes a geographic adjustment factor which compares the relative costs of goods and services in a specific service region with the national average of such costs. This factor is reviewed at least every 3 years. As a result of the geographic adjustment factor, two physicians in the same specialty performing the same procedure in different parts of the country could be paid different fees.

In addition, cost sharing is required in the Medicare system. After an initial annual deductible of $100 is paid by the patient, Medicare pays 80% of the Medicare-approved payment and the patient is responsible for paying the remaining 20%. "Writing off" the coinsurance due from the patient without making an attempt to collect it is generally prohibited and may cause Medicare to penalize the provider and/or exclude the provider from the program.

Generally, physicians have the option of: 1) billing the patient and attempting to collect from the patient, and having the patient seek reimbursement from Medicare, or 2) billing Medicare directly and collecting only the coinsurance from the patient. Medicare encourages physicians to take the claim on assignment (bill Medicare and accept its payment as payment in full without the coinsurance) by creating a participating physician program. Participating physicians get reimbursed at a higher rate than nonparticipating physicians. Medicare also publishes a directory of participating physicians and notifies Medicare patients that if they use participating physicians, they will not be subject to balance billing (billing the difference between actual charges and Medicare reimbursement). Since September 1, 1990, all claims submitted to Medicare for payment must be submitted within 1 year from the date the service was provided to the patient. Claims may be submitted either electronically by computer or by paper on claims forms designated by Medicare. The Secretary encourages electronic filing by providing expedited payment for electronically submitted claims.

Physicians are prohibited from assigning or selling their Medicare claims to a third party who would bill and collect. They are, however, allowed to use Medicare and/or Medicaid accounts receivable as collateral to obtain a loan. There are computer programs designed to assist providers and their staff with Medicare billing and reimbursement calculations. The programs are designed to help code Medicare claims quickly and accurately, thus decreasing the number of claims rejected on the first submission.[20]

Medicaid Reimbursement

Because the Medicaid program is governed by each state's Medicaid plan, there are numerous methods of calculation used to determine physician reimbursement in the Medicaid program. The four basic methods of reimbursement calculation are: a percentage of the prevailing charges, an established fee schedule, a relative value scale, and Medicaid as a managed-care program. Again, it is important to consult an expert in the state in which one practices to determine that state's method of reimbursement calculation.

Medicare/Medicaid Fraud and Abuse

Providers may be terminated from the Medicare and/or Medicaid programs if the Secretary of Health and Human Services determines that: 1) the provider made false statements or misrepresented material facts while applying for payment, or 2) submitted claims for services or supplies in excess of the patient's medical needs or of a quality below the professionally recognized standards.[6] There are also civil money penalties payable for each fraudulent claim submitted.[8]

In December 1995, the Clinical Practices of the University of Pennsylvania entered into a settlement agreement with the U.S. Government to pay $30 million after a federal audit disclosed the fact that false (as defined by the False Claims Act) Medicare bills were submitted for faculty physician services from 1989 to 1994. The audit disclosed that faculty physicians were billing for services actually performed by residents, bills were coded at the highest service level regardless of the services actually provided, and there was inadequate documentation for many bills submitted.[23]

In another suit, the Secretary of the Health and Human Services ruled Dr. Bruce Erickson would be excluded from Medicare, Medicaid, and other federally funded health care programs for 15 years following the determination that he submitted false claims to Medicare. Dr. Erickson appealed this decision to the federal court, and the Ninth Circuit Court of Appeals found Dr. Erickson was properly excluded from the program.[14] The 10th Circuit agreed, upholding provider exclusion from participating in Medicare and Medicaid for improper conduct by a provider.

Medicare Reform Proposals

No Medicare/Medicaid reform bill was passed by the U.S. Congress in 1996, although numerous Medicare reform packages have been debated. It is impossible to predict when or if restructuring will occur. On the positive side, without reform there will not be large reductions in Medicare/Medicaid funding. However, without reform, the programs will most likely be insolvent in the not-too-distant future. One of the current Medicare reform proposals would reduce spending by $45.5 billion on hospital care and $12.6 billion on physician care. Physician fees would be reduced by lowering the current conversion factor to $36 for each unit of service. This would decrease the surgery unit by 9.6% and decrease the primary care unit by 1.1% while increasing other nonsurgical procedures. As long as volume of services continues to grow in the Medicare program, this conversion unit could continue to drop until the year 2005. This particular package also includes oversight and licensure of provider-sponsored Medicare managed-care organizations, antitrust provisions designed to allow hospitals and physicians to form working networks, and tort reform.[15]

In addition, a reform bill could enact significant changes in fraud and abuse laws and physician self-referral. First, the criminal and civil antifraud and abuse statutes currently apply only to the Medicare and Medicaid programs. It is proposed that this be expanded to include all federally-funded health care programs. Second, a reform package might establish required exclusionary time frames from the federal program for fraud and abuse, as well as significantly increased monetary civil penalties for certain violations of the fraud and abuse statutes. Third, self-referral prohibitions might be limited to the following five areas: clinical laboratory services; radiology services, specifically magnetic resonance images and computed tomography scans; parenteral and enteral nutrition, equipment, and supplies; outpatient physical therapy services; and outpatient occupational therapy services. This aspect of the proposed legislation is less restrictive than current federal law.[28]

Another potential area of Medicare reform is malpractice liability. Reform packages include a uniform 2-year statute of limitations with no cases being filed more than 5 years after the date of the injury. Non-economic damages would be limited to $250,000 per case. Punitive damages would be limited to the greater of $250,000 or treble the economic damages, and punitive damages could be awarded only after a finding by clear and convincing evidence that the injury resulted from conduct intended to cause harm or conduct that demonstrated a conscious, flagrant indifference for the rights and/or safety of others.[28]

Medicaid Reform Proposals

Passage of a Budget Reconciliation Act could totally revamp the Medicaid program. One reform package calls for current Medicaid law to be repealed in its entirety and would allow each state to dictate virtually every aspect of the Medicaid program. Moneys would be appropriated in a block grant approach; federal funds would go to each state to use as the state sees fit. Generally, each state would determine who is eligible for benefits and also what benefits would be provided. States would only be required to provide health care coverage to pregnant women and children age 12 years or younger whose income was below the poverty level. The only mandatory benefits would be family planning and immunizations. Federal aid to states would be reduced by $182 billion over the next 7 years.

In addition to federal Medicaid reform, a significant number of states are currently considering or have recently passed Medicaid reform at the state level. A number of states have applied for a Section 1115 waiver from HCFA to develop Medicaid managed-care demonstration projects. These projects are designed to demonstrate that using a managed-care approach in the Medicaid population can control costs and improve outcomes while expanding the scope of coverage. As of March, 1996, 13 Section 1115 waivers have been granted. In addition, 38 states have received Section 1915(b) waivers which allow the states more flexibility in their Medicaid programs.[22] Other states (New York, Oregon, New Hampshire, and Louisiana) recently enacted Medicaid reform legislation designed to reduce state spending in the Medicaid programs. This is achieved by reducing payments to physicians, hospitals, and nursing homes; tightening eligibility standards, which reduces the number of people eligible for Medicaid; and implementing a monthly premium for participants.[22] Finally, several states recently passed Patient Protection Acts or Patient Access Acts that give patients and providers additional rights when dealing with health maintenance organizations and health care plans.[22]

Physicians can expect Medicare and Medicaid reform proposals to be reintroduced to Congress in 1997. The goal of reform will remain the same: reduction in spending. Thus, the theories, if not the specifics, of the 1996 reform proposals are likely to resurface. Only time will reveal what the future holds for Medicare and Medicaid patients and providers in the United States.

REFERENCES

1. 31 USC 3729-33
2. 42 CFR Part 2
3. 42 USC 1320c-9
4. 42 USC 1395 et seq
5. 42 USC 1395 y(a)
6. 42 USC 1395cc(b)(2)(D), (E), and (F)
7. 42 USC 1396 et seq
8. 45 CFR 1003
9. 52 Federal Register 21809 (June 9, 1987); 52 Fed Regis 41977 (Nov 2, 1987)
10. Alabama Code §22-8-(1-9)
11. California Family Code, Chapter 3, §6920-6929
12. Dentzer S: The war over the other M program. **US News World Report 119:**71, Oct 9, 1995
13. *Enaw v Dowling,* 632 NYS 715 (1995)
14. *Erickson v US,* 75 F3d 470 (9th Cir)
15. Gardner J: Congressional leaders inch toward Medicare reform. **Modern Healthcare 26:**2, Feb 12, 1996
16. Gardner J: Wrestling with Medicare doc fee schedules. **Modern Healthcare 25:**88, Oct 2, 1995
17. Idaho Code §39-3801
18. *McIntyre v WVU Medical Corporation,* #95-C-175 (Monongahelia County, WV, filed June 1995)
19. McNamee M: Smashing "the beast of medical inflations." **Business Week 85.** Jan 9, 1995
20. Montague J, Pitman H: Currents: payments. **Hospitals Health Networks 70:**16, Feb 5, 1996
21. Rosenbaum D: In the war of politics, Medicare spending has become the latest battlefield. **New York Times.** May 2, 1995, p A14 (Late New York Edition)
22. Seward W: Health systems reform: 1995 state legislative wrap up. **Bull Am Coll Surg 81:**41, March 1996
23. *US v Clinical Practices of the University of Pennsylvania,* ED Pa, Dec 12, 1995
24. WV Code §16-4-10
25. WV Code §16-29-1(b)
26. WV Code §60-6-23
27. WV Code §60A-5-504
28. Yale K: The Medicare Preservation Act of 1995—review and analysis of key issues. **Health Law Digest 23:** 3, Nov 1995

CHAPTER 25

SOCIAL SECURITY DISABILITY: THE ROLE OF THE PHYSICIAN

JANIE R. VALE, MD, MSPH

> *The American people want some safeguard against misfortunes which cannot be wholly eliminated in this man-made world of ours. . . . I am looking for a sound means which I can recommend to provide at once security against several of the great disturbing factors in life—especially those which relate to unemployment and old age.*

These were the words of President Franklin D. Roosevelt in his message to the United States Congress on June 8, 1934.[6]

In response, Congress enacted the Social Security Act of 1935, which provided a pension program for the elderly. President Roosevelt's historic words were to be followed by the Beveridge Report, prepared by the British government in 1941 during the midst of World War II.[8] The report outlined a comprehensive social security policy to make "want" unnecessary under any circumstance. The aim of a national social security plan was to extend protection to the greatest portion of the total population. It was understood that a comprehensive range of benefits' protection would provide against income loss (temporary and long-term) as well as health care protection and family benefits. The benefits were to be considered a right, but with compulsory participation. The plan called for a mix or sharing of responsibility by the state, private sector, and individuals. This concept was well addressed in the following quotation from the report.

Social Security must be achieved by cooperation between the State and the individual. The State should offer security for service and contribution. The State in organizing security should not stifle incentive, opportunity, responsibility: in establishing a national minimum, it should leave room and encouragement for voluntary action by each individual to provide more than that minimum for himself and his family.[5]

Consistent with the principles of the Beveridge Report, the Social Security Disability Insurance (SSDI) plan, which provided for a federally created and regulated insurance plan, was established by Congress in 1954. The SSDI is funded from the Federal Insurance Contributions Act (FICA) taxes, which are assessed on wages paid to workers. The SSDI program assists primarily the working population and survivors of workers. Two independent elements must be met for an individual to qualify for SSDI benefits. These are: 1) the person's prior earning capacity, and 2) the magnitude of the impairment. The specific requirements for how much and for how long a worker must contribute to the fund to be eligible for benefits have changed over the years and will continue to change. Workers may become work disabled after contributing for variable time periods.

Obviously, some individuals who have never contributed to the fund are unable to work. In 1973, the federal government assumed administration of the Supplemental Security Income (SSI) program, which provides a minimum income level for the needy aged, blind, and disabled who have had minimal or no significant labor force participation. SSI draws on general tax revenues. Of note, disabled workers covered under SSDI receive monthly benefit amounts that are more than twice the amount received by SSI-only recipients.[9]

The Social Security Administration (SSA) has the mandated responsibility for the administration of both the SSDI program Title II and the SSI program Title XVI. On August 15, 1994, President Bill Clinton signed a law making the SSA an independent agency. As of March 31, 1995, the SSA was separated from the Department of Health and Human Services. The goal was to ensure the agency freedom from political control.

To qualify for benefits under either program, SSDI or SSI, an individual must have a medically determinable severe impairment. This medical informant requirement defines the role of the physician and/or psychologist. The health care professional must provide the medical evidence upon which impairments will be evaluated. The individual seeking disability compensation first must file a claim with an SSA district or branch office. The claim undergoes an initial review and processing, and then is referred for the next review phase. Under federal contract and regulation, there is a Disability Determination Service (DDS) agency in every state. Evaluation teams, consisting of a physician and a disability evaluation specialist, are responsible for making individual disability determinations. Quality control procedures are initiated by SSA and are reviewed periodically.[9] Medical evidence forms the "backbone" for disability claim review and determination. The physician providing medical information on his or her patient filing disability claims must have a working knowledge of the following terminology. Without such knowledge the physician may unknowingly provide the patient and his or her family with unrealistic expectations for the outcome of their claim.

SOCIAL SECURITY TERMINOLOGY[14]

Activities of Daily Living—activities learned by the time of reaching adulthood, taken for granted and which do not require specialized training.[3]

Disability Determination—"primary consideration is given to the severity of the individual's impairment . . . age, education, and work experience. Medical considerations alone (including the physiological and psychological manifestations of aging) can . . . justify a finding that the individual is under a disability where his impairment is one that meets the duration and is listed."[6]

Disability—the inability to engage in any substantial gainful activity by reason of a medically determinable physical or mental impairment that can be expected to result in death, or has lasted or can be expected to last, for a continuous period of not less than 12 months.

Laboratory Findings—manifestations of anatomical, physiological, or psychological phenomena demonstrable by replacing or extending the perceptiveness of the observer's senses. Includes chemical, electrophysiological, roentgenological, or psychological tests.

Listing of Impairments—as defined by the SSA. Published in the Federal Register, this listing comprises evaluation criteria. Tabulation of medical impairments which, ipso facto, are considered severe enough to prevent a person from doing any gainful activity. Lists are applicable to the evaluation of adults and children. Listings of impairments include the following categories: musculoskeletal system, special senses and speech, respiratory system, cardiovascular system, digestive system, genitourinary system, hemic and lymphatic system, skin, endocrine system, multiple body systems, neurological disorders, mental disorders, and neoplastic diseases (malignant).

Qualifying Impairment—medically demonstrable anatomical, physiological, or psychological abnormality. Medically determinable if manifested in signs or laboratory findings apart from symptoms.

Signs—anatomical, physiological, or psychological abnormalities that can be observed through the use of medically acceptable clinical techniques. In psychiatric impairment, signs are medically demonstrable abnormalities of behavior, affect, thought, memory, orientation, and contact with reality.

Statutory Blindness—a person having 20/200 or less vision in the better eye with the use of corrective lenses, or with tunnel vision of 20 degrees or less. The latter represents the loss of visual efficiency.[13]

Substantial Gainful Activity—is defined as any work of a nature generally performed for remuneration or profit involving the performance of significant physical or mental duties or a combination of both. Work may be considered substantial, even if performed part time, and even if it is less demanding or less responsible than the individual's former work. It may be considered gainful even if it pays less than the individual's former work.

Symptoms—claimant's own perception of his/her physical or mental impairments. Abnormalities that manifest themselves only as symptoms are not medically determinable.

Physician's Role in Disability Determination

The operating principle in Social Security disability claims review is that with sufficient disease the individual ought to experience illness. If the disease is of sufficient magnitude, the illness should manifest itself as incapacity in the workplace. The weight to be given to the medical evidence provided depends on how specific and complete the clinical findings are and how consistent the clinical findings are with severity and probable duration of the impairment.

The physician will best serve his or her patient and the SSA by providing medical records promptly when requested. The records should be of sufficient detail to permit determination of the severity and duration of the condition. The records should be signed by the physician or the copies certified as accurate by the custodian or the medical records administrator.

Ideally, reports should contain the medical history relating to the impairment(s) which prevent work. Physical examination findings should be described and supporting laboratory data should be provided. Review of the evaluation criteria in the listing of impairments can provide guidance as to what information will be most useful to the DDS review team. All symptoms, signs, and laboratory findings, however, should be provided. Clinical judgment without supporting data is given little probative weight.

Physician reports should cover the period of time requested or the actual period the condition was covered in the records. The medical history should address when the impairment began to interfere with activities of daily living and work capacity, in addition to questions routinely covered in a patient encounter. It is necessary to report response, lack of response, or adverse reaction to treatments to help determine if the condition is reversible or is expected to continue. A medical source statement should outline what activities the patient can and cannot perform. A statement with supporting documentation as to progress and future prognosis is extremely helpful. Most importantly, the physician or psychologist should indicate the functional capacity limitations. Specific performance capabilities (i.e., sit, stand, walk, climb, bend, lift, carry, push, pull, kneel, crawl, and squat) are critical. A statement from the testing physician that the patient can lift and carry "very little" is useless. The preferred response should clearly spell out the exact limitations (e.g., "Mr. Jones can lift and carry weights not in excess of 20 pounds on an occasional basis, and 10 pounds frequently").

The SSA allows for the payment of a fee for medical reports used for disability determination. Fees are set by the state DDS and usually are comparable to the fees paid for reports for other state medical programs. The treating physician usually is asked if he/she would be willing to provide additional medical evidence about the patient if requested by the review process. This request usually will accompany the request for medical records. It is often the practice of the busy treating physician to not personally review these letters. It may be left up to the office staff to forward the patient's medical records.

If the treating physician does not indicate his/her willingness to further evaluate or provide additional medical information about the patient, the SSA evaluation team must then refer the patient to a consulting examiner. The review physician of the SSA evaluation team will not examine the applicant. Despite SSA guidelines recommending the additional medical opinion and documentation on claims be obtained from the treating physician, the majority of cases are eventually referred to consulting examiners.

The consulting examination will be scheduled at the expense of the federal government. Prior to the examination, a letter is sent to the consulting physician from the SSA review team detailing what additional medical documentation or testing is needed to resolve the issue of disability. Consulting examiners are also requested to render opinion as to residual functional capacity as a measure of physical fitness. The consultative medical source statement is to provide further opinion as to the claimant's ability to do work-related activities or to function in a work setting. Data provided by consulting physicians has a profound effect on the economic and medical well being of millions of disability applicants. However, studies have shown that these physicians often feel ill-prepared for their task by inadequate training, and also feel that it is almost impossible to determine impairment based on a single office visit. In addition, many of the consultants were found to be skeptical of claims, thought applicants could work, and believed that patients exaggerated their symptoms.[2]

The consulting physician's conduct and reputation must be such as to avoid any negative reflection that would erode public trust in the federal government's administration of the Social Security programs. The physician must not be an employee of the state or any component of the SSA, unless there is no other qualified physician available. Obviously, the physician must not have any familial, financial, or other relationship to the applicant.[14] Any physician having questions about the role of a consulting physician performing disability examinations should contact the Chief Medical Consultant for the SSA, who can be identified through the Social Security office in the local area.

The consulting physician should understand that he/she should not release a consultative report, or information used to prepare the report, to anyone—including the applicant examined. Requests for records should be directed to the office that arranged for the consultative services. Under the Privacy Act, effective September 27, 1975, an individual has the right to request the medical evidence used to make a disability determination under the Social Security disability programs. However, these records are not available to the general public. When requests for medical evidence are received by the SSA, the claim file is reviewed to determine if release of the information could have any possible adverse effect on the applicant. If so, the information will be released only to an authorized representative designated by the applicant. The consulting physician also should notify the office that arranged for the examination if records or testimony are requested by court order. The assistance of the office and, if necessary, the Regional Attorney for the DDS will be made available to assist in actions seeking disclosure of information.

A determination will be made by the SSA review team as to whether an individual is able to return to his or her past work or "perform other jobs that exist in the economy in significant numbers." Claims are not denied solely because the claimant's impairment is unlisted. The Code of Federal Regulations does provide that "An impairment . . . shall be determined to be medically equivalent to an impairment listed . . . only if the medical findings with respect thereto are at least equivalent in severity and duration to the listed findings. . . . A decision . . . shall be based on medical evidence."[5]

Prior to 1971, the treating physician's opinion as to the claimant's ability to work and his or her functional capabilities had minimal if any impact on disability determination. This determination was relegated to governmental administrators. However, in 1971 *Richardson v. Perales*[12] resulted in the treating physician's opinion having substantial impact on the patient's disability claim.[10] The courts ordered SSA to pay closer attention to the opinion of the treating physician in these matters. The assessment of the patient's ability to perform sustained activity such as sitting, standing, and walking in an 8-hour day, as well as the ability or inability to lift and carry weights (occasionally or frequently), was given increased importance. However, again the importance of objective physician reporting documentation was emphasized.

The physician's role in Social Security disability determination should become proactive rather than reactive, as discussed above. All too often, physicians involved in the care of patients who have chronic progressive conditions or injuries and who are not expected to have complete functional recoveries wait until the individual is faced with either returning to work or continuing to work with difficulties before addressing impairment and disability options. More importantly, physicians often wait too long before addressing short-term and long-term functional capabilities with their patients. Though high-quality research in the area of disease, illness, and work capacity is limited, physicians should provide guidance to their patients based on what is known.

Musculoskeletal conditions are the most common cause of activity limitation in the U.S.[16] As of the end of l992, they accounted for 20% of individuals receiving SSDI benefits.[13] Individuals with musculoskeletal conditions that cause them to stop working have been found to have poorer overall health status. Often, they have one or more comorbidity factors, decreased function, more frequent use of physical aids, lower reported levels of commitment to work, and problematic working conditions. Actually, the demands of work have been found to have the most significant effect upon disability status. Individuals who were self-employed, had white collar jobs, and had greater control over their job's activities were less likely to be disabled. But individuals in jobs with less employment security, where the functional demands of the work and the functional limitations of the individual were incongruous, had a greater likelihood of work incapacity as the outcome. The physician must always remember that the medical signs and symptoms of an illness, particularly of mild or moderate severity, are much poorer predictors of work capacity than the work conditions themselves.

In medically managing the condition of impairment, the concerned clinician must consider how the patient's function fits with his/her work requirements over time. The physician should encourage job modification or moving the patient into more appropriate positions whenever possible. If not possible, the patient should be directed toward alternative employment or vocational rehabilitative services. Although the strategies are not clear, the physician should also strive to enhance, rather than erode, the patient's commitment to a positive work ethic and commitment to family. Research in work capacity and general health status consistently shows improved outcomes for married individuals and employed individuals. When the severity of the impairment(s) precludes work capacity, the physician is obligated to assist the patient in disability application.

When disability is being pursued, the physician must further understand that the patient is then entering an adjudicatory environment in which illness and impairment must be proven. The physician must be prepared to handle increased symptomatology and possibly even decreased compliance with the medical and self-directed care plan. The necessity to remain ill during the claim review process may, in and of itself, contribute to the development of other impairing conditions, including cardiovascular, gastrointestinal, or psychiatric problems.[4]

Although the physician is not expected to be an expert in SSD programs, a basic understanding of the claims review process and the general benefits of SSDI and SSI can aid the physician in caring for patients with chronic functionally limiting conditions. It should be conveyed to the patient that approximately 70% of claims are denied by DDS.[6] The claimant can file an appeal, though the decision is seldom altered unless additional objective medical evidence is provided. The next recourse is to request a review of the case by an administrative law judge. At this stage of the process, the patient may have legal representation by an attorney knowledgeable and experienced in Social Security matters. It is well documented that the unrepresented patient is less likely to receive a favorable verdict than one with legal representation.

The administrative law judge has considerably more freedom in claims review than the DDS. The administrative law judge determines whether the claimant can engage in substantial gainful activity. Approximately 50% of denied

TABLE 1

COMPARISON OF BENEFITS PROVIDED BY SOCIAL SECURITY DISABILITY
INSURANCE AND SUPPLEMENTAL SECURITY INCOME

Social Security Disability Insurance

- Disabled workers under the age of 65 years who have sufficient quarters of Social Security covered employment. In general, workers need work credit for at least 5 of the 10 years preceding disability onset. If disabled before the age of 31, the requirements can be reduced to as little as 1.5 years of work.

- Individuals disabled since childhood, if before the age of 22 a parent covered by Social Security retires, becomes disabled, or dies. These "childhood disability" payments will continue as long as the individual is disabled. The individual need not have worked to qualify.

- A disabled widow or widower, if the deceased spouse was covered under Social Security. The disabled widow or widower need not have worked under Social Security. The disability, however, must have occurred before or within 7 years of the spouse's death. Benefits will be paid also to a nondisabled mother or father caring for an entitled child.

Supplemental Security Income

- A disabled adult over the age of 18 years, meeting defined income and assets tests.

- An adult meeting the definition of statutory blindness (see Terminology section).

- A disabled child under the age of 18. Since a child is not normally considered to engage in work activity, vocational factors are not considered. Instead, interference with normal growth and development is a prime consideration.

- A blind child meeting the definition of statutory blindness. There is no duration requirement for benefits on the basis of blindness.

---

claims go to the administrative law judge review and about 50% of these claims are allowed. In addition, an increasing number of the denied claims are being taken to federal courts of appeal. These claims often focus on pain as a functionally limiting factor and on issues of discontinuation of benefits based on demonstration of "medical impairment."[4]

Under SSDI Program Title II and SSI Program Title XVI, basic categories of individuals can quality for disability benefits. These are summarized in Table 1.

SSI allows for "presumptive disability." If an individual is found to be "pre-emptively disabled," he or she may be paid for as many as 6 months while the formal disability determination process proceeds. This allows for a needy individual to meet his or her basic living expenses. If an adverse decision is reached, the individual does not have to refund the overpayment. There is no similar "presumptive disability" under the SSDI program.[14]

Physicians should always encourage functional and vocational rehabilitation. Physicians should be aware that Social Security disability claimants may be eligible for vocational rehabilitation services. Public Law 97-35 authorizes payment for rehabilitation services that would result in the individual returning to work at a level of "substantial gainful activity." These services are not limited to improving vocational skills only, but can include counseling, prosthetics and training in the use of prosthetics, and job placement services. Physicians must understand that information from the treating and/or consulting physician is most important in determining if an individual would benefit from vocational rehabilitative services.

Title II disability beneficiaries are eligible for Medicare coverage after 24 months of eligibility for disability. It must be understood that Medicare is a federal-state partnership and can vary in benefits from state to state.

The Social Security disability programs do allow for a trial work period. A beneficiary will continue to receive benefits for up to 9 months when he or she returns to work. If successful in the return to work, benefits will continue for an additional 3 months beyond the 9-month period and then will be terminated. Of interest, an individual with statutory blindness is not eligible for a trial work period. However, if the individual is engaged in substantial gainful activity, his or her benefits may be adjusted according to earned income. If, after a successful trial work period, the individual impairment(s) again prevents him or her from working, he or she will automatically receive benefits if work incapacity occurs within 15 months of the trial work period. Physicians should frequently encourage their patients receiving Social Security disability benefits to seek options for entry or re-entry into the workforce. If an individual understands that he or she actually has a two-year grace period, and with physician encouragement and attention to close medical management during the adjustment phase of the trial work period, it certainly would be feasible for many disabled individuals to achieve financial independence. A successful trial work period for individuals previously considered disabled from the work force is also facilitated by mandates for workplace accommodations under the Americans With Disabilities Act. Physicians should become knowledgeable in the provisions of this act in order to further assist their patients in maximizing their functional capabilities.

Although this chapter does not allow for an in-depth discussion of the Black Lung program, physicians involved in the care of miners with pneumoconiosis should realize that some, but not all, cases are administrated under the SSA. The Black Lung program was established in 1969 by the Federal Coal Mine Health and Safety Act. Claims through 1973 and some survivor benefits through 1983 are administered through the SSA and are financed from general U.S. Treasury funds. Benefits for later claims are administered by the U.S. Department of Labor.[11] Table 2 provides data regarding benefits that reflect the impact of implementation of safety programs to prevent and control exposure to miners, as well as the impact of a decreasing employment population in traditional mining jobs.

CONCLUSION

The financial burden of disability in the U.S. is alarming. Under SSI alone, there has been a 43% increase in beneficiaries between 1978 and 1993. In 1993, 4.08% of the working-age population (ages 18 to 64) was receiving benefits. This represented 6.7 million individuals, compared to 3.37% and 4.7 million, respectively, in 1978. SSI benefits paid in 1992 were over $22 billion. It is of significance that over 50% of beneficiaries in 1993 were receiving benefits because of mental disorders. In 1992, 3.5 million disabled workers received SSDI benefits at a cost of over $31 billion. Approximately 25% of claimants received benefits for mental disorders other than mental retardation, 20% for musculoskeletal conditions, and 15% for diseases of the circulatory system. It should be understood that disabled workers receiving benefits under SSDI, upon reaching the age of 65, are automatically switched to retired worker benefit status. This does not apply to individuals covered under SSI.[9,13] These trends are consistent with the U.S. moving from a manufacturing to a service-based economy. One of the greatest, if not the greatest, increases in labor costs during these decades has been in disability benefits.

In view of the above data, it is not surprising that on April 11, 1994, the trustees of the Social Security system advised that funds for the payment of Social Security benefits would run out in 2029, seven years earlier than predicted in 1993.[15] Physicians must realize that, as the number of contributors to Social Security financing decreases while increasing numbers of previously employed persons seek income replacement via the Social Security rolls, much more stringent scrutiny will be applied to the evaluation of disability claims. At the same time, it is likely that limitations in resources will be imposed for those approved for benefits. This will require even greater expertise on the part of the medical community to prevent and manage

TABLE 2

EXAMPLE OF BENEFITS ADMINISTERED BY THE SSA

Benefits paid to miners, widows, and dependents:

Year	No. Miners	No. Widows	No. Dependents	Total	Benefits (in thousands)
1970	43,921	24,889	43,166	111,976	$111,000
1975	165,405	139,407	177,499	482,311	$947,700
1980	120,235	146,603	132,639	399,477	$1,032,000
1985	77,836	138,328	78,682	294,846	$1,025,000
1990	45,643	118,705	46,330	210,678	$863,400
1992	35,971	109,091	37,334	182,396	$882,500

Benefits paid to miners, widows, and dependents for the five states with the greatest number of individuals covered as of 1992:

State	No. Miners	No. Widows	No. Dependents	Total	Monthly Amount (in thousands)
Kentucky	5,553	11,657	6,289	23,499	$8,229
Ohio	1,791	7,358	1,989	11,138	$4,085
Pennsylvania	9,542	31,125	8,529	49,196	$18,407
Virginia	2,802	6,349	3,021	12,172	$4,343
West Virginia	7,656	17,948	8,660	34,264	$12,023

trauma and chronic conditions and their resultant impairments. Training in impairment and disability prevention and medical management must receive greater emphasis and time, not only in medical school, but also in postgraduate and continuing medical education courses. Clinical investigations following rigorous research methodologies are needed to establish valid criteria for disability determination. However, this may be an unobtainable goal in a nation that directs only 1.1% of health care dollars spent annually to the study of illness, disability, and disease while spending 14% of the U.S. Department of Defense budget on research and development.[7]

As legislative and public debate continues over the future viability of a national Social Security system, physicians must remain committed to individual and community health and the financial needs of the truly vulnerable members of society who cannot be gainfully employed. A "safety net" for these individuals simply cannot be eliminated. Physicians must balance the needs of this segment of our population with active participation at the individual and aggregate levels to encourage current and future disability beneficiaries to leave the benefits rosters and to become actively employed, thus returning to society an otherwise enormous loss of human potential. This latter effort also requires active research on incentives and disincentives for productivity.

Social Security disability reform is inevitable. "The challenge is that of forging a social contract among the citizens which reflects the consensus of the population concerned about the issues of social solidarity and the redistribution of resources."[5] During this period of debate and change, physicians would be well served to hold onto a simple thought in their daily interaction with all of their patients:

"People don't hurt as much if they have something better to do."[1]

REFERENCES

1. Bigos SJ, Baker R, Lee S, et al: Back injury compensation: overcoming an adversarial system. **J Musculoskeletal Med** 2:17-24, June 1994
2. Carey TS, Fletcher SW, Fletcher R, et al: Social Security disability determinations—knowledge and attitudes of consultative physicians. **Med Care** 25:

267-274, 1987

3. Engelberg AL: Disability and workers' compensation. **Prim Care 21:**275-288, 1994

4. Fawley IL: A historical perspective on health reform. **MGM J.** March/April 1992, pp 44-49

5. Hadler NM: Criteria for screening workers for the establishment of disability. **J Occup Med 28:**940-945, 1986

6. Hadler NM: Medical ramifications of the federal regulation of the Social Security Disability Insurance program, Social Security and medicine. **Ann Intern Med 96:**665-669, 1982

7. Hatfield MO: The war against disease and disability. **JAMA 274:**1077, 1995

8. Hoskins DD: Developments and trends in Social Security, 1990-92: overview of principal trends. **Social Security Bull 55:**36-43, Winter 1992

9. McCoy JL, Weems K: Disabled-worker beneficiaries and disabled SSI recipients: A profile of demographic and program characteristics. **Social Security Bull 52:**

16-28, May 1989

10. Miller KA: Court orders Social Security Administration to give treating physicians' opinions greater weight. **J Tenn Med Assoc 81:**581, 1988

11. Nelson WJ Jr: Workers' compensation: 1980-1984 benchmark revisions. **Social Security Bull 51:**4-21, July 1988

12. *Richardson v Perales*, 402 US 389 (1971)

13. US Department of Health and Human Services Social Security Administration: **Annual Statistical Supplement, 1993,** to the **Social Security Bulletin**

14. US Department of Health and Human Services Social Security Administration: **Disability Evaluation Under Social Security,** May 1992 (SSA Publication No. 64-039)

15. **The World Book Year Book 1995.** Chicago, Ill: World Book, Inc, 1995

16. Yelin EH, Henke CJ, Epstein WV: Work disability among persons with musculoskeletal conditions. **Arthr Rheum 29:**1322-1333, 1986

CHAPTER 26

WORKERS' COMPENSATION: THE ROLE OF THE PHYSICIAN

JANIE R. VALE, MD, MSPH

Protecting the health and safety of the worker and the community is the primary concern.

The role of the physician engaged in a workers' compensation claim is to provide medical evaluation, treatment, and direction of rehabilitative services for the employee who has sustained a work-related injury or illness. In general, state and federal workers' compensation laws require the physician to provide care within his or her scope of training, clinical experience, and as covered by licensure. Further, it is the physician's responsibility to monitor the worker on a periodic basis to assess and document compliance and response to the treatment plan and to revise the diagnosis and treatment plan as clinically indicated.

In addition to providing medical care, the physician should determine and document whether the employee is able to work in his or her regular position, is able to work in a modified duty or capacity, or is entirely unable to work. The physician should also provide a "best guess" as to the projected period of time that the injured/ill employee will be not able to work or will be on restricted duty. In general, an employee cannot return to work when any of the following conditions are present: the patient is hospitalized, confined to bed rest, or taking medication required for treatment which affects functional capacities (e.g., narcotics, mood-altering drugs, or medications with adverse side effects such as chemotherapy agents used in the treatment of occupational cancers); driving or riding to get to and from work is contraindicated by the nature of the medical condition; the patient is infectious to others or is so compromised that exposure to others would be potentially harmful (e.g., burns, infected wounds, or some occupational lung diseases); or when working even in a modified capacity could adversely affect the results of medical and/or surgical treatment, or if the injured/ill worker presents a safety risk to self or others. It must be realized that in some environmental exposure cases simply re-entering the offending work environment could result in exacerbation or progression of the occupational illness.

The physician must document the worker's description of the mechanism of the reported injury or illness. The physician must also state whether there is a linkage between the workplace and the condition diagnosed "within a reasonable degree of medical certainty" (which implies a 90% or greater level of confidence) or "within a reasonable degree of medical probability" (which requires a decision accuracy of only 51%). Therefore, the physician must carefully qualify their written or verbal responses concerning causality with quantitative differences in mind. Determining this linkage is a unique physician responsibility when caring for a patient in the workers' compensation system. A causality determination, as this linkage is often termed, should never be taken lightly as it may have a profound impact on the medical care provided to the worker and on economic, legal, and vocational outcomes for the worker, as well as for the employer and society.[23]

The determination of whether the medical complaint or finding is truly derived from or aggravated by factors in the workplace is the causality determination. The physician must correlate or exclude the relationship of probable or certain effect of the workplace exposure with the probable or certain diagnosis. In many cases that do not involve straightforward, witnessed trauma, the worker/patient history is simply not adequate. Quantitative information, in addition to qualitative information, must be obtained. There must be corroboration of the workplace exposure(s) by the employer, or, if not available in a timely manner, by review of the accident/incident investigation findings, by review of previous industrial hygiene data, by review of the essential job functions, or by direct physician worksite evaluation. Put more simply: If A is an exposure cause or aggravation, and if B is a medical condition or diagnosis, are A and B related? And if A and B are related, did A exist in the workplace? The physician must rely on his or her training to make the causality determination and to render opinions in the framework of decision accuracy (e.g., a 90% confidence level is *certain*, 51% is *probable*, and a confidence level lower than 51% is *possible*).

If the physician makes a false positive causality determination, the worker may be deprived of or be directed away from further indicated nonworkplace-related medical evaluation. If a false negative determination is made, the worker may continue in a job and experience resultant continuing injury and aggravation which may have been preventable. The physician can standardize his or her approach to causality determination by answering the "Work-Relatedness Criteria Questions" in Table 1.[14] Obtaining the information necessary to answer these questions will provide direction in those cases where cause and effect are unclear or may be challenged at some future date.

If the physician is unable to render an opinion as to causality because of lack of objective information or individual expertise or experience, he or she should request the needed information and/or make the appropriate referrals. In the interim, it is always best to render the opinion of "undetermined" causality rather than having to explain or justify a change of opinion at a later time. All information about the workplace used in causality determinations should be reviewed with the injured or ill worker before rendering an opinion in order to feel confident that all parties are in agreement with the accuracy of the information.[14] The physician, however, must be prepared to use his

TABLE 1

WORK-RELATEDNESS CRITERIA QUESTIONS

Injury
1. Are the symptoms consistent with the history of the mechanism of injury?
2. Are signs and diagnostic studies consistent with the injury?
3. Does workplace incident investigation support the history and diagnosis?
4. Is there a lack of non-workplace activities and incidents to cause injury?

Illness
1. Are the symptoms consistent with the diagnosis?
2. Are the signs consistent with the diagnosis?
3. Do diagnostic studies confirm/support the diagnosis?
4. Is the temporal relationship of exposure and disease clear?
5. Do fellow workers with similar exposures have similar symptoms?
6. Is workplace monitoring data available and indicative of suspected exposure?
7. Is the condition biologically plausible and confirmed?
8. Is there a lack of non-occupational exposure to the toxin?

or her best judgment in those situations where there is disagreement among the involved parties as to what is and is not factual. Significant misunderstanding and lack of expertise exist as relates to causality determination. Educational courses are needed not only for physicians who have the primary responsibility in rendering opinions as to causation, but also for adjusters, adjudicators, attorneys, and legislators.[15]

When caring for a patient in the workers' compensation system, it is the physician's responsibility to determine when no further medical treatment is indicated. At the time of maximum medical improvement, the physician must address the worker's permanent functional capabilities. The physician must also render a knowledgeable opinion as to whether or not a permanent impairment has been sustained and whether or not special or accommodated work conditions need to be considered. The complexities of the physician's role in impairment determination will be discussed in greater detail later, in the impairment section. Opinion is also to be given as to whether or not future medical care or monitoring is indicated to maintain function or to minimize projected future functional change associated with progression of the condition. The physician must possess expertise in ergonomic assessment and management of the workplace, worker accommodation options, and vocational rehabilitation to optimally address these issues. As in all professional settings, if the physician is not comfortable in such decision-making, the specific reasons for needing more information should be outlined and recommendations be made for referral to the appropriately skilled resource.[3]

During all phases of the physician's care of the workplace-injured or ill worker, communication and documentation are critical. Any delays in transmitting objective information in terms that are understandable to the non-physician will only guarantee delays in authorization for treatment, delays in delivery of compensation benefits to the worker, and "delayed recovery" of the worker. Ideally, in our current technological age, it is best to send reports via secured fax to all parties as quickly as possible. Whatever method is selected for report sending, the physician should have an operational system for notification of receipt of information. The ability to document

TABLE 2

EMPLOYER CHECK LIST FOR SELECTING AND EVALUATING A PHYSICIAN PROVIDER IN WORKERS' COMPENSATION CASES

1. Credentials for provision of services that are anticipated to be needed.
2. Experience and familiarity with the workers' compensation system.
3. Accountability for what happens to the worker when he or she enters the provider system and continued accountability if referred.
4. Thorough workups to establish differential diagnoses and etiology(ies).
5. Cooperation of the provider and support staff in the flow of information. This includes timely reporting and communication of pertinent medical information, and the willingness to address issues of noncompliance and specific return to work planning.
6. Cost-effective case management.
7. Quality of care and ethical practice style.
8. Established provider networks for anticipated needed expertise.

the timely delivery of medical opinion confirms the physician's commitment to meet the professional and ethical responsibilities as a "patient advocate." Such documentation also prevents the physician from being the target of allegations of not cooperating or of adding costs to the system because of not communicating. All too often, forwarded physician reports are misplaced or lost within the system.[3]

Physicians choosing to provide services to occupationally injured or ill patients should evaluate themselves through the eyes of the employer before entering what is, and will continue to be, a complex medical-legal-administrative system. The physician must be able to respond positively, without reservation or hesitation, to the "Employer Check List for Selecting and Evaluating a Physician Provider in Workers' Compensation Cases" (Table 2). If the physician is unable to respond positively to the eight points covered, he or she should elect nonparticipation or obtain the necessary additional training, skills, and experience.

It is important for the physician to remember

that his or her professional activities in a workers' compensation claim must be accomplished in a legislated administrative system in which multiple parties have an interest. The parties include not only the patient/worker and the physician, but also the employer, insurance representatives, lawyers, union representatives, the worker's family, coworkers, workers' compensation administrators, and society as a whole.[34] It goes without saying that these parties more often than not have varying goals and expectations for case resolution. The physician practicing within this arena must constantly remember that the long-term goal is prevention of workplace injury and illness and the delivery of the highest quality of medical care in a cost-effective manner. In addition, the physician should be proactive in workers' compensation legal reform.

Once the physician becomes a service provider within the workers' compensation system, he or she must strive to provide input regarding prevention strategies that may decrease or eliminate the risk of workplace injury and illness. Although this activity would appear on the surface to be obvious and respected, it can be fraught with controversy. Primary and secondary workplace prevention requires employers and their representatives to accept that the workplace does present potentially adverse health and safety exposures to the workforce. To implement corrective actions requires commitment of financial resources and management time. Also, during the improvement phase, employers may increase their potential "exposure" to citations and litigation, as well as experience increased reporting of workers' compensation claims.

For the physician to make an informed decision about whether or not to enter or to continue professional participation in the various workers' compensation systems, it is helpful to understand the historical perspectives and basic internal workings of workers' compensation. It is also necessary to appreciate the relationship of workers' compensation to other "systems" directly affecting physician practice, such as the Americans With Disabilities Act, the Family and Medical Leave Act, and the Occupational Safety and Health Act. The following section provides an overview of these topics.

WORKERS' COMPENSATION: A HISTORICAL OVERVIEW

Throughout history, various societies have formed their own unique workers' compensation systems.

Workers' compensation systems actually predate the time of Hippocrates (460-377BC), the father of modern medicine.[33] The first Workers' Compensation system was recorded between 1945BC and 1902BC during the reign of Hammurabi. The Code of Hammurabi included monetary payments for injuries plus an "eye for an eye and a tooth for a tooth" reimbursement formula. The Bible outlines that payment must be made for loss of time due to injury (Exodus 21:18-19). In addition, the responsible party "shall have him [the injured party] thoroughly healed." The Romans required employers and slave owners to care for their injured workers. In about 1000AD, guilds were formed to protect workers. By the 1700s, pirates had implemented a payment system for the loss of body parts. Of interest, the loss of a hand by a pirate was not considered compensable, as a hook was perceived to enhance the pirate's ability to engage in battle and did not represent a loss for generating income.[5]

A comprehensive social insurance system that included workers' compensation was introduced in Germany in the 1880s by Otto Von Bismarck. The workers' compensation component was compulsory and was administered by the government. In contrast to current practice in the United States, workers contributed financially to the fund. At the same time in England, the Employer's Liability Act, which eliminated the issues of contributory negligence and assumption of risk, set the framework for the British Workers' Compensation Law of 1887. Interestingly, in 1907, Russia implemented a schedule relating injuries and physical impairment to a percentage of total disability; disability was determined based on lost earning capacity and was adjusted based upon specific job requirements. This system served as the model for the California Industrial Accident Act of 1914.

The growth of industrialization in America during the late 19th and early 20th centuries resulted in ever-increasing numbers and severity of injuries and fatalities in the workplaces of the U.S. Legal remedies for workers and their dependents were limited to tort or breach-of-contract lawsuits. The tort system, by this time, was viewed as unsatisfactory for dispute resolution in work injury cases by almost all parties involved. Adequate legal recourse for workers was further limited by the following common law tort rules:[8,35]

1. The "Fellow Servant" rule created an exception to the general rule that the master is liable for the wrongful acts of a servant if the servant's action resulted in injury to a fellow servant. The injured servant was to obtain redress from the offending servant. Therefore, the employer was not legally responsible if the actions of one employee resulted in injury to a coworker.
2. The "Assumption of Risk" doctrine prevented the recovery of damages if the injured party accepted the risk of foreseeable injury. This was interpreted by the courts to mean that the worker could not recover for injuries from unknown hazards in the workplace, because he or she was free not to enter a potentially hazardous work environment.
3. Under the "Contributory Negligence" defense rule, if the worker's action in any way contributed to his or her injury, the employer was free of responsibility.

The courts' interpretation of these rules, at that time, placed the significant time and financial burden of proving that the employer was negligent on the worker or his or her survivor.[36] If, by luck or chance, the worker was granted a favorable ruling it was not unusual for the worker's lawyer to receive over half of any award as the fee for services provided.[12] Even in modern times, it is often shown that the legally represented worker will receive lower net recoveries than the nonrepresented worker.[29]

In 1910, New York became the first state to pass workers' compensation legislation. Other states followed suit only to have their efforts blocked by the courts, which ruled that these bills blocked the employers' right to property without due process of the law, a violation of the Fourteenth Amendment. The opinions of the courts were changed dramatically by public outcry after 145 workers died from a tragic workplace fire at the Triangle Shirt Waist Com-

pany in 1917. Following this incident, the U.S. Supreme Court ruled that it was within the constitutional interpretation that states may balance the workers' right to health and welfare and the employers' right to due process.

Between 1910 and 1949, all states passed legislation defining a "no fault" worker compensation system with benefits to all parties. The worker no longer had to prove employer negligence and was provided with assurance of some financial recovery. The employer was no longer at risk of being found "at fault," and no longer at risk of having to pay large awards for such things as pain and suffering. Finally, society was no longer left with the burden of providing medical and financial support for injured workers and their dependents. However, it must be understood that employers do pass the cost of supporting a mandated compensation system on to society through increased costs of products and services. Also, those states that do not legislate for the provision of retraining or vocational placement of the permanently impaired worker leave a costly burden to society.

Funding for state workers' compensation is legislated to be the employer's responsibility. In general, employers are required by state law to assure that they can meet the financial responsibilities of workers' compensation, as a matter of doing business in a given state. Employers can purchase insurance policies or become self-insured. In both situations, they are required to maintain adequate reserves and solvency.[8]

Over time, case law and legislation expanded the scope of workers' compensation. In addition to covering workplace traumatic injuries, benefits were extended to workplace aggravation of pre-existing medical conditions if the aggravation was deemed related to workplace activities. States also began to recognize occupational diseases as compensable, as epidemiology proved that workplace exposures did, in fact, result in specific illnesses. In 1917, Massachusetts and California were the first states to acknowledge occupational disease. By 1976, all states provided at least some occupational disease coverage. States usually publish a list of covered occupational diseases and, in addition, will provide compensation benefits if it can be shown that the condition is "peculiar to an industrial trade or process." However, there continues to be a gross under-reporting of occupational diseases because of lack of physician understanding of workplace exposure and the often long latencies for disease development. Also, workers' compensation reports provide very inadequate tools for workplace exposure surveillance. In addition, there are significant deficiencies in case definitions.[4,26]

The adjudication of occupational disease cases also reflects a deficient legal-administrative knowledge base. Of interest, 60% of disease claims are initially denied, while only 10% of injury claims are denied.[26]

The Missouri Court of Appeals has ruled that a "disorder is compensable if the employee has had exposure at work greater than or different from that of the general public, and if there is a recognizable link between the disorder and some distinctive feature of the employee's job that is common to all jobs of that type." Further, most states have adopted a "discovery rule" that allows claims if filed in a timely manner within a certain number of years of the occupational disease diagnosis and the determination of the potential work relatedness.[19] Although not accepted in all states, workers' compensation coverage for the cumulative development of conditions, particularly of the upper extremities, has emerged over the past decade. The current reporting of repetitive motion disorders represented nearly 63% of the occupational illnesses reported in 1992. In addition, repetitive motion disorders led all conditions in lost days from work and length of recuperation.[32]

Federal legislation has been passed to cover special groups of workers. Although most physicians deal with state workers' compensation systems on a more regular basis, the first official national program in the U.S. was passed in 1908. The Federal Employees' Compensation Act (FECA) of 1916 was a no-fault system covering employees of common carriers engaged in interstate and foreign commerce. Employees of the U.S. government are still covered under this law.[36] Under this act, workers found guilty of violating safety statutes lose their right to compensation.

Additional legislation covers other special groups of workers. The Longshoremen's and Harbor Workers' Compensation Act, passed in 1927, applies to private and public maritime workers. It is commonly known as the Jones Act.[6] The Federal Mine Safety and Health Act of 1977 provides workers' compensation coverage to the nation's miners, millers, and ancillary personnel.[26] Railroad workers are covered under the Federal Employees Liability Act (FELA).[23]

Physicians should be aware that, in the federal workers' compensation system, the employee has the burden of proving that the disability claim is causally related to an injury sustained in the performance of duty or that an occupational disease is causally related to employment. This is strikingly different than state-legislated systems where, in general, the laws are supportive of the employee and the employer must effectively challenge a claim to deny responsibility. A federal employee must submit reliable and substantial medical evidence for his or her claim. Medical evidence must be in writing, and the quality of the documentation of the injury or illness, not the quantity of the report, is essential. Claims are routinely denied if the medical evidence is absent or weak in causation determination. Also, medical evidence plays a key role in the continuation of benefits.

Today only about 12% to 14% of the civilian workforce is not covered by some type of workers' compensation. The three main categories of workers not covered include: agricultural workers, domestic workers, and employees of firms with fewer than three employees. It is basically impossible to review or comment on the workers' compensation law of each individual state, because legislation and adjudication decisions result in annual or even more frequent minor and, at times, fundamental changes.[21] The "Analysis of Workers' Compensation Laws" is published by the U.S. Chamber of Commerce and provides a concise summary of each state's benefits. This resource can be ordered from the following address: Publications, U.S. Chamber of Commerce, 1615 H Street NW, Washington, DC 20062 (telephone 1-800-638-6582 or 1-202-659-6000).

In 1970, nearly 14,000 workers were killed on the job annually, and it is reported that over 2 million workers annually suffered a disabling injury. This represented a 29% increase in workplace accident rates between 1961 and 1970.[18] In response, the U.S. Congress overwhelmingly passed the Occupational Safety and Health Act

TABLE 3

THE IDEAL WORKERS' COMPENSATION SYSTEM

1. Provides sure, prompt, and reasonable income and medical benefits to work-accident victims, or income benefits to their dependents, regardless of fault.
2. Provides a single remedy and reduces court delays, costs, and workloads arising out of personal injury litigation.
3. Relieves public and private charities of financial drains (incidental to uncompensated industrial accidents).
4. Eliminates payment of fees to lawyers and witnesses, as well as time-consuming trials and appeals.
5. Encourages maximum employer interest in safety and rehabilitation through an appropriate experience-rating mechanism.
6. Promotes frank study of causes of accidents (rather than concealment of fault), reducing preventable accidents and human suffering.

of 1970, establishing the Occupational Safety and Health Administration (OSHA). The "general duty clause" of the act required employers to provide "a place of employment which is free from recognized hazards that are causing or are likely to cause death or serious physical harm to employees."

In 1972, OSHA formed a National Commission to study workers' compensation systems in the United States.[35] The Commission recommended full coverage for all work-related injuries and illnesses, medical and rehabilitation services, and increased levels of compensation. The impact of the commission's report was to move workers' compensation into an era of legal redefinition. The ideal system for states required the six basic considerations outlined in Table 3.[3]

The physician must understand that despite workers' compensation systems in general being "no fault," employers convicted of willful violation involving the death or serious injury of a worker or workers may face criminal charges with fines and/or imprisonment.[4,26] Also, the workers' compensation remedy is not exclusive and tort liability is possible if the worker's injury was caused by a deliberate and intentional act by the employer. This situation pro-

vides the employee recourse under the "intentional tort exception."[19] More recent legislation in many states also relieves the employer of responsibility to the injured worker if injury occurred during the act of violating a law or if the employee was functionally impaired by the use of illegal drugs or alcohol. Special denial categories apply in some states if injuries result from willful misconduct, self-inflicted injury, or if the injury occurred during horseplay.

WORKERS' COMPENSATION TERMINOLOGY

Effective communication is the key to successful professional participation in the various workers' compensation systems. Physicians must translate and communicate medical terminology and concepts to the many nonmedically trained participants in the workers' compensation system. However, the physician must also have a clear understanding of the terminology of the workers' compensation system. If the physician does not have a clear understanding of the following terms and does not use them correctly, significant confusion will result which can adversely affect injured or ill workers and the equitable resolution of their workers' compensation cases. Not understanding what these terms mean can also result in delay, even nonpayment, for physician services.

Accident—a sudden, traumatic, and unexpected incident.

Accommodation—a legal and administrative term referring to modifications in a job, the workplace, or the environment. Accommodation allows a disabled individual to meet the same job demands and conditions of employment required of any other employee in the same or similar job.[2]

Apportionment—concerns the decision regarding the degree to which an occupational disorder is affected by either workplace or nonworkplace exposures or conditions.[10] Thus, there is a division of responsibility between different employers/insurers or between one employer/insurer and the private resources of the affected worker. Only impairment, NOT causation, is apportioned.

Medical decision-making, as it relates to apportionment, is extremely difficult, particularly if the current treating physician or the physician rendering an opinion has not examined the worker prior to the recent accident or exposure, does not have access to previous medical documentation of the pre-existing findings and functional status of the worker, or if the medical records are of insufficient detail to be of assistance.

Causation—a term involving the determination of whether a job activity or work injury actually caused an impairment.[8]

Disability—a legal and administrative term. As defined by the American Medical Association (AMA), disability is "a decrease in, or the loss or absence of the capacity of an individual to meet personal, social or occupational demands, or to meet statutory or regulatory requirements."[2] Disability represents the gap between what an individual can do physically and what a specific job requires. As a legal term, its determination is unique to a given workers' compensation jurisdiction. In addition to medical findings, other factors that can affect disability include age, gender, education, and training, as well as the economic and social environments.

"Permanent Partial Disability"—a term used to describe a person able to return to work but functionally limited as a result of the injury.[24] Although state laws vary, benefits generally provide a percentage of the difference between pre-injury wages and the wages of the functionally modified position if those wages are lower. Scheduled compensation is also provided in many states for permanent loss of a body part. Permanent partial disability will usually take into consideration the worker's age, education, training, vocational experience, transferable skills, and general health in addition to functional limitations resulting from a specific occupational injury or illness.

"Permanent Total Disability"—a term used to describe a person who is unable to return to any gainful employment as a result of the occupational injury.[24] Benefits may include a percentage of wages for the worker's lifetime or a maximum settlement. Examples of permanent total disability injuries include total loss of vision, loss of two or more limbs, and quadriplegia.

"Temporary Partial Disability"—a term used to define a person as temporarily unable to perform full duties, but one who can perform some work.[24] It is important for the physician to understand that, depending on the laws applying to a given case, compensation payments can be terminated to the worker if he or she is released to modified duty, even if such modified duty is not provided by the employer. The physician must be knowledgeable about the laws of the individual state.

"Temporary Total Disability"—a term describing a person who is temporarily unable to work, but for whom full recovery and return to work is anticipated. Most states pay a percentage of full pay up to a maximum amount determined by laws. Many states require a three to seven day period of lost time before benefits are initiated.[24]

Employability—a term used to indicate that an individual is capable of meeting the demands of a job as defined by the employer, with or without accommodation.[2]

Exacerbation—most commonly a term used to imply a temporary appearance or manifestation of previous injury, while "reinjury" or "aggravation" usually implies a new or different exposure producing additional impairment to the previously affected anatomic region. The impairment will be compensable if the work put the individual at a risk greater than the general public. The physician may be presented with the phrase "aroused into disabling reality" as applied to a work-related injury that results in a pre-existing dormant or active condition becoming disabling.[8,19]

Fraud and *Abuse*—"fraud" is a false statement, willfully made for material gain, with the intent to deceive. "Abuse" is an exaggerated statement, willfully made for material gain, with the intent to confuse.[27] Each year, more states pass legislation related to fraud and abuse within the workers' compensation system. The penalties for fraud and abuse apply to all parties involved in the system and are generally severe. Physicians should be cognizant of this and at all times practice and bill in accordance with the standards and ethics of their profession. Physicians should be aware that the courts are permitting plaintiffs to sue physicians who are knowledgeable of the presence of workplace-related disease and fraudulently conceal that fact from workers.[19]

Functional Capacity Evaluation—a systematic process of measuring an individual's capacity to dependably sustain performance in response to broadly defined work demands. A functional capacity evaluation requires maximum voluntary effort on the part of the individual being tested. If the effort is less than necessary for task performance, it must be determined if the effort is because of a biomechanical, cardiovascular, metabolic limit, or the individual's own voluntary limits.

Handicap—an "impairment that substantially limits one or more of life's activities."[2] An individual is also considered handicapped if there is a record of an activity-limiting impairment or the individual is regarded as having such an impairment.

Impairment—a medical term which is to be assessed by medical means. According to the AMA *Guides,*[2] an impairment is "a deviation from normal in a body part or organ system and its functioning." Impairment is further defined by the World Health Organization as "any loss or abnormality of psychological, physiological, or anatomical structure or function." It is, in general, assumed that an impairment will have an affect on activities of daily living. According to the AMA *Guides*, a "permanent impairment" is one that "has become static or stabilized during a period of time sufficient to allow optimal tissue repair and that is unlikely to change in spite of further medical or surgical therapy."

Maximum Medical Improvement—the point in time when the physician determines that further medical evaluation and treatment will not significantly affect the further recovery of the injured or ill worker. Basically, it is the time of stabilization of the medical condition.[24]

Probative Value—applies primarily to FECA claims. It is the "value" of evidence in serving to prove a particular fact or contention. Determination of probative value requires physician opinion and sound medical reasoning. The terms "might be," "may be," and "could be" lack probative value since they are considered speculative or conjecture and so are essentially worthless when used in medical opinions.

Second Injury Fund—a term used in non-apportionment states. It allows a worker who previously was partially disabled and then is further disabled by a work-related injury or illness to receive additional compensation to make up for the level of overall or actual total disability. For example, if a worker had previously lost vision in one eye and had been determined to have 24% impairment of the total body and then lost sight in the other eye, he or she would be eligible to receive an additional 24% impairment rating. However, in most states, the worker would now be considered at permanent total disability. The Second Injury Fund would make up the difference between the 24% + 24 % = 48% and the (actual) 100% award. The philosophical goal of the Second Injury Fund is to encourage employers to hire individuals with existing disabilities by decreasing the associated potential financial risk.[23]

Weight of the Evidence—applies primarily to FECA claims. This implies that the "quality" of the medical specialist's report has more weight than that of the general practitioner.

Workers' Compensation Disease—medical evidence must show that the disease was caused by the duties of the affected worker's employment and that it did not result from conditions or activities to which the worker was exposed outside of his or her employment.[10] This condition usually develops over time. If possible, it is extremely important for the physician to provide information concerning the source, amount, volume, density, and duration of the exposure(s) as well as the time frame for onset of signs and symptoms.

Workers' Compensation Injury—injury or death that "arises out of and in the course of employment."[36] It is of interest that this phrase dates back to the British Workers' Compensation Act of 1887.[10] In general, the injury must have occurred within the time of employment, at a place where the employee should reasonably be during work, and while performing a task that was the duty of employment or something incidental to it.[30]

Work Disability—as defined by the Centers for Disease Control, it is the inability to perform work due to a physical, mental, or other health condition of six months duration or longer. If severe, no work of any type can be performed, while if non-severe, it limits the amount and type of work that can be performed. In general, incidences of work disability declined between 1980 and 1990. However there were significant prevalence rate and trend differences among states.[22]

RELATIONSHIP OF WORKERS' COMPENSATION TO OTHER LEGISLATION

The physician involved in medical management of the worker who has sustained a work-related injury or illness must be familiar with the Americans With Disabilities Act of 1990 and the Family and Medical Leave Act of 1993.

Americans With Disabilities Act

The purpose of the Americans With Disabilies Act (ADA) of 1990 is to mainstream persons with impairments into society. Title 1 of the ADA applies specifically to employment and prohibits discrimination in employment against "qualified individuals with disabilities." The Equal Employment Opportunity Commission (EEOC) is responsible for the enforcement of the Act. Individuals are defined as having disabilities if they have:[10]

1. a physical or mental impairment that substantially; limits one or more of the major life activities;
2. a record of such an impairment; and
3. have been regarded as having an impairment.

The EEOC defines a physical impairment as a "physiologic disorder or condition, cosmetic disfiguration, or an anatomical loss affecting one or more of the following body systems: neurological, musculoskeletal, special sense organ, respiratory including speech organs, cardiovascular, reproductive, digestive, genitourinary, hematological or lymphatic, skin and endocrine." Mental impairment is defined as any mental or psychological disorder such as mental retardation, organic brain syndrome, emotional or mental illness, or specific learning disabilities.

It is imperative for physicians to understand that when the patient/worker they treated under workers' compensation reaches maximum medical improvement and is determined to have a residual impairment rating, he or she may then also be deemed by the EEOC to be a "qualified individual" under the ADA. In fact, in the first year of experience under the ADA, 80% of ADA claims involved injured workers rather than individuals seeking employment.[35] Having been awarded an impairment/disability determination does not guarantee coverage under this legislation. This is obviously confusing to the physician, as well as the worker. The impairment must limit *substantially* one or more major life activities. These major life activities include hearing, seeing, walking, breathing, performing manual tasks, caring for oneself, learning, or working. Being unable to perform one specific job or the job that the worker was performing at the time of the incident or exposure does not necessarily mean that the worker cannot work. A unique twist to workers' compensation cases has occurred in that, "An injured employee who claims to be totally and permanently disabled for purposes of determining the amount of workers' compensation benefits due may still be capable (or be made capable with a reasonable accommodation) of performing all the essential job functions of the employee's current job or a vacant position."[16] Reasonable accommodation is only required if making the accommodation would not result in an "undue hardship" to the employer. Although undue hardship is left up to case-by-case ruling, the accommodation will be considered necessary unless it is unduly costly, extensive, substantial, disruptive, or would alter the nature or the operation of the business.

Therefore, the physician must have the clinical competency to render an objective opinion as to the worker's ability to perform the essential job functions of a given position or positions. The employer must define the essential job functions, not the employee or the physician. The physician should expect to have more than a job description when requested to render a professional opinion as to an individual's ability or inability to perform an essential job function. Ideally, the physician should know the MET level (MET level is defined as multiples of resting metabolic energy used for any given activity; one MET equals 3.5 ml [/kg/min] oxygen consumption) or equivalent requirement of the task, the postures involved, the spine and extremity exertional limits, and be aware of known or possible emergency situations in which the individual's impairment might prevent or delay his or her safe escape. The ADA does allow for evaluations to be performed to determine the worker's current "fitness" to perform specific essential job functions. Such evaluations and their associated functional measurements can assist the physician in rendering opinions as to impairment and the necessity for accommodation.

In addition, the physician may be asked by the worker or the employer for accommodation recommendations. A unique component of the ADA is the opportunity for the qualified individual to make his or her own suggestions as to how the essential job functions could be modified to allow successful employment, as well as to participate in the cost of the accommodation.

A final responsibility of the physician under the ADA is to determine and record when a "direct threat" situation exists. A direct threat is defined as a significant risk of substantial harm to the health and safety of the individual or others which cannot be eliminated or reduced by accommodation. The physician must be able to identify the specific risk and state that the risk is current and is not based on general fears about the risk. The physician may be required to address the nature and severity of the potential harm, the imminence of the harm, and the expected duration of the risk.[1]

Although confidentiality of medical records is a usual consideration, the ADA does allow for medical information obtained in the course of a post-offer, pre-placement examination to be made available in order to make employment decisions otherwise within the scope of the ADA requirements. Under the ADA, medical examinations can only be performed after an offer of employment has been made. The medical records, however, must be kept separate from general personnel records and in confidential medical files. The ADA does, however, allow these medical files to be provided to state workers' compensation administrators, state Second Injury Fund offices, and workers' compensation insurance carriers if this is also in accordance with individual state workers' compensation laws.[13]

TABLE 4

ADA RESOURCES

The President's Committee on
 Employment of People with Disabilities
1331 F Street NW
Washington, DC 20004
(telephone 202-376-6200)

The U.S. Equal Employment
 Opportunity Commission
1801 L Street NW
Washington, DC 20507
(telephone 800-669-3362)

Job Accommodation Network
West Virginia University
918 Chestnut Ridge Road, Suite 1
P.O. Box 6080
Morgantown, WV 26506-6080
(telephone 800-232-9675)

Physicians providing care to injured and ill workers should keep up-to-date information as to the trends in adjudication relating to ADA claims. They should also have resources available to inform their patients of their rights under the ADA and how to seek assistance in learning about accommodation options. Table 4 provides a listing of such resources.[13]

Family and Medical Leave Act

The Family and Medical Leave Act (FMLA) of 1993 applies to employers with 50 or more employees. The FMLA mandates job protection for 12 weeks of unpaid leave per year for eligible employees to care for a newborn; care for a newly adopted or foster child; care for a sick parent, spouse, or child; or for the employee's own serious health conditions. The FMLA can complicate the medical, legal and administrative management of a workers' compensation case in that it exempts the worker from having to work with or without restrictions while on FMLA-covered leave. It also may exempt the worker from keeping medical appointments or participating in the rehabilitation plan for his or her work-related injury or illness.

Physicians increasingly are requested by their patients to provide medical documentation stating the necessity for them to provide care to family members, often when it is unclear that the medical situation demands the worker to be off work to provide care or that their own medical conditions are of a severity to preclude the performance of work activities. At the end of their FMLA-covered leave period, workers may make demands upon the workers' compensation system for additional time off from work, modified work, and/or resumption of medical care for the work-related injuries or illnesses.

Mental Stress Claims

In the 1980s, prior to the enactment of the ADA and FMLA legislation, other new issues were beginning to have a significant impact on work-related claims. For example, in California, "mental stress" claims doubled between 1980 and 1982, while other claims decreased by 10%.[9] As was the situation in occupational disease claims, there were and continue to be variances in the interpretation and acceptance of stress claims on a state-by-state basis. These claims were soon categorized as follows: mental-physical, physical-mental, and mental-mental (vide infra).[35]

"Mental-physical" claims allege that various job stressors such as prolonged mandatory overtime, frequent lay-offs, management-union conflict, or worker nonparticipation in decision-making result in physical illness such as hypertension, coronary artery disease, alcoholism, and ulcer disease. The Occupational Health and Safety Act of 1970, in Sections 20 (a)(1) and 20(a)(4), directed the National Institute for Occupational Safety and Health (NIOSH), an agency of the U.S. Department of Health and Human Services, to include psychological, behavioral, and motivational factors in worker health and safety research. NIOSH responded not only by conducting extensive research on workplace stress, but also by proposing national strategies for the prevention of work-related psychological disorders. The research of NIOSH and others has resulted in the majority of states accepting mental-physical claims.

The physician involved in the care of the worker who experiences an occupational mental-physical disorder must understand that acceptance of such claims by the employer and/or its representative may be challenged despite state workers' compensation laws that allow for such coverage. The physician may expect multiple inquiries as to causality, as well as challenges to the physician's ability to understand the organizational structure and production demands of the workplace. While challenging the diagnostic impression of the physician, the employer may also block access to the necessary information to substantiate the diagnosis, leaving the physician with only the history as provided by the worker. In these and the other types of stress claims to be discussed, the physician must never lose sight of the responsibility to function as a "patient advocate." Also, the physician must realize that if stressors in the workplace are not addressed, the ill worker may have unnecessary progression of his or her medical condition(s) or other workers may suffer a similar fate.

A "physical-mental" claim is based on the assumption that a physical injury results in a mental disorder. A post-traumatic stress disorder is one of the best examples. In most cases, a particularly traumatic event (such as being shot during a robbery while working as a convenience store clerk) results in obvious objective injury (for instance, the gunshot resulting in a splenic laceration necessitating surgical splenectomy). As the worker begins to recover from the physical injuries, he or she experiences profound emotional difficulties including sleep disturbance and dreams about the event, is afraid of returning to the scene, and has altered relationships with friends, relatives, and the employer. In these situations, the medical care needed to appropriately diagnosis and treat the psychological injury may be far more extensive and costly than the physical injuries, and often produces less satisfactory "healing." In less dramatic scenarios, the worker will have sustained a workplace injury, and recovery will be delayed by mood disorders such as depression or anxiety or the exacerbation or progression of a pre-existing personality disorder or psychosis. The physician caring for such an injured worker may meet firm opposition to requests for psychological testing and treatment. The physician may then be confronted with the almost impossible situation of directing the rehabilitation of the worker who does not have the psychological stability to comply with and achieve treatment and return-to-work goals. In these situations, the physician must fully document diagnostic impressions and how these impressions were reached, as well as pursue avenues available within the system to assist the worker. If all efforts fail, it may be in the best interest of the patient to suggest that the patient obtain legal representation, if not already secured. During the case review process, the physician must be willing to review any and all medical or other documentation of pre-existing medical conditions and other potential nonwork-related etiologies of the observed mental status changes.

A "mental-mental" claim alleges that job-related stressors have resulted in an emotional disorder which, in turn, exacerbates or less frequently results in the worker being diagnosed with new psychopathology. Mental-mental claims are extremely difficult for the nonmedical community to understand and are almost never accepted without significant challenge by employers, their representatives, and often the workers' compensation administration. In these cases, the nonpsychiatric physician will best serve the medical care needs of the patient by early referral to a psychiatrist or psychologist with special interests and expertise in rendering objective opinions in such cases. Again, the needs of the ill worker are best served by meticulous attention to documentation.

Psychiatric Illness

In considering the implications of each of these three categories, the physician treating the injured or ill worker must be aware that in a published review of workers' compensation care that could not be resolved in the usual and customary time frame, 86% of the workers involved were found to have psychiatric illness. These workers had been off work for an average of 41.5 months, yet the original work incident had been considered "minor" in the majority of cases. Interestingly, a mean of 32 months had elapsed before a psychological assessment had been requested.

The diagnosis of depression was found to be the most common emotional illness.[16]

Additional studies suggest that a small group of workers' compensation patients suffer from pre-existing mental illness and account for substantial expenditures through increased claims and lost time from work. Physicians involved in these time- and energy-consuming cases must remember that, in most situations, the impaired worker will have demonstrated job performance problems or difficulties in interacting with coworkers and management prior to the claim for compensation. The physician must always remember that a pill, a shot, a diagnostic study, or even the most carefully and compassionately outlined and delivered care plan will not turn a bad worker into a good worker.

The use and abuse of alcohol and illicit drugs is obviously a psychological dysfunction. Injured and ill workers covered under workers' compensation are in no way immune from these problems. The physician involved in the care of the ill and injured worker must be cognizant of the possible impact of alcohol and /or illicit drug use contributing to the work-related injury. Despite many states having legislated limitations on employer workers' compensation responsibility if substance use contributes to a workplace injury, if the employer does not have a written and conspicuously-posted policy on substance use, the use of restricted substances by an injured employee usually will not be enough to reduce or relieve the financial responsibilities of the employer under workers' compensation. In addition, most state laws require the employer to demonstrate that the worker was observed to be impaired and not adequately performing essential job functions at the time of the incident and that the substance usage was contributory to the incident. The physician must therefore be prepared and willing to obtain or appropriately refer the injured or ill worker for drug and alcohol testing, often even prior to the initial examination, unless delay would result in further harm to the worker. The physician, however, must be knowledgeable of the specific requirements and coverage for such testing under the workers' compensation system applicable to the situation.

The same significant difficulties arise in the medical management of a worker's compensation case if there are psychosocial factors contributing to delayed recovery or noncompliance with the medical care plan. Employers and insurers often do not want to accept the costs of evaluation and treatment of these co-morbidity conditions. Therefore, it is up to the physician to educate and convince all parties involved that if these factors are not dealt with, the resolution of the case will be adversely affected. A very important and often overlooked issue is the responsibility of the physician to protect public safety if the chemically or psychologically impaired worker's essential job function affects the welfare of the public (e.g., bus drivers, police and firefighters, and nuclear plant workers).

Table 5 outlines "red flags" that, if noted by physicians in their interactions with injured or ill workers, should alert them promptly to consider problems with case resolution far greater than anticipated based on the objective findings in the case.[7,21,31] In addition, these red flags should alert physicians to carefully and comprehensively address the possibility of psychosocial dysfunction in the history and in the physical and mental status examinations.

MAXIMUM MEDICAL IMPROVEMENT AND IMPAIRMENT DETERMINATION

Once the worker has reached maximum medical improvement (MMI), the treating physician has the responsibility to render an opinion as to any impairment associated with the workplace injury or illness or recommend that the worker be referred for such determination. MMI is actually a misnomer in that a worker is never truly at MMI, unless the injury was very straightforward, such as a small laceration or contusion which healed. Basically, there are no medical or legal guidelines for MMI. There is always the possibility of another test, another treatment, or a new symptom.

As in all aspects of medical practice, it is best to refer a patient to another physician if one is lacking in training or experience in impairment determination. However, treating physicians must understand that they are probably better qualified than anyone else to render impair-

TABLE 5
RED FLAGS FOR PROBLEM CASES*

Worker Profile Factors
- has low pride in work product or performance
- has family members with disabilities, especially if work related
- makes what seems to be excessive demands on the physician and the administrative system
- is making plans for retirement or job change
- has had recent disciplinary action
- has multiple addresses and phone numbers
- has less than a ninth-grade education
- is a smoker
- has frequently cancelled or was a no-show for appointments
- has experienced divorce or other crisis recently
- has a lower paying job with few opportunities for advancement
- has changing shift

Workplace Profile Factors
- has unstable employment patterns, (i.e., layoffs, excessive overtime)
- is experiencing labor/management conflict or contested negotiations
- has impending plant closure or sale
- has deteriorating work ethic
- has monotonous, repetitive jobs, requiring little concentration
- has an unpleasant work environment

Injury Profile Factors
- was not witnessed
- was caused by the worker's actions
- is subjective in presentation
- is reported by worker's legal representative
- has widely varying medical findings and opinions
- is associated with doctor shopping

*Reproduced from Derebery and Tullis[7] and Nelson.[21]

ment opinions, as they have witnessed the objective impact of the injury and illness on the worker and also may have known the functional capabilities of the worker prior to presentation. As defined under the terminology section, impairment is medically determined based on any loss or abnormality of psychological, physiological, or anatomical structure or function. In the earliest years of workers' compensation, impairment and subsequent disability determinations were limited to profound loss of bodily function, such as amputations, loss of vision, or death. Percentages were legislated, and the physician really had very little to do other than provide the medical documentation of the loss. Most states continue to contain such disability schedules within their laws. Figure 1 is an example of the Missouri Workers' Compensation Permanent Partial Disability Schedule.

Impairment determination must never be taken lightly. The human and economic costs associated with impairment determinations are significant. Many employers' payrolls include from 6% to 12% in direct disability costs. The majority of physicians receive little or no training in impairment determination during their medical school and residency training. It is therefore recommended that physicians involved in the care of injured and ill workers attend impairment and disability evaluation courses, such as those offered by the American College of Occupational and Environmental Medicine. Certification in impairment determination is now available through the American Board of Independent Medical Examiners.

Although various guides and references are available to assist the physician in impairment determination, the most widely accepted is the AMA's *Guides to the Evaluation of Permanent Impairment*, currently in its fourth edition. If followed in all final impairment determination reports, the four steps from the AMA's *Guides*, outlined in Table 6, would provide administrators of the various compensation systems with the information needed to establish financial awards and permanent disability payments. The impact of these awards on the impaired worker's future behaviors and productivity, as well as on the future of society as a whole, are truly incalculable and impose great responsibility on the physician providing a rating. It is therefore incumbent upon the physician to provide as comprehensive a report as possible, as well as to be knowledgeable in the detailed use of the *Guides* itself. The physician, however, must not use the AMA's *Guides* if it is not accepted by the workers' compensation laws covering the case. The physician must be knowledgeable of the laws that apply.

If the treating physician does not render an opinion as to maximum medical improvement and impairment determination or in situations of pending litigation or disputed claims, an independent medical examination (IME) often will be requested by the employer or its representative, the workers' compensation administration, or a representative, usually legal, of the worker whose case is at issue. The purpose of the IME is to obtain a thorough and complete opinion, based on detailed review of medical records and diagnostic studies obtained to date, as well as comprehensive patient history-taking and physical examination, including testing if clinically indicated. In the past, these examinations usually were referred to as adverse opinion examinations. This is certainly no longer the accepted trend, and the physician selected to perform the IME is expected by all parties to be non-biased and friendly. However, it serves the best interests of all parties for the IME examiner to carefully explain to the injured or ill worker that the role of the IME is to provide an opinion only and not to be actively involved in the medical care of the patient. The straightforward explanation of the role of the IME physician will go a long way toward preventing unrealistic patient expectations and possible lack of patient cooperation during the evaluation. The IME will serve the medical-legal-administrative parties by preparing a report in a manner similar to the example outlined in Figure 2.[2]

Often, the IME physician will be asked to render an opinion as to apportionment as well as to the cost of future medical treatment. In these cases, the physician will need to carefully detail whether the future treatments or their related costs are "probable" (i.e., expected to be needed in greater than 50% of such cases) or are only "possible" (i.e., having less than a 50% chance of being needed).

THE FUTURE

Workers' compensation laws and the system in which they are administered influence the "cause" of injury and illness, access to medical care, patterns of workplace injury and disease, diagnostic evaluations, treatment, treatment response, and residual disability. For example, sciatica in the U.S. is considered injury-related 92% of the time, and in Great Britain and Swe-

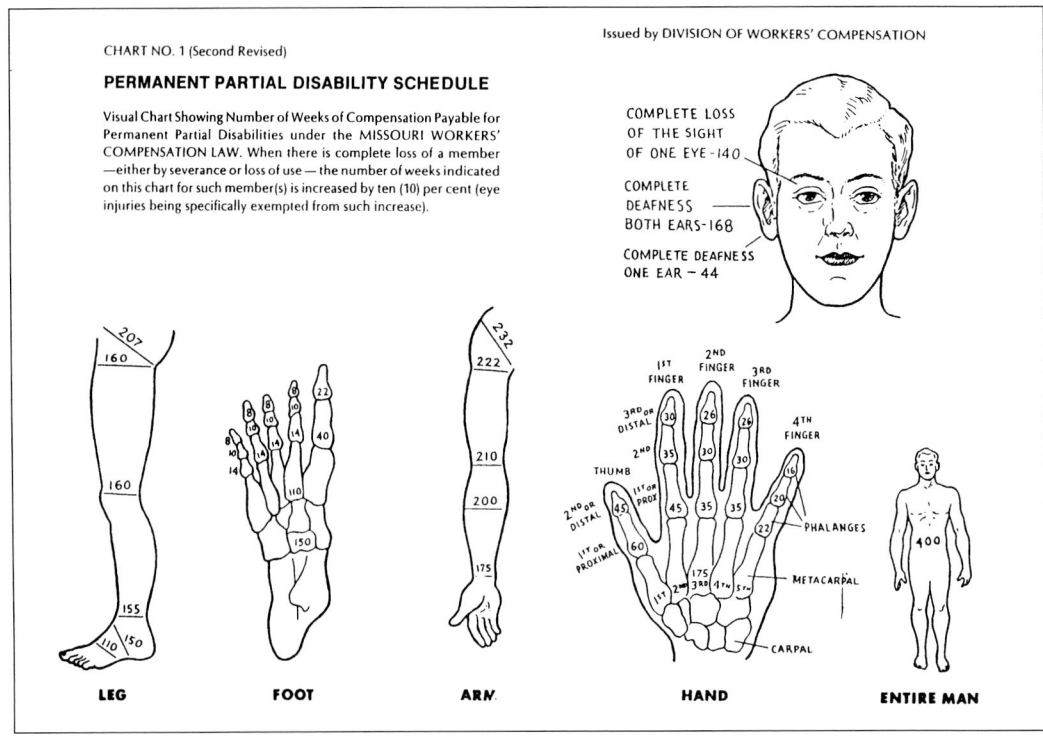

Figure 1: Missouri Worker's Compensation Permanent Partial Disability Schedule.

Report of Medical Evaluation (Permanent Medical Impairment)

To:

Re:

Case number:

Report date:

Onset of injury or illness:

1. Medical history		Yes	No
a. Medical office records	Reviewed		
	Enclosed		
b. Hospital records	Reviewed		
	Enclosed		
c. From other source (describe)			
d. From patient			

2. Clinical evaluation		Yes	No
a. Physical examination	Reports enclosed		
b. Laboratory tests	Reports enclosed		
c. Special tests and diagnostic procedures	Reports enclosed		
d. Specialist's evaluation	Reports enclosed		

3. Diagnoses

a.

b.

c.

d.

4. Stability of the medical condition	Yes	No
a. The clinical condition is stabilized and not likely to improve with surgical intervention or active medical treatment; medical maintenance care only is warranted.		
b. The degree of impairment is not likely to change substantially within the next year.		
c. The patient is not likely to suffer sudden or subtle incapacitation.		

Report of Medical Evaluation (Permanent Medical Impairment) Page 2

5. Other analyses

a. Explain briefly the impact(s) of the medical condition(s) on the patient's activities of daily living, including occupation (see Chapter 1 and Glossary, p. 315)

List types of daily activities affected

1

2

3

4

5

6

b. Is there a medical reason to believe the patient is likely to suffer injury, harm, or further medical impairment by engaging in usual activities of living or other activities necessary to meet personal, social, or occupational demands? Explain briefly.

_____Yes No_____

c. Is there a medical reason to believe restrictions, accommodations, or assistive devices are necessary to help the patient carry out usual activities or meet personal, social, and occupational demands? If so, briefly describe them and explain their therapeutic, risk-avoidance, or other kind of value.

_____Yes No_____

6. Impairment evaluation according to *Guides*–Attach a complete report of findings and narrative comments for each body part or system. Each organ system impairment estimate should be expressed in terms of percent impairment of the whole person.

Body part or system	**Chapter No.**	**Table No.**	**% Impairment of the whole person**
a			
b			
c			
d			

7. Final estimated whole-person impairment: _______________%.

8. _____ This patient has been under my care from _______________ to _______________

_____ I have not provided care for this patient. I have seen this patient _______ time(s) for the purpose of evaluating medical impairment.

9. I (do) (do not) believe there is inconsistency among the history, physical examination, laboratory finding, and other studies (cross out the nonapplicable verb phrase). If an inconsistency exists, explain it in writing.

_______________________________, MD
(Signature)

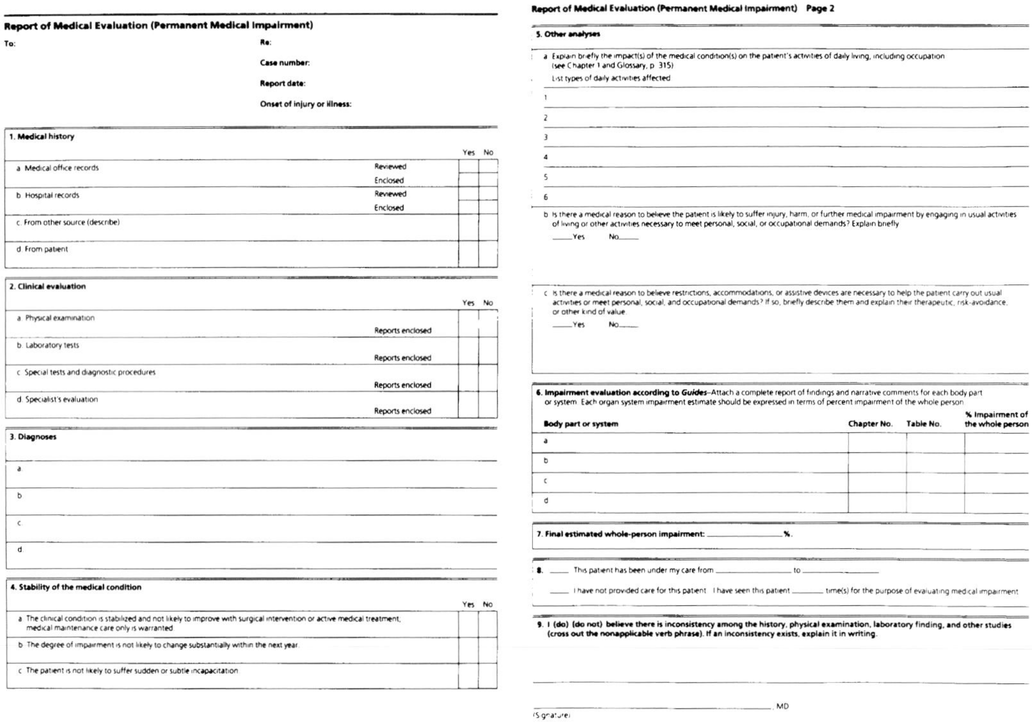

Figure 2: Example of report form used for medical evaluation for permanent medical impairment.

TABLE 6

PERMANENT MEDICAL IMPAIRMENT EVALUATION REPORTING*

Step 1

Collect the complete medical history and information on the condition(s) being considered for impairment determination. This is followed by completion of a comprehensive medical evaluation supported by appropriate tests and diagnostic procedures.

If the evaluation findings are consistent with the previous medical records it is appropriate to go to Step 2. However, if inconsistencies are found, then further clinical evaluation must be undertaken.

Step 2

Analyze the history, clinical, and diagnostic findings to determine the nature and extent of the impairment or dysfunction of the individual worker.

Step 3

Compare the findings in Step 2 with the criteria in the AMA Guides *to determine the impairment rating.*

The physician should use good clinical judgment to determine if a rating should be higher or lower than the rating as defined by the AMA *Guides.* The reasons for such rating modification should be given in writing in as much detail as necessary to be understandable by those reviewing and acting upon the reports.

On occasion, the physician will need to provide an opinion as to impairment in a situation in which the worker refused a specific medically recommended treatment or surgery. The individual's decision should not affect the impairment rating as based on the findings of the outlined steps. However, the physician may comment on the anticipated benefits and risks of the interventions refused and the basis of and impact on the impairment determined.

Step 4

Prepare the report.

A clear and comprehensive report is indicated. The report example in Figure 2 can be used "without permission from the AMA" and covers the content areas suggested for a standardized comprehensive rating report.

* From AMA's *Guides to the Evaluation of Permanent Impairment.*[2]

den only 59% and 22% of the time, respectively. In the U.S., work-related injuries to the spine receive 200% more therapy than nonwork-related conditions with the same findings. Even if physicians have a thorough understanding of the workers' compensation systems under which they practice and a clear vision of their role, there will always be difficult and complex issues. The following discusses some of the most common of these issues. These issues provide challenges for active physician participation in reform of this medical-legal-administrative system for the welfare of the injured/ill workers and for the enrichment of society as a whole.

Problem 1

The physician is always to be the "patient advocate." The physician must respond to the total patient, not just that part of the individual that is the "worker." In many situations there is not a clear separation of the work-related injury/illness from the complexities of the patient's other medical conditions, habits, coping mechanisms, and past medical experiences. If effective interventions for managing the total patient cannot be realized, the worker often will enter a period of confusion and dysfunctional processes, searching endlessly for "the answer." This often results in a progressive pattern of self-imposed and/or health care-imposed and/or legal system-imposed limitations that result in a generalized deconditioned status which becomes a disability in its own right. All too often, the worker becomes increasingly angry at everyone involved in the situation and is left with "getting even" rather than "getting well."

Problem 2

In a seemingly ever-increasing number of workers' compensation cases, after the injured/ill worker has had an evaluation by the physician and treatment initiated, an inquiry will be made by the employer or the insurer questioning whether the presenting signs and symptoms are or are not work-related. Interestingly, in the majority of these claims, the information provided to the physician from any sources other than the involved worker history is either non-existent or very limited. In these scenarios, it must be understood that the physician is left only with what the worker tells him or her in the way of history, including the description of the mechanism of injury, the workplace exposures, and the job tasks. Unless the employer or its representative provides incident investigation information, such as a written description or videotaping of the job tasks and specific industrial hygiene monitoring information on the workplace, the physician is left to render a medical opinion based solely on the worker history. Certainly the physician can state in the clinical records "assuming that the patient's history is correct, my opinion regarding causation is. . . ." In and of itself, this does not prevent the decision to be made at some future point that the claim is not going to be accepted. The physician is then left with services delivered but with a question about reimbursement and an even more important patient-physician commitment to an individual who may see the physician and every one else involved in the claim as being "out to get him."[28]

Problem 3

The physician who is truly committed to improving the health and safety of workers must have access to the workplace environment. Lack of access limits the physician's ability to provide thoughtful opinions as to causality and return to work with or without accommodation, and it certainly blocks effective strategies for prevention. Though physician and employer scheduling can be a problem, every effort must be made for the physician to perform a workplace walkthrough. In addition, those employers not providing a modified duty return to work program are tying the hands of the health care team. Several studies support the conclusion that modified duty programs result in less adversarial and controversial case management situations, less confusion and depression on the part of workers, and definitely less indemnity and medical expenses. The injured or ill worker who is back in the workplace does not become distanced from the employer. The worker who feels rejected, even if this is perception only, will manifest measurable physical symptoms. Once the injured worker becomes a cog in the workers' compensation system, it is easy "to become seduced by the benefits. Some benefits are very high, and an injured worker often can adapt to them."[20] The physiological and psychological needs of workers are best met by return to work in an environment where they can develop good work habits, build strength, and acquire agility.[20]

Problem 4

Chronic pain and disability syndromes must be better defined and accepted by all parties involved in the workers' compensation system. In large measure, disability is behavioral and behavior is learned. Behavior reflects the motivation and perceived success in return to work, as well as the perceived outcomes of not returning to work. Therefore, some workers with minimal impairment are greatly disabled and others with great impairment are minimally disabled. The total financial compensation for not working must not equal or exceed the real income associated with returning to work. For when it does, any form of treatment is doomed to failure. It must always be remembered that the workplace-injured worker who does not meet anticipated recovery goals often lacks appropriate social skills and job-seeking skills. It must also be remembered that the adversarial nature of the workers' compensation system often is the etiology of the operant rather than the actual injury. Many workers cannot or will not let loose of their pain complaints, especially if they are chronic, until case closure and settlement.

CONCLUSION

The problems in workers' compensation will only be resolved when the medical-legal-administrative components of the system move away from giving lip service and paper programs to true efforts at workplace prevention of injury and illness. The first step is the development of policy statements and enthusiastic management support of health and safety. It must be demonstrated that prevention is a management/employee cooperative venture. Management must develop and require goal-oriented and goal-measurable programs for success. Those in management must also be trained and updated frequently in positive acceptance of the risk and occurrence of workplace injury and understand that there are real occupational illness exposure issues in the workplace. The second step involves effective strategies to eliminate hazards, isolate hazards from the employees, and, as a last resort, isolate the worker from the hazards. The third step involves the safety and health training of workers. It must be presented in a sincere and ongoing process. Training activities must be routine, not just accident/incident triggered. The management of these programs should be placed in the hands of those who know the workplace, the employees, the machines, the material, the standard practices, and the usual hazards. Following these steps will allow for progression from the current state of employee dependency and unilateral legal responsibility on the part of the employer, to a more cooperative environment with increased self responsibility on the part of employees for workplace health and safety.

Physicians must continue to strive to identify safe, reliable, and valid quantification measurements of function to match the individual worker with the essential functions of work. Work is the most powerful means of binding an individual to reality. An individual's self esteem and economic security are directly related to his or her productive capacity. In addition, the economic health of society is dependent on an optimally healthy workforce.

There are currently significant variances in the diagnosis and management of work-related injuries and illnesses in the various regions of the U.S. as well as within individual medical communities. Physicians must accept that this results in significant confusion and mistrust of medical providers in general and may cause significant delays in approval for testing and treatment for the affected workers. It is critical for physicians to participate in the development and implementation of guidelines for causation determination and for the diagnosis and treatment of the most common workplace conditions covered under workers' compensation.[17] In addition, physicians must assist in the development and clinical use of outcome measurement tools for the guidelines. It is necessary to work with the legal, administrative, and legislative bodies involved in workers' compensation for consensus building in order to develop "objective and uniform methods to evaluate medical impairment and disability."[34] Further, physicians should participate in the determination of education, competency, and licensure standards for all parties involved in workers' compensation. The greater challenge for the physician is to participate in research efforts to identify effective clinical skills and interventions to optimize workers' self responsibility and their active participation in their own functional restoration.

Physicians in their daily activities must encourage society as a whole and its individual members to value what people can do, rather than what they cannot do. The physician should practice with a style that " coddles people a little, but aims to keep them active and productive."[25]

REFERENCES

1. 56 **Federal Register** 144 (July 7, 1991)
2. American Medical Association: **Guides to the Evaluation of Permanent Impairment.** Chicago, Ill: American Medical Association, 1993
3. **An Orthopaedic Primer on Workers' Compensation.** Chicago, Ill: American Academy of Orthopaedic Sur-

geons, 1991 (Draft)

4. Bale A: The American compensation phenomenon. **Int J Health Serv 20:**253-275, 1990

5. Colledge A: Is splitting up booty turning into a mutiny? **Occup Health Safety 64:**32-33, June 1995

6. DeCarlo DT, Minkowitz M: **Workers' Compensation Insurance and Law Practice: The Next Generation.** Fort Washington, Pa: LRP Publications, 1989

7. Derebery VJ, Tullis WH: Delayed recovery in the patient with a work compensable injury. **J Occup Med 25:**829-835, 1983

8. Diorio PG, Fallon LF Jr: **Workers' Compensation Impairment and Disability. Occupational Medicine, State of the Art Reviews.** Philadelphia, Pa: Hanley and Belfus, Vol 4, January-March 1989

9. **Emotional Stress in the Workplace—New Legal Rights in the Eighties.** Deerfield Beach, Fla: National Council on Compensation Insurance, 1985

10. Engelberg AL: Disability and Workers' Compensation. **Prim Care 21:**275-288, p9ch25, 1994

11. Equal Employment Opportunity Commission Notice, No. 915.002:45 (May 19, 1994)

12. Fawley IL: A historical perspective on health reform. **MGM J.** March/April 1992, pp 44-49

13. Forger G: Using materials handling to help the disabled. **Modern Materials Handling.** Boston, Mass: Cahners Publishing, October 1993, pp 40-45

14. Greenwood J, Taricco A: **Workers' Compensation Health Care Cost Containment.** Horsham, Pa: LRT Publications, 1992

15. Hadler NM: Occupational illness: the issue of causality. **J Occup Med 26:**587-593, 1984

16. Koslow SM: **CCH Workers' Compensation Business Management Guide.** December 3, 1993, Vol 5, pp 33-34

17. Leavenworth G: Setting standards for Workers' Compensation. **Business and Health.** Washington, DC: Vol 10, Washington Business Group on Health, October 1994, pp 49-50, 52, 54

18. Levy BS, Wegman DH**: Occupational Health: Recognizing and Preventing Work-Related Disease.** 2nd ed. Boston, Mass: Little, Brown, & Co, 1988

19. McCunney RJ: **A Practical Approach to Occupational and Environmental Medicine.** 2nd ed. Boston, Mass: Little, Brown, & Co, 1994

20. **Morbidity and Mortality Weekly Report 35:**613-620

21. Nelson N J Jr: Workers' compensation: 1980-1984 benchmark revisions. **Social Security Bull 51:**41-58, July 1988

22. Nelson N J Jr: Workers' compensation: coverage, benefits, and costs, 1990–91. **Social Security Bull 56:** 68-74, Fall 1993

23. Norris CRL: Understanding Workers' Compensation law. **Hand Clinics 9:**231-239, 1993

24. **Physicians' Guide: Medical Practice in the California Workers' Compensation System.** State of California: Industrial Medical Council, March 1994

25. Remeny AG, et al: **New Developments in Worker Rehabilitation: The Workcase Model in Australia.** New York, NY: World Rehabilitation Fund, 1987

26. Rom WN: **Environmental and Occupational Medicine.** 2nd ed. Boston, Mass: Little, Brown, & Co, 1992

27. Taricco A: **Medical Issues of Fraud and Abuse in Workers' Compensation.** Horsham, Pa: LRP Publications, 1995

28. Telles CA: An overview of medical cost containment in Workers' Compensation. **Benefits Quarterly. Fourth Quarter.** 1993, pp 42-50

29. Thomason T: Are attorneys paid what they're worth? Contingency fees and the settlement process. **J Legal Studies 20:**187-223, 1991

30. **Workers' Compensation Guide for Employees.** Richmond, Va: Virginia Workers' Compensation Claims Division

31. **Workers' Compensation Manual for Managers and Supervisors.** Commerce Clearing House, 1992

32. **Work Injuries and Illnesses by Selected Characteristics, 1992.** NEWS, US Department of Labor, Bureau of Labor Statistics USDL-94-213, April 26, 1994

33. **The World Book Encyclopedia 1986.** Chicago, Ill: World Book, Inc, 1986, Sect H, p 226

34. Wyman ET, Cats-Baril WL: Working it out: recommendations from a multidisciplinary national consensus panel on medical problems in Workers' Compensation. **J Occup Med 36:**144-154, 1994

35. Yorker B: Workers' compensation law: an overview. **AAOHN J 42:**420-424, September 1994

36. Yospe J: US industries director: "claim" vs. "condition" in the analysis of Workers' Compensation cases. **J Law Med 12:**273-303, 1986

CHAPTER 27

MEDICAL MALPRACTICE

G. ROBERT NUGENT, MD

You and your colleagues face a choice. If you do nothing, the current situation will worsen from the perspective of all relevant interests: physicians and health care institutions will experience more litigation, a small percentage of victims of medical injuries will receive compensation, and the cost to the health care and judicial systems will grow higher and higher. On the other hand, if you take steps to streamline and improve malpractice litigation, to enhance and encourage institutional responsibility and injury reduction, and to develop a scheme of decent, accessible compensation for all those suffering significant avoidable health care injuries, we have the possibility of fewer injuries, fewer wasted costs, a higher level of social justice and a crisis averted.[148]

This comment by Mr. Robert Prichard was made in 1990 in a report by the Committee on Liability and Compensation Issues in Health Care to the Minister responsible for National Health and Welfare in Canada. It sums up succinctly the situation we also face in the United States.

One's perspective about medical malpractice and the malpractice problem is colored by one's profession, one's interpretation of the facts, and one's past experience. To the doctor there is a "crisis" because of the increasing number of cases and escalating awards. On the other hand, medicine is by its very nature an inexact science with inexact rules and uncertain outcomes. To others, including some patients, social scientists, and those in the legal profession, there are too many negligently injured patients who never get into the tort system. To them the "crisis" is one of too few suits, not too many. An additional issue is the cost of the current system. A study by the RAND Corporation indicates that more than

50% of providers' liability insurance premium dollars are spent in paying the costs of the claims resolution system as opposed to paying awards to persons injured by medical malpractice. Much of this money goes to resolve the many suits in which no malpractice occurred in the first place.[65,67]

Thus there is a major concern about the ability of the present tort system to equitably meet the needs of anyone concerned. Indeed, Daniel Creasey, President of the Risk Management Foundation of the Harvard Medical Institutions, has said: "It would be a tremendous abrogation of intellectual responsibility to look at a system with this many problems, that costs this much and serves the public this poorly, and say that it is the best we can do."[36] This chapter attempts to provide an overview of these issues along with a look at the proposed alternatives to the tort system. However, it is obvious that there is no easy answer to this problem and there is no certainty that another system could do better.

THE LAW OF MALPRACTICE

Negligence and Malpractice Defined

Negligence is a tort or legal wrong. It is an action, or failure of action, that a reasonably prudent person would not commit. It is a departure from the standard of care, particularly a careless or incautious departure, that is the actual and proximate cause of the patient's injuries. Negligence occurs not merely when there is error, but when the degree of error exceeds an accepted norm or standard of care. The Secretary's Commission on Medical Malpractice defines malpractice as an injury to a patient caused by the negligence of a health care worker.[115] Thus malpractice requires two things, negligence and injury. The mere demonstration of negligence or a breach of the standard of care is not malpractice.

The definition of *malpractice* can be further elaborated to include four elements: 1) an established *duty* of the physician to the care of the patient (doctor-patient relationship); 2) a *breach* of that duty (negligence); 3) a defined *injury* to the patient; and 4) the breach being the proximate *cause* of the injury.[147]

An economic concept of malpractice considers that negligent behavior is the failure to invest resources up to a level that equals the anticipated savings in damage. Or, negligence occurs whenever it would cost less to prevent a mishap than to pay for the damages predicted to result from it. This is the Learned Hand Rule and tells potentially negligent people that it will cost them more to be careless than to invest in appropriate prevention.[165]

Physician Liability

There are a variety of situations in which the physician is considered negligent and liable for breaching the standard of care. They include:[147]

Abandonment—This occurs when medical care was unreasonably discontinued, when the termination of care was against the patient's will, when the physician failed to arrange for care by another physician, and when actual harm was suffered by the patient because of the abandonment.

Aggravation of a Pre-existing Condition—the physician is liable only for the aggravation, not the original injury.

Alternative Procedures—unusual or new procedures are considered in this definition. The physician is not liable if he or she follows a course of treatment supported by reputable and reasonable medical experts.

Battery—in battery, the patient does not consent to surgery or the patient consents to surgery by one physician but is operated upon by another.

Breach of Confidentiality—the physician is obligated to maintain the confidentiality of each patient's communications. There is an implied right for the physician to release patient information to others also treating the patient.

Delay in Treatment—if a delay in treatment leads to the patient's death or injury, the physician is liable (e.g., failure to act promptly on a lung lesion visualized on x-ray to be cancer renders the physician liable).

Failure to Follow Up—it is the physician's obligation to follow up on such things as a breast lump in a patient (that is ultimately cancerous), on suspicious lesions on chest x-rays, or upon x-rays read by an emergency department physician as normal but later read by a radiologist as showing a fracture.

Failure to Obtain Informed Consent—discussed below.

Failure to Respond to an Emergency Department Call—the emergency department physician and the hospital may both be liable in this instance.

Failure to Seek Consultation—consultation with an expert (as with an infectious disease expert) is often necessary and should be timely. Failure to act upon a consultant's advice can also be a problem. If the physician is in doubt and the patient requests consultation, it should be provided.

Fraud—this occurs when there is a representation to a patient with the intent that he or she rely on it, when there is knowledge on the part of the defendant that the representation is false, when there is belief by the plaintiff that the representation is true, and when reliance on such representation results in injury to the plaintiff.

Infection—this pertains only when there is proven departure from the standard of care and infection results.

Lack of Documentation—the requirement for office and hospital chart documentation is broad and is often a major issue in malpractice litigation.

Medications—overmedication, undermedication, misprescription, failure to consider side effects, or use in patients with contraindications. The physician should document periodically the reason for continuation of medication.

Misdiagnosis or Failure to Diagnose—this is the most frequently cited cause of a malpractice action. A multitude of situations fall under this heading.

Mistaken Identity—this is especially a problem when it leads to such things as operating upon the wrong person or the wrong extremity or organ.

Premature Discharge—discharge should be based upon the medical factors and not economic factors.

Treatment Outside the Field of Competence—this is at times a problem for nonboard-certified physicians. Separate areas of liability have been defined for high-risk specialties such as anesthesiology, obstetrics/gynecology, psychiatry, surgery, and radiology.

Informed Consent

Previously, the *physician* decided what a patient should know about a procedure and its risks.[201] This has changed not only due to a better appreciation of patients' rights but also to legal developments. In 1972, the Court of Appeals of the District of Columbia in *Canterbury v. Spence*[28] applied a new concept of informed consent, holding the physician responsible for disclosing what a *reasonable person* would want to know before providing or declining consent.

States vary in their requirements for informed consent. For the proper administration of informed consent, guidelines mandate that the patient be provided with the following:

- the diagnosis of the condition requiring treatment;
- the nature and purpose of the treatment;
- the risks generally recognized as a consequence of the treatment;
- the likelihood of success of the treatment;

- practical alternatives to the treatment and their risks and benefits; and
- the prognosis if no treatment is rendered.

In practice, it would appear that some courts do not demand strict adherence to all aspects of informed consent, particularly those concerning the disclosure of alternatives, and the major issue comes down to whether there was indeed good communication between the doctor and patient concerning the treatment.

There have been several studies showing that patients frequently have a very poor memory and understanding of the information conveyed to them in the informed consent process, even when documented that this has been given in an adequate fashion.[127,149,158] However, one study of informed consent showed that patients were more interested in the diagnosis and the surgical technique to be used than in the risks involved; in addition, the concepts of the goals and benefits of a proposed treatment were poorly comprehended.[70] Patients recall an average of only 29% to 35% of what they have been told in the preoperative interview, and even when the correct responses were suggested, one study revealed that they recalled an average of only 42% of the information. The errors of recall fell into the categories of failure to recall, positive denial of the truth, the ascertainment of an untruth or falsehood, and attributing to the informed consent interview information received from another source.[93,149,158]

Most important is documentation of the preoperative/preprocedure dialogue between physician and patient in which the situation is discussed in some detail. The physician must speak in lay terms, using as little medical terminology as possible. There should be documentation showing that the patient understood what he/she was told.[147] Documentation of this dialog may take the form of a written statement detailing the risks, etc., which is signed by the patient. Some document the process by videotaping the interview. The author (G.R.N.) records in the patient's medical record any specific details (e.g., which family members were present and what questions were asked) that make it apparent that the physician interacted with the patient and was directly involved in the process. It is generally not acceptable for consent to be obtained by nurses or other surrogates, regardless of their competency.

Forms have been developed by hospitals, physicians, and commercial sources to document that informed consent has been provided. Specific forms for special procedures are useful. However, not all forms are adequate. Hopper and others[75] analyzed 549 consent forms from 156 institutions and found that one would need to have completed at least one year of college to understand the average clinical consent form. A Johns Hopkins study of oncology research protocols had similar findings.[58] Numerous other studies have confirmed that consent forms, especially those for research, require a level of reading ability well beyond that of the average patient.[5,59,62,75,114,129,133,184]

Recently it has been suggested that physicians should know and offer their personal experience and results in describing a procedure so that patients can use this additional relevant information in the decision-making process. In a recent Wisconsin case, a plaintiff obtained a $6.2 million settlement on the basis that she was not informed of the surgeon's inexperience in performing difficult aneurysm surgery which rendered her quadriplegic. There may be increasing demands by patients along these lines.[204]

There are times when the law recognizes that formal informed consent is not required. These include the following:[160]

- The risk not disclosed is too commonly known to warrant disclosure.
- The patient assured the physician that he/she would undergo the procedure regardless of the risk involved, or the patient assured the physician that he/she did not want to be informed of the matters to which he/she would be entitled to be informed.
- Consent by or on behalf of the patient was not reasonably possible because of an emergency situation.
- The physician, after considering all of the attendant facts and circumstances, used reasonable discretion as to the matter and extent to which such alternatives or risks were disclosed to the patient because of a belief that the manner and extent of such disclosure could be expected to adversely and substantially affect the patient's condition.

Plaintiffs suing on the basis of a failure to provide informed consent must prove that:[147]

- The defendant physician failed to adequately inform them of a material risk before securing consent to a proposed treatment.
- If they had been informed of the risk, they would not have consented to the treatment.
- The adverse consequences that were not made known did in fact occur.
- The plaintiff was injured as a result of the treatment.

There are other obvious and well-known aspects of informed consent. No guarantee of cure should be offered. When appropriate, the patient should be informed that the operation is not being offered to reverse or cure a process, but to halt the progression of the disease. The patient should also be warned of the worst that could happen (e.g., blindness after eye surgery, paraplegia after spinal cord surgery, foot-drop after surgery for an L4-5 ruptured disc, or complications from hemorrhage). Surgical patients must always be warned of the possibility of postoperative infection.

Although informed consent is one of the more well-defined aspects of a malpractice suit, informed consent is a minor issue in most liability claims and is the primary claim in only 2% of cases. Since it is the doctor's word against the plaintiff's and since most doctors are respected individuals by patients, their word that informed consent was indeed given often prevails. Plaintiff attorneys, however, may claim an absence of informed consent in an attempt to show that this is an additional area in the case where the doctor failed to meet the standard of care, and it may be an additional factor the jury considers in reaching their decision.

The problematic aspects of informed consent are apparent in such instances as patients who claim they would not have had intravenous contrast enhancement for a radiological study had they known there was a fatal reaction in 1:20,000 to 1:75,000 such examinations.[64,168] It is reasonable to believe that a patient would usually not be dissuaded by such a low risk. The "prudent man" concept is applicable here. If a prudent person in the plaintiff's circumstances would undergo the procedure regardless of whether the person were informed of the risk, the physician may not be held liable if he or she did not present the risk to the patient. It may be negligent to fail to disclose, but liability is not imposed because the negligence did not cause any injury since the patient would have given consent regardless. Juries, however, may make the final determination as to whether this concept applies to a particular patient in a particular situation.[88] Several states have accepted this concept.

The computerization of records introduces new problems about informed consent, including storage and access.[33]

Damages Awarded for Malpractice

Monetary damages generally are awarded to individuals in cases of personal injury and wrongful death resulting from malpractice. They are usually initially set by the jury but are subject to judicial review and change if they are "excessive" or are not supported by the evidence. Plaintiffs seek recovery for a variety of damages.[147]

Economic damages include loss of earnings, medical costs, and loss of financial support. For example: loss of child's services when a minor child is injured in the accident; medical and other health expenses reasonably paid or incurred, or to be incurred in the future; past and future loss of earnings sustained and to be sustained; and permanent diminution in the plaintiff's earning capacity.

Noneconomic damages (hedonic damages) are awarded to compensate for the loss of the enjoyment of life and pain and suffering. For example: permanent physical disabilities; permanent mental disabilities; past and future physical and mental pain and suffering; loss of enjoyment of life; and loss of consortium when a spouse is injured in the incident.

Punitive damages are unusual in medical malpractice cases, but they are awarded in cases of gross carelessness or reckless disregard for the safety of others.[147]

The Tort System— Compensation and Deterrence

As it relates to medical malpractice, the central objectives of the tort system are 1) to *com-*

pensate the negligently injured for their losses, and 2) by deterrence, to *prevent* injuries caused by physician negligence. Some might add emotional vindication for the injured as a third objective.

The majority of adverse events due to malpractice are never pursued. About eight times as many patients suffer an injury from medical negligence as there are malpractice claims.[99] Only one in 10 legitimate malpractice incidents reach the tort system, only 40% of these receive payment, and two out of three claims are closed without any payment to the claimant although incurring significant cost along the way. Thus, the system does not promote adequate compensation.[20, 145] In addition, only 43% of each dollar spent on medical liability reaches injured patients. Furthermore, time to resolve litigation is tremendous. Professional liability litigation typically lasts 25 to 27 months, or 40 to 46 months if the case goes to trial.[170,172] On the other hand, negligence was not proved in 82% of filed cases.[99] Even when the physician defendant wins a case, as is true 81% of the time in some areas,[83] the physician loses a great deal, including community reputation and social position which are important socioeconomic assets for a physician.[137]

To some, malpractice litigation is justified as a deterrent.[197] However, there is little significant economic loss by tort action insofar as malpractice insurance covers most of the award and an increase in patient fees may offset any increase in premiums. It is the anguish and agony of a time-consuming, income-reducing process of litigation which threatens the physician's reputation that is an emotionally devastating ordeal. Therefore, fear of malpractice action, along with the stress and anguish it involves, does have a significant deterrent effect on the physician and influences the way doctors manage and react to their patients.[17,142,170] It is this fear that acts as a deterrent without regard to the existence of economic deterrence.[8] The best estimate from the Harvard study is that, at least in New York state, the various influences on a physician's practice brought by the threat of a malpractice suit probably reduced the risk of patient injury (deterrence effect) by about 11%.[196] However, another opinion asserts that: "There is virtually no conclusive empirical evidence on the deterrent effect of tort law in any field . . . [and] it is difficult to be at all confident that tort law can accomplish its objective of deterring adverse outcomes."[172] Others agree that there is no research showing that malpractice litigation reduces iatrogenic injury.[174]

The problems of inadequate compensation and flawed deterrence could be addressed by altering the current law. One legal scholar recommended that there be an uncoupling of compensation from deterrence and that the benefits to tort victims then be readdressed as part of the function of our regular social insurance and employee-benefit systems.[179] In the opinion of some, the punishment the physician receives for an error should be carried out by the state medical licensing board and not the tort system.

The History of Medical Malpractice

Reports from the first millennium reveal that a bad result from physician error sometimes led to execution of the physician.[55,60] Physicians of the Middle Ages and Renaissance, as today, were sued for the failure to cure, for overcharging, and for neglect, as well as for a variety of other problems.[34] Court action was similar to that of today. Cases were tried before judge and jury, testimony was sworn by plaintiff and defendant, and expert witnesses were called to testify. Physicians have been liable for malpractice suits since the 14th century in England and the late 18th century in the United States.[42]

The first case of malpractice in this country leading to appeal (the only records available are from appellate cases) was probably in 1794.[176] Between then and 1940 there were only 1,513 appellate malpractice cases recorded. Probably fewer than 500 medical malpractice actions were brought in American courts prior to 1835.[125] A pivotal year was 1840. A "deluge" of malpractice cases around that time led Frank Hamilton, a New York physician, to claim that between 1833 and 1856 "suits for malpractice were so very frequent in the Northern states" that many men "abandoned the practice of surgery, leaving it to those who, with less skill and experience, had less reputation and property to

lose."[43,61] At that time public attitudes were changing, with greater expectation of cure often encouraged by the exaggerated claims prevalent in medical advertising of the time. New technical rules of legal pleading also facilitated the bringing of a suit. As now, technological advances often were related to malpractice actions. Prior to that time, for instance, most compound fractures were treated by amputation, but newer techniques often saved the extremity albeit with complications of infection, shortening, and malalignment, which led to suit. The contingent fee system also was established about this time.

Starting in the 1950s, an attitude of increasing social liberalism in association with more liberal interpretation of the law and a less antiplaintiff trend in common law doctrines made it easier to initiate malpractice suits.[42] A series of changes in the court system came about in an attempt to replace the prevailing restrictive rules. Appellate jurists and legal academicians by and large encouraged the expansion of tort liability.[12] Courts of appeal, acting on changes in societal thinking, expanded the grounds under which injured parties may be compensated for noneconomic damages.[18] The new Federal Rules of Evidence enacted by the United States Congress in 1975 relaxed previous rules of evidence.[140] Plaintiffs had access to more and varied expert witnesses than was previously allowed.[83] The abolition of the locality rule and of charitable and government immunity and the development of the doctrine of *respondeat superior*, which made hospitals responsible for the actions of their employees, made it easier to bring and manage malpractice suits. The effects of these changes have been felt particularly since the 1970s. The American Bar Association ethical cannon #28, which forbids attorneys from "stirring up litigation," was abandoned and a new interpretation of litigation offered that lawyers, by their actions, were now protecting and changing society for the better, and as such were public servants. This involves the "invisible fist" concept, directed toward deterrence of negligence as a result of the threat of a malpractice suit.

A "crisis" occurred in the mid-1970s when increasing malpractice litigation precipitated the mass withdrawal from the market of commercial insurers writing medical liability coverage. This led to physicians establishing not-for-profit physician-owned insurance companies. In addition, 43 states enacted various tort reforms.[6] These reforms were designed to reduce access to the courts and limit the amount of recovery, "improving" the malpractice system primarily from the perspective of providers and insurers. However, it appears that these reforms have further undermined compensation and deterrence goals of tort law.[86]

Another "crisis" occurred in the mid-1980s. Between 1975 and 1986, inflation-adjusted mean-paid claims rose five-fold, while inflation-adjusted median-paid claims rose nearly three-fold.[138] Premiums doubled over a 3-year period, claim frequency rose by 12% per year, and the magnitude of awards increased, leading to another flurry of tort reform action on the part of the states.[42,65] In 1981 the St. Paul Fire and Marine Insurance Co. paid out $56 million in claims, but in 1985 its paid claims exceeded $173 million. By 1986 the average malpractice verdict had soared to $1.4 million.[38] It has been argued that judges and juries were holding the physician to higher liability standards, amounting to strict liability, instead of the traditional fault-based negligence standard of care, and this does seem to be an explanation for some of the current trends in malpractice attitudes.[83]

Coverage was available in the mid-1980s but at a marked increase in rates. The insurance industry at this time was accused of egregiously raising premiums and even manipulating the facts to permit the increase in rates, although these complaints have not been confirmed.[171] A study by Harrington and Litan[63] found that the increase in premiums since 1980 related to the fact that premiums failed to keep pace with losses through 1984, with the result that especially large increases were needed in 1985 and 1986 to catch up with the increase in losses. The growth in premiums also was aggravated by reductions in interest rates that led to even greater increases in the discounted value of losses. Furthermore, collusion among insurers was not found to be an underlying problem.[63] However, by 1985 the tort reforms enacted by many states did indeed reduce claim frequency. Especially effective were caps on awards and collateral source offsets (see below).[41]

In the early 1990s the *frequency* of professional liability claims moderated and remained stable. The number of payment awards decreased by 8.7%, from 19,999 in 1994 to 18,257 in 1995.[178] Still, a 1995 *Medical Economics* poll of 349 surgeons revealed that three-fifths of the surgeons reported they had been sued for malpractice at least once, and one-third had been named in multiple suits.[104] On the other hand, the *severity* of claims (amount paid out) over this same time period is about double the 1985 rate.[119] The median malpractice payment reported during 1995 was $65,000—a 9.4% increase over the 1994 median payment of $59,429.[178] The number of million-dollar awards given by juries in 1995 was 35% of verdicts, up from 27% in 1994.[103] There was also an increase in the number of "failure to diagnose" suits, where the current payouts amount to 25% of all payouts.[187]

A new development is the increase in suits related to managed care situations, where there are uncertainties about the contract liability of physicians. "Gatekeeper malpractice," where cost concerns may outweigh clinical choices, has entered the picture, along with problems related to "denial and delay of care" and restricted access to specialists and diagnostic technology, all in the interest of cost containment.[106] Additional risk to physicians results from plans that use economic data, as opposed to quality data, in determining physician status. There is a real question as to whether the legal system can change or accommodate to the new cost-sensitive management decisions. Fortunately, it must be proved that the physician involved knew their cost-cutting actions would put patients at risk and willfully disregarded that risk, which may be difficult.[3]

Another development is the use of malpractice awards as a surrogate social insurance program. Some juries and judges seem to feel an obligation to give awards to aid the injured even when malpractice has not been proved.

A major concern for physicians is the large number of suits brought where no malpractice was ultimately proved. The Harvard University study shows that in only 17% of claims filed was there evidence of negligence, and in 55% of these there was no evidence of an injury.[21] A Massachusetts study found about 50% of its cases to be unfortunate medical results rather than examples of negligence.[113] There is no mechanism to deter inappropriate filing of suits.

MALPRACTICE LITIGATION TODAY

Today, nearly 22% of cases are dropped without settlement. About 30% are settled after the suit but before the trial is scheduled. Six percent of cases are decided by court decision prior to trial. Another 22% are settled after the trial is scheduled but before the jury is seated. Slightly over 5% are settled during the trial. Only about 10% of claims go to a jury decision. Just over 4% of court decisions are settled on appeal.[98] Therefore, the major activity of the malpractice legal process occurs in depositions to determine the facts of the case and in pretrial negotiations to resolve questions of liability, magnitude of damages, and costs of settlement. The final judgment and award is then not usually made by a judge or jury but independently "in the shadow of the law" by the plaintiff and defense attorneys. Their decision is usually based on the likelihood of liability, the magnitude of damages, and the financial and intangible costs to the parties from going to trial. In some cases, it is not the client or attorneys who make the decision as to settlement but the insurance company. The final decision is often determined by the testimony of the expert witnesses who establish the all-important standard of care and identify the medical facts of the case. This phase of the case may be tainted by biased statements of "professional" expert witnesses compounded by the reluctance of reputable physicians to expend their time to serve as experts, particularly for plaintiffs.

The nature of the law must be understood. Federal judge Henry Friendly has stated, "Under our adversary system the role of counsel is not to make sure the truth is ascertained but to advance his client's cause by any ethical means. . . . Causing delay and sowing confusion not only are his right but may be his duty."[52] Judge Rothwax has noted, "In reality, the law is not necessarily a search for the truth. . . . Our system is a carefully crafted maze, constructed of elaborate and impenetrable barriers to the truth."[159] This is difficult for the physician to understand and accept,

and its usefulness could be argued.

The unpredictability of juries (and some judges), and their propensity to reward on the basis of emotional and sympathetic factors rather than fact and reason, is often cited as a problem leading attorneys on both sides to procure settlements that may be out of proportion and against their better judgment. For example, in California cases are often settled for $30,000 because only awards above that amount are required to be reported to the Board of Medical Quality Assurance. This is the cost to avoid bringing a nuisance case to the risks of trial.[203]

It has been reported that of the cases settled before trial, 54% result in no payment to the plaintiff, and, of those that do go to trial, in 77% the judgment was in favor of the physician.[81] In another study, 8,231 closed cases were reviewed by the physician-reviewer, the claims representative, the defense attorney, and the defending physician; in 62% of cases, the physicians' care was considered defensible. However, a payment was made in 21% of these cases. In 25% of cases, in almost half of which the physician admitted error, the review process considered the error indefensible, and payment was made in 91% of these. In another study, only one quarter of the 12% of cases going to a jury resulted in payment to the plaintiff. The severity of the injury was not related to the frequency of payment.[183]

There are some regional differences. Peterson[144] found that plaintiff victories in medical malpractice cases increased during a 20-year period from 27% to 53% in San Francisco and from 25% to 49% in Cook County (Illinois), although the reason is not clear.

Posttrial reductions in awards occur in 33% of cases. Awards between $1 million and $10 million were reduced by judicial or other review by an average of 39%.[166] These posttrial reductions must be considered when discussing average malpractice verdicts for recent years.

THE SCOPE OF THE MALPRACTICE PROBLEM

Frequency and Severity of Claims

Malpractice activity is often measured in terms of both the increased *frequency* of claims and the increase in *severity* of claims (i.e., the amount paid out).

In the late 1950s there was approximately one claim per 100 physicians per year. By the mid-1980s there were 17 claims per 100 physicians per year.[195] Malpractice suits in New York increased 300-fold in the past two decades. Of all malpractice suits filed in the United States since 1944, 80% have been brought during the second half of this period.[47] Presently, one of every eight physicians will be sued each year. Medical malpractice claims are filed ten times more frequently in the U.S. than they are in Great Britain and 30 times more than in Japan.[56,121] However, the number of plaintiffs recovering damages has remained steady over the past four years, with plaintiffs prevailing 53% of the time in 1995.[80]

The severity of claims is more difficult to accurately quantitate and more subject to variability in interpretation. A report in 1986 on tort policy produced by the U. S. Department of Justice stated that between 1975 and 1985 the average medical malpractice jury award had increased from $220,108 to $1,017,716.[195] The average medical malpractice jury verdict in Chicago increased from $50,000 in the early 1960s to $1,294,000 in the early 1980s. In San Francisco, there was a similar experience.[144] These figures have been challenged on the basis of an invalid sampling scheme by the reviewing agency.[192]

A study in 1991 by Jury Verdict Research, Inc., of Solon, Ohio on the size of plaintiff verdicts alleging doctor and/or hospital negligence found that verdicts of $1 million and above accounted for the largest proportion of awards (23%); 43% of the total number of verdicts were for $500,000 and above. These awards were significantly higher than other kinds of personal injury liabilities.[116] Another study by Jury Verdict Research of Horsham, Pennsylvania showed that awards for medical malpractice rose 40% from a median of $356,000 in 1994 to $500,000 in 1995. In cases with more serious injuries, such as quadriplegia, median verdicts more than doubled, from $2.4 million in 1994 to $6.5 million in 1995. At the same time, there was a drop of 32% in product liability verdicts. A study by Tillinghast-Towers Perrin shows medical liability costs totaled $12.7 billion in 1994, up from $8.54 billion in 1990.[117]

The National Practitioner Data Bank's records show that the frequency of lawsuits increased in 1994 over the year before, and malpractice payments in 1994 totaled $3.3 billion —8.4% greater than in 1993.[102] The 1995 Data Bank showed a 9.4% increase in median malpractice payments over 1994, but the number of payments decreased 8.7% over the same time period.[178]

In the 1980s malpractice insurers raised their rates as much as 500% and denied coverage to certain high-risk specialties.[146] By the mid-1980s the number of companies offering professional liability insurance had decreased from 39 to eight.[107] From 1960 to 1990, malpractice premiums increased from $60 million to more than $7 billion.[195] (A decrease in claims frequency in the late 1980s resulted in handsome profits for some insurance companies.) The insurance premium costs in high-risk areas for those in high-risk specialties such as neurosurgery, ortho-pedic surgery, and obstetrics ranged between $150,000 to $200,000 a year.[196] A concomitant increase in physician fees, however, matched this increase in premium costs.

As of 1987, 12.4% of obstetrician-gynecologists had given up obstetrics because of liability concerns and 27% had decreased performing high-risk care. In Florida, liability insurance costs add $1,119 to the cost of each delivery.[65] In 1995 the largest jury awards cited in medical malpractice cases involved obstetrical cases. The awards in those suits ranged from $42 million to $98 million.[118]

The California and Harvard Studies

The California study was initiated in 1974 by the California Medical Association to evaluate the feasibility of a no-fault system of compensation for medical injuries. The records of 23 California hospitals were examined. They found that one in 126 patients admitted to the hospital suffered a negligent injury (0.8%), but only one in 10 filed a claim and only 40% of these claims resulted in payment to the plaintiff. In other words, only one in 25 negligent injuries resulted in compensation to the patient.[27]

As part of a major legislative reform of its medical liability laws, New York state commissioned a multidisciplinary group from Harvard to acquire information on malpractice in that state. For the year 1984 they reviewed 30,121 randomly selected records from 51 randomly selected hospitals in the state.[20, 92, 99] This extensive, well-designed, well-conducted research project provided, for the first time, valid factual information about medical malpractice, although the information may now be somewhat outdated. The fundamental findings of this study in terms of adverse events, negligence, and the incidence of suits are the following.

- Adverse events occurred in 3.7% of hospitalizations. Of these, only 27.6% were due to negligence, which thus occurred in approximately 1% of the hospitalizations. Most of these injuries were relatively minor.
- The percentage of adverse events attributable to negligence increased in the more severe injuries, in the elderly, in the uninsured, and in hospitals which served a large minority population and patients below the poverty level.
- Many of the adverse events identified were neither preventable nor predictable given the current state of medical knowledge. Fortunately, 70% of adverse events led only to short-term disability.
- Drug complications were the most common type of adverse event (19%), followed by wound infections (14%) and technical complications (13%). Twenty-nine percent of surgical adverse events were due to wound infection, and 13% of these were deemed negligent.
- Nearly half the adverse events were associated with an operation. Thirty-six percent of the "surgical failures" were commonly related to such things as persistent back pain that responded to a second operation to correct a problem that had not been treated adequately in the first place.
- Only 3% of adverse events occurred in the emergency department, but 70% of these were due to negligence—often due to diagnostic errors.
- In only 17% of claims filed was there evidence of an actual negligent adverse event, and in 55% of these there was no evidence of a medical injury in the first place. Many of these claims were dropped early on.
- Ninety-eight percent of all adverse events due to negligence did not result in malpractice claims. Within this group, 58% of the patients had only moderately incapacitating injuries and recovered within 6 months.
- In other words, for every 7.5 negligent medical actions, only one malpractice claim was filed. On the other hand, only one malpractice claim was paid for every 15 torts inflicted on hospitals. However, when the more serious injuries are considered in patients under age 70, one claim was paid for every three negligent injuries.

Other information emerging from the Harvard study indicates that race, gender, income, and the characteristics of the hospital were not independently associated with risk for medical injury or substandard care, but the study found that the uninsured patient was indeed at a greater risk for negligent care.[25] The complexity of the care, the number of procedures performed, and the number of doctors involved in the care of the patient do not seem to be a major factor in suit initiation.[122] A recent follow-up of the 46 malpractice claims filed in the Harvard study showed that it was the permanence of the disability, not the fact of negligence, that was the major factor influencing the size of the malpractice payout in those cases.[21]

It might seem that adverse events occurring in only 3.7% of all hospital admissions with a 1% incidence of negligence is not too bad, and few if any comparable activities probably do as well.[16] But the Harvard study also tells us that there is too much *preventable* negligence and that the malpractice system is too inaccessible to the victims of negligent medical treatment. On the other hand, the Harvard study tells us that a substantial majority of malpractice claims filed are unassociated with negligent injury or any injury at all. Thus, the tort system does not adequately protect the patient but at the same time it leads to many unwarranted suits.[196]

Guidelines and Practice Parameters

The terms "guidelines" and "practice parameters" usually are used synonymously. However, to some, guidelines are less rigid and aimed at assisting the practitioner in making health care decisions, whereas practice parameters are somewhat more binding. "Guidelines" is probably the more acceptable and safer term to use.

To resolve conflicting concepts and terminology, the Institute of Medicine in 1990 recommended the following definitions:[32]

- *Practice Guidelines* are systematically developed statements to assist practitioner and patient decisions about appropriate health care for specific clinical circumstances.

- *Medical Review Criteria* are systematically developed statements that can be used to assess the appropriateness of specific health care decisions, services, and outcomes.

- *Standards of Quality* are authoritative statements of: 1) minimum levels of acceptable performance or results; 2) excellent levels of performance of results; or 3) the range of acceptable performance or results.

- *Performance Measures (Provisional)* are methods or instruments to estimate or monitor the extent to which the actions of a health care practitioner or provider conform to practice guidelines, medical review criteria, or standards of quality.

Many guidelines have been developed and adopted in the United States. Over 1,600 guidelines have been written by more than 60 organizations, and more are being produced all the time.[4] They relate to the malpractice problem in that they speak to the standard of care and to the extent that they may be used to confirm or deny adherence to the standard of care.

Guidelines have been developed by various agencies, states, and physician groups, but those developed by the federal Agency for Health Care Policy and Research perhaps come closest to representing standards of care. However, the existing rules of evidence limit the use of guidelines in establishing the legal standard of care, which still rests upon expert testimony. Under the "hearsay rule," courts generally allow guidelines to be admitted as evidence, but only in conjunction with expert testimony.[87,100]

Guidelines for patient management received a boost in 1989 when the Federal Omnibus Budget Reconciliation Act (OBRA) supported the concept of practice guidelines to help control

costs and waste and utilize only effective procedures.[51] The success of the anesthesiology practice parameters, as well as the parameters set up to define who should or should not receive a pacemaker, has stimulated interest in the more widespread development of practice parameters. The Agency for Health Care Policy and Research has sponsored guidelines on postoperative pain management, bedsores, urinary incontinence, cataracts, benign prostatic hypertrophy, low back pain, and sickle cell disease, and others are being developed. Also, the AMA [American Medical Association] Practice Parameters Partnership and Forum is preparing a CD-ROM that will allow access to the entire collection. These have been created by a group of experts who by consensus used their best judgment in developing the statements. Health insurers, health maintenance organizations (HMOs), and utilization management firms have also prepared their own versions of criteria or guidelines which may be used for refusing payment for "inappropriate" care.[51] Many medical specialty groups are actively developing their own set of guidelines. State workers' compensation agencies have also created such guidelines.

Specific problems with guidelines include: the inherent complexity of the practice of medicine, the variability in treatment options, the difficulty of using guidelines in the patient with multiple problems, the uncertainty of the best management courses, and particularly, rapid outdating. Some clinical situations lend easily to parameters and guidelines, but many do not.

Despite these problems, the concept of guidelines makes sense to many, and it is the hope that good guidelines, if widely accepted, will help alleviate the malpractice problem by: 1) reducing the number of claims by improving the quality of care; 2) reducing the number of suits by outlining what is appropriate care; 3) providing protection for the practitioner who could demonstrate adherence to these norms; 4) satisfying insurance companies and funding agencies that management and treatment are quality and cost controlled; 5) reducing the time and cost of litigation; and 6) reducing the costs of defensive medicine by defining what tests and procedures are truly indicated. However, the true effect of guidelines will not be known until they have been more widely used.[30]

The expanded use of guidelines has been considered by some to be a more legally acceptable alternative to reform than such proposed changes as no-fault programs, pretrial screening, or the limiting of the size of awards. On the other hand, if (as the Harvard study has shown) there are many more cases of negligent injury than reach the courts, there is a concern that guidelines may suggest inadequate care and therefore increase the number of claims filed.

Guidelines have met with some success in the malpractice arena. According to the American College of Physicians, they have resulted in decreased numbers of malpractice claims and lower insurance premiums.[54] Harvard's anesthesia malpractice losses were significantly lower following implementation of the standards set up to monitor for hypoxia during anesthesia. The professional liability premiums for the Harvard hospitals, other Massachusetts physicians, and anesthesiologists nationwide have been reduced.[54,74,97,131]

Under the common law of most states, to admit practice guidelines as evidence, a party must demonstrate that they are relevant and that they meet some exception to the hearsay rule. Relevancy is more easily documented for guidelines, and the common law has evolved an exception to the hearsay rule that allows experts to testify regarding the contents of "learned treatises" which would be applicable to the admittance of guidelines if the scientific validity of the guidelines can be demonstrated. Once the guidelines are admitted into evidence, the jury may consider them as evidence of the standard of care. In some states, the written document may be placed directly into evidence, while in other states, following the federal approach, a written document containing guidelines or practice parameters is not received as an exhibit. Instead, it can only be read into evidence in conjunction with the testimony of the expert.[11,19]

In the face of guidelines, if negligence is claimed, expert witnesses will still be needed to show that the guidelines are indeed authoritative and accepted by the medical profession, to confirm that the guidelines are current and correct, to propose alternate standards of care, to justify why a defendant did not follow the guidelines, or to show that the guideline was not applicable to the case at hand.[54]

In November 1993, Blue Cross and Blue Shield of Illinois introduced a provision into its contracts with specialists that required them to follow established practice guidelines developed by national medical specialty organizations. About 925 of the 1,300 specialists who received the contracts had signed and returned them by the end of February 1994.[26]

As part of a 5-year demonstration project, the state of Maine developed practice parameters and risk management protocols for four specialties: anesthesiology, obstetrics and gynecology, emergency medicine, and radiology. These are admissible as a defense in malpractice cases. To prevent them from being used against physicians, the law prohibits their being introduced by the plaintiff.[131,187] Although it was the hope that the Maine guidelines would aid the defense of malpractice cases, after 3 years into this experience there has been no instance in which the guidelines have been introduced as a defense at trial or at a pretrial screening panel. This may relate to the complexity of the cases in which claims have been filed.[131]

Minnesota allows its state-developed guidelines to be used as an absolute defense in malpractice litigation.[124] Vermont will allow a wide variety of guidelines but makes them available to both the plaintiff and defendant. The guidelines hold no more legal weight than other expert testimony.[187]

A survey of 578 attorneys revealed that 27% reported that a guideline had influenced their decision to settle a case. Twenty-six percent stated that guidelines had been influential at least once in the previous year in a decision not to take a case, and 40% reported that a guideline influenced their decision to accept at least one case in the previous year. The same study found that practice guidelines are likely to be used for inculpatory purposes (implicating the defendant physician) twice as frequently as for exculpatory purposes (exonerating the physician).[78] A report to the Physician Payment Review Commission entitled "Practice Guidelines and Medical Litigation in 1994" noted that the guidelines have more often been used to cite error and attach blame rather than to clear the physician from guilt. They have not been useful as an aid for defendant physicians in medical malpractice.[131]

Despite the widespread dissemination and

enthusiasm for guidelines, caution is required when considering them as "standards of care." Although guidelines represent another factor to be added to the equation for the evaluation of patient care, further experience will be required to determine their place as an adjunct to medical practice.

Not to be confused with practice guidelines, "practice profiles" have been developed by numerous sources and are performance-based assessments attempting to evaluate the quality of physician care. They are part of the "need to know" attitude about the accountability and capability of the physician and thus indirectly relate to malpractice. Most are based on patterns of care and billing experience rather than specific clinical decisions, physician performance, or outcome assessment and they may be more oriented to cost considerations than patient care.[199] They have already been used in decisions about hiring, firing, disciplining, and paying physicians and they may be used in such instances as granting clinical privileges and certifying physicians.[85] They are currently in use by half of all hospitals in the U.S.[136] The general feeling is that these profiles must be much more accurate than they are now to be valid indicators of patient care, and, when used, an appeals mechanism must be in place to ensure fairness to the practitioner.

Another mechanism for reviewing the physician is the Uniform Clinical Data Set developed by the Health Care Financing Administration (HCFA) to evaluate the management of Medicare patients. The Data Set is used to look at physician practice patterns (such as the number of admissions, average length of stay, malpractice claims, and volume of procedures), to compare them with practice patterns of other physicians, and to identify physicians who deviate from the norm.[72]

Costs and Cost Controls Through Tort Reform

Malpractice law alters health care costs in two ways: 1) directly, through the costs of administering the malpractice system (these direct costs may be hard to measure), and 2) indirectly, through the effects of the malpractice system on physician and hospital behavior by such things as the effect of deterrence and defensive medicine on cost—either up or down.

A background study entitled *Impact of Legal Reforms on Medical Malpractice Costs* was prepared by the Office of Technology Assessment (OTA).[189] This study pointed out, as have other studies, that the direct costs of medical malpractice measured by insurance premiums paid by physicians, hospitals, HMOs, and other providers account for less than 1% of the health care budget. The OTA study showed that there was a steady increase in the number of claims per 100 physicians over the period 1980-1984 in every state.

On the other hand, more recent data from the St. Paul Fire and Marine Insurance Co. indicate that claim frequency was stable from 1990 through the first half of 1992. Also, total direct insurance losses, a measure that combines trends in both payment per paid claim and the probability of a claim resulting in payment, have declined in both current and constant dollars in recent years. Malpractice insurance premiums declined 10% between 1989 and 1991.[208]

Another factor in the equation is the increase in costs related to alterations in a physician's practice due to fear of liability. As a result of this fear, in 1984 the average physician increased record-keeping costs by 2.9%, prescribed 3.2% more tests and treatment procedures, increased follow-up visits by 2.6%, and spent 2.4% more time with patients. The total increase was approximately $5,900 per physician or $10.6 billion, a cost that was passed on to the system by increased fees.[18]

One way to reduce costs is to limit access to the courts. Access to the courts can be limited by the requirement of *pretrial screening panels*. The purpose of this panel is to weed out the frivolous claims and bring about a speedy settlement of the meritorious claims. The panel often consists of an attorney and/or judge, a doctor or other health care provider, and a lay person.[188] Of the 22 states with some form of pretrial screening, it is mandatory in 16. Screening panels have produced a large backlog of cases in some states. These panels have been overturned in six states on the grounds that they infringe on the state constitutional rights of trial or access to the courts.[189]

Costs also can be reduced by limiting malpractice awards. Thirty states rescinded the *collateral source rule* and permit the disclosure of other sources of monetary reward such as health and disability insurance, Medicare and Medicare reimbursements, Social Security, workers' compensation benefits, and Blue Cross and Blue Shield, which may be subtracted from the jury award through either a discretionary or mandatory offset.

A cap on *damage awards* has been initiated in several states. These caps are usually imposed on noneconomic damages, which often translates into pain and suffering awards. These damages, broadly defined, now make up nearly 50% of total tort damages paid for medical cases.[195] The amount most often proposed as a cap is $250,000 on noneconomic damages, which would seem to be reasonable.[82]

Alternate proposals recommend the development of a *scale* of damages to prevent the more minor injuries from being compensated to the same degree as major injuries, or a *schedule* of injuries that would fix a precise damage amount for each type of injury.[195]

A cap on damage awards is the one reform that consistently has been shown to decrease the malpractice cost indicators. As a result of the Medical Injury Compensation Recovery Act (MICRA) enacted in California in 1975, the limit of $250,000 has stabilized malpractice premiums, and physicians feel that cases are less likely to be pursued because of their emotional value alone.[185] But such caps have been controversial, and at least 15 state supreme courts have declared them unconstitutional.[189]

A cap on *punitive damages,* except where malice can be established, has also been proposed. Some would have the punitive award payable to the state medical disciplinary board to improve risk management rather than to the patient.[141] Others believe all or part of the punitive award should be converted to a societal benefit.

Periodic payments may reduce the impact of a large award on the payor. Fourteen states mandate periodic payments if damages exceed a threshold level which usually ranges from $100,000 to $250,000. Another 16 states allow for but do not mandate court-awarded periodic payments.

Joint liability permits a plaintiff to sue several defendants and recover from each one. In *several liability*, the plaintiff may also sue any one defendant and recover the total amount of damages, even if the defendant is only partially responsible. This does not mean the defendant will ultimately pay the entire amount, because he or she can sue the other defendants for their share.[189] Assistant surgeons may find themselves involved in a lawsuit even though they were only remotely connected to an untoward event. Approximately two-thirds of the states have modified this rule to some extent.[190] In some states, several liability has been eliminated. More often, however, the statutes require that several liability be limited depending upon the degree of the defendant's or plaintiff's fault or the ability of other defendants to pay the claim. A number of states make several liability conditional on the defendant's meeting a certain threshold of responsibility.[189,190]

Most states have *statutes of limitations,* usually 2 years. The statute of limitations begins at the time that the plaintiff knew or should have known about the injury. The "discovery rule" allows the judge to determine if a longer period is allowable in those cases where it was not reasonable to discover the injury earlier than 2 years. For minors, the statute of limitations is usually extended until a specified time after the child has reached the age of 18 years.

Only a few studies exist on the efficacy of these reforms as they relate to claim frequency and payment per claim. Two studies showed that pretrial screening panels had little or no effect on the frequency of malpractice claims, but one study showed that these panels did significantly increase payment per paid claim.[42,207] Two studies reviewing the effect of collateral source offsets showed that although mandatory offsets had no significant effect on frequency of claims, these offsets significantly reduced payment per paid claim.[40,207] Limits on attorney fees produced a significant effect on frequency of claims but no impact on malpractice premiums.[40, 208] Another study found no significant effect on either payment per paid claim or the probability that the claim would result in payment.[174] The evidence regarding the effect of limitation of the statute of limitations on malpractice claim frequency is mixed. These reforms showed no effect on payment per paid claim.

OTA's "tentative conclusions" based on an analysis of tort reform proposals are that caps on intangible (non-economic) damage awards (most frequently recommended at $250,000) and mandatory collateral source effects were the only reforms that showed a consistent and significant effect in reducing malpractice costs.[189] Surprisingly, mandatory or discretionary periodic payments showed no significant impact either on payment per paid claim or on the probability that the claim would result in payment.[13,173] The OTA study also raises the question of whether the reduction of medical malpractice costs mitigates the deterrent effect on physician behavior by removing the incentive for more thorough diagnostic workup of patients, thus jeopardizing the overall quality of patient care.

Tort reform is occurring. Over half the states have amended the traditional collateral source rule, allowed for periodic payments, shortened or modified the statute of limitations, implemented pretrial screening, and/or placed some type of limit on attorney fees. Some of these have been voluntary and some state mandated. In addition, almost half the states have set statutory caps on noneconomic or total damage awards. There is increasing interest in using practice guidelines in reducing costs.

A liability reform bill, the Common Sense Product Liability and Legal Reform Act (H.R. 956), recently passed in the U.S. House includes amendments that would: 1) extend the bill's joint and several liability (i.e., "fair share") provisions to medical liability lawsuits; and 2) limit non-economic damage awards to $250,000. The Senate passed a modified version of this bill which does not include any provisions that directly deal with medical liability. Through conference reconciliation, Congress may resolve the differences in these two versions. Medical liability provisions are included in the House's Medicare reform bill, the Medicare Preservation Act (H.R. 2425), which was released in September 1995. This bill includes a $250,000 cap on non-economic damage awards, joint and several liability reforms, and a statute of limitations on filing of claims. The Senate Medicare reform plan provided no medical liability reform provisions.[163]

The Contingency Fee Question

The arguments on behalf of contingency fees are straightforward. These arrangements allow individuals who might otherwise be unable to afford legal vindication of their rights to gain access to justice and fulfill the fundamental ideal of equality before the law. The current contingency fee system is effective in weeding out a significant number of non-meritorious claims, once the facts are learned, because it is not worth the time and effort for most attorneys to take a case that does not predict a favorable outcome for the plaintiff. A figure of $50,000 is often cited as a starting consideration for many lawyers.[187] Other justifications for the contingency fee consider that: 1) it widens access to the legal profession; 2) it permits persons, regardless of their poverty, to spread the risk of defeat in litigation; and 3) the lawyer, theoretically at least, becomes a strong advocate of the plaintiff.

The arguments against contingency fees are that they lead to an increase in the volume of litigation and comprise and encourage opportunistic, vexatious, and frivolous claims.[101,205] Elimination of the contingency fee and the limitation of attorney fees has been a popular proposal, especially among physicians. The English common law, the French and German civil law, and the Roman law all hold that it is unethical for lawyers to accept contingency fees and such fees are not accepted anywhere in the world except the United States and a few Canadian provinces.[101,140]

Cases taken on a contingency basis involve a risk to the attorney (the risk of losing), and because of this risk successful clients pay their lawyers more than they would under alternative fee arrangements. Unfortunately, the percentage fee may be set at a figure that bears little relationship to the time and money that lawyers must put at risk. Indeed, there may be a high contingency fee in situations when there is no risk of failure, when perhaps a flat fee should be charged.[23] About one-half of the states either specify a limit on attorney fees or authorize the courts to set these fees.[189]

Revisions of the contingency fee system include staging the fee (e.g., 15% if settled at a pretrial screening, and up to 35% if the case goes to a trial verdict). This arrangement would provide a more rational relationship to the actual amount of work involved, the expenditures, and risk undertaken by the attorney. It also would encourage defendants to consider early settlement because they will pay a smaller proportion to their attorney.[197]

Perhaps a cap on defense attorney fees should also be considered.

Problem Areas

In 25% to 30% of all malpractice cases, a missed or delayed diagnosis is the basis of the suit.[49,191] Related to this, a 1991 study found that the most frequently reported claim in medical malpractice cases was wrongful death (37%).[116] A 1995 study by the Physician Insurers Association of America revealed that the single most common source of malpractice claims is the failure to timely diagnose breast cancer. This same association in their evaluation of 78,712 claims found that 36% of all medical "misadventures" leading to claims were due to improper physician performance. Errors in diagnosis accounted for 24% of misadventures, with the diagnosis of breast cancer, cancer of the lung, appendicitis, acute myocardial infarction, and ectopic pregnancy being the most common. Other areas with common problems included improper prescription of medication, consultations, interview and evaluation, and abdominal hysterectomy. The most frequently occurring misadventures leading to a high average indemnity were related to delay in performing a procedure or not performing it at all. Cesarean section was most often cited here. Failure to postpone a case had the single highest average indemnity, but problems monitoring a patient during surgery or recovery, failure to properly respond, and improper performance of resuscitation were not far behind.[73]

Other in-house areas with problems frequently encountered included patient falls, burns or pressure neuropathy (often in operating room situations), and poor management of cardiac arrest where excellent records are required.

Additional problem areas that bear on malpractice relate to unnecessary surgery, which unquestionably does occur. This is suggested by the variation in the frequency of procedures.

Angioplasty is done three times more often in Connecticut than in Boston. Tonsils are removed in Maine at eight times the national average.[139] The U.S. Value Health Sciences cites as unnecessary: 27% of hysterectomies, 14% of laminectomies, 17% of carpal tunnel surgeries, and 16% of tonsillectomies. In one area of Maine, 50% of men had prostate surgery by the age of 85, whereas in another city in the state just 10% did.[194] However, local standards of care as well as academic training and requirements of hospitals and managed care facilities may determine why a physician performed a particular service.[2]

In the Harvard study, almost 75% of the claims originated in the following areas in the hospital setting:[196]

- *Emergency Department:* Although only 3% of all adverse events occurred in the emergency department, 70% of the injuries were due to negligence, often a failure to diagnose.
- *Surgery:* The highest number of adverse events occurred here (48%), but these were less likely to be judged negligent than the nonsurgical adverse events (17% vs. 37%, respectively).
- *Diagnostic Errors:* Although making up only 8% of adverse events, 75% were considered due to negligence.
- *Medication Errors:* These amounted to 19% of all adverse events but in most the impact was relatively minor. However, 14% of these resulted in permanent disability or death. Medication injuries were less likely to be due to negligence than almost any other type, and most often were due to the fact that many were related to unpredictable and nonpreventable side effects or allergic reactions. Antibiotics were a frequent cause.

Complications arise as a problem when: it cannot be shown that the physician (surgeon) anticipated the complication or made plans to prevent, neutralize, or reverse it; the physician did not provide adequate informed consent; the physician did not properly respond to the complication; or the physician did not explain the problem to the family's satisfaction.[112]

A high risk of claims is to be expected in catastrophic incidents such as paralysis (e.g., from neurosurgical procedures, anesthetic accidents, or improper use of casts), brain damage (e.g., obstetric cases, neurosurgical procedures, or cardiac arrest), blindness (e.g., from ophthalmological procedures or neurosurgical operations), loss of a limb (e.g., from arterial injury or improper use of casts), and unexpected death.

Defensive Medicine

Any consideration of the malpractice problem also involves the issue of defensive medicine. Defensive medicine unquestionably is a response to the physician's fear of "failing to diagnose," a most common cause for suits.[49,187] The AMA definition considers defensive medicine to be "the performance of diagnostic tests and treatment procedures which, but for the threat of malpractice action, would not have been done."[151] The unnecessary performance of tests and procedures for defensive purposes is considered to be "positive defensive medicine." The avoidance of high-risk patients and procedures for defensive purposes is "negative defensive medicine."

Often cited as excessive are such practices as overutilization of skull x-rays and computed tomography scans in head trauma, elective fetal monitoring, cesarean sections, and pre-anesthesia laboratory testing. In the past, defensive medicine was encouraged by the presence of a readily available funding source—health insurance. It can be argued that the performance of unnecessary services is immoral, unethical, and even fraudulent, and therefore in itself is a form of medical malpractice.[143] However, some defensive medicine may be beneficial (e.g., spending more time to communicate with patients or keeping better records). In addition, unexpected findings from tests performed defensively may improve patient care. These multiple and various factors cannot be completely calculated, making it impossible to determine the true cost of defensive medicine.

A 1983 study by the AMA of 1,240 physicians revealed that the following occurred because of litigation threats: 41% prescribed more than the usual diagnostic tests; 27% said they provided additional treatment procedures; 36% said they spent more time with patients; 45% referred more cases; 35% refused to accept certain kinds of cases; and 57% kept better records.[154] A 1992 Gallup poll found that 93% of physicians practice defensive medicine.[198] However, there has been no reliable hard data to indicate the true cost of defensive medicine to the health care system. Estimates of this cost range from $9 billion a year to the often quoted $36 billion for 5 years recently estimated by the research firm of Lewin-VHI, Inc.[96,155]

To help resolve this dilemma and arrive at a useful estimate of the cost of defensive medicine, the U.S. House Committee on Ways and Means and the Senate Committee on Labor and Human Resources requested that the OTA provide an in-depth study of defensive medicine. This was initiated in February 1992.[187] Because of the complexity of the issues and despite the thoroughness of the study, OTA declared that the accurate measurement of the extent and cost of defensive medicine was "virtually impossible" to achieve. The OTA study did uncover some interesting aspects of the problem. There is a wide disparity in physicians' concepts of defensive medicine. The number of physicians who cited malpractice concerns as a primary reason for choosing certain clinical actions varied between 5% and 29%. Physician respondents indicating restrictions in their practices due to malpractice concerns varied from 1% to 64%, and from 20% to 81% stated that malpractice liability concerns had led them to order additional tests and procedures. One study ranked malpractice concerns last out of 19 reasons for excessive testing,[202] and, according to the OTA study, less than 8% of diagnostic procedures were performed because of the fear of malpractice. This is perhaps the most significant finding of the OTA study. There were two clinical areas where defensive medicine was more clearly a problem. The cost of "defensive" cesarean deliveries in 1991 was $8.7 million, and the cost of diagnostic radiology of the head in minor head injury was $45 million. In addition, general practitioners and nurse-midwives in high liability areas have reduced their obstetric practices with the result that obstetricians have a greater volume of cases. The OTA study indicated that the usual malpractice "reforms" would most likely have little or no effect on the practice of defensive medicine.

The OTA study has been criticized by U.S. Rep. J. Dennis Hastert (R-Illinois) on the basis that it was "designed to intentionally underestimate the phenomenon of defensive medicine," and several American College of Surgeons members of the advisory panel for the study took exception to some of the conclusions of the report.[163] In general, however, the costs and extent of defensive medicine are probably overestimated and amount to only a small fraction of the overall national health care costs.

Future changes in the way medicine is practiced, including malpractice reform, clinical practice guidelines, alternate dispute resolution, health care reform, managed competition, and risk management, will further confound the defensive medicine issue.

The Impaired Physician

The AMA identifies the "impaired physician" as someone whose professional performance is adversely affected by reason of mental illness, alcoholism, or drug dependence.[1] Another definition considers that the impaired physician is unable to practice medicine with reasonable skill and safety by reason of physical or mental illness, including the results of stress and aging. On the other hand, the incompetent physician is not ill, but ignorant or unskillful, and the unethical physician knowingly and willingly violates fundamental norms of conduct toward others, especially his or her own patients. These often overlap.[128]

A British study of disciplinary problems in physicians found, in the order of frequency, the following forms of disruptive or irresponsible behavior: lack of commitment to duties; poor skills and inadequate knowledge; dishonesty, sexual misbehavior; disorganized practice; and poor communication with peers. This study found these problems in 6% of the senior medical staff.[45]

A spectrum of causes of physician-related adverse patient outcomes can be identified and some relate to impairment. The first is the complete accident in which the physician is in no way responsible, as with a sudden power failure or equipment malfunction. The second is the well-justified action or decision by the physician that unexpectedly turns out badly. The third involves those decisions and actions of the physician where there is disagreement or uncertainty in the medical community as to the best course of action. The fourth is where the physician exercises poor, although not outrageously bad, judgment or skill. The fifth involves those actions that are egregious or outrageous violations of the expected quality of care. Knowledge of these categories, the last two indicating an impaired physician, along with a measure of the seriousness of the violation in each area, can be of value to committees evaluating physician actions and behavior.[128]

A major cause of physician impairment is substance abuse, including alcoholism and drug dependence. The AMA and the American Psychiatric Association consider alcoholism to be a primary, chronic disease with genetic, psychological, and environmental factors influencing its development and manifestations.[14] The AMA estimates a lifetime prevalence for physicians of 6%-8% for alcoholism and 1%-2% for drug dependency.[76]

The drug addiction rate among physicians probably compares with that in the general population.[22,111] Certain specialties have an increased problem, namely family practitioners, anesthesiologists, psychiatrists, and those in emergency medicine.[29,169,181] Patterns include cannabis and cocaine abuse in medical students, the use of benzodiazepines by the practicing physician, and the use of a pure opiate (often fentanyl) by the anesthesiologist.[206] The New Jersey Commission of Investigation in 1992 reported that up to 13% of that state's doctors may be addicted to drugs or alcohol.[193]

Etiology and Detection of Chemical Dependency. Several investigators have attempted to define the etiological factors for chemical dependency in physicians.[84,111,156,180,206] Although no certain or well-defined cause is apparent, suggestions include genetic predisposition, parental deprivation, associated depressive reaction, poor coping skills, drug availability, chronic fatigue, stress factors, and high-risk specialties. Because of the risk, 25 states now prohibit physicians from prescribing for themselves or their families.[29]

The early discovery of chemical dependency in a physician may be difficult. The hallmark of dependency is denial. This, along with family and colleague acceptance of the problem, often allows the matter to progress to a point where work is affected. Because most persons agree

TABLE 1

PROBLEMS OF THE DRUG- OR ALCOHOL-IMPAIRED PHYSICIAN IN
SIX AREAS OF BEHAVIORAL PATTERNS*

Community
- Isolation and withdrawal from community activities, leisure pursuits, hobbies, church, friends, or peers
- Embarrassing behavior at club or parties
- Arrests for driving while intoxicated; legal problems
- Unreliability and unpredictability in community and social activities
- Unpredictable behavior (e.g., inappropriate spending, or excessive involvement in political activities)

Family
- Withdrawal from family activities, unexplained absences from home
- Fights; child abuse
- Development in spouse of disease of "spousaholism"
- Abnormal, antisocial, illegal behavior by children
- Sexual problems—impotence, extramarital affairs, contracultural sexual behavior
- Assumption of surrogate role by spouse and children
- Institution of geographic separation or divorce proceedings by spouse

Employment
- Numerous job changes in past 5 years
- Frequent geographic relocations for unexplained reasons
- Frequent hospitalizations
- Complicated and elaborate medical history (often obtained from employment applications)
- Unexplained intervals between jobs
- Indefinite or inappropriate references
- Working in job inappropriate for qualifications
- Reluctance of job applicant to let spouse and children be interviewed

- Reluctance to undergo immediate pre-employment physical examination

Physical Status
- Deterioration in personal hygiene
- Deterioration in clothing and dressing habits
- Multiple physical signs and complaints
- Numerous prescriptions and drug use
- Accidents
- Emotional crises

Office
- Disruption of appointment schedule
- Hostile, withdrawn, unreasonable behavior to staff and patients
- "Locked-door syndrome"
- Excessive ordering of supplies of drugs from local druggists or by mail
- Complaints by patients to staff about doctor's behavior
- Absence from office (unexplained or due to frequent illness)

Hospital
- Making rounds late or inappropriately abnormal behavior during rounds
- Decreasing quality of performance (e.g., in staff presentations or writing in chart)
- Inappropriate orders or overprescription of medications
- Reports of behavioral changes from hospital personnel ("hospital gossip")
- Involvement in malpractice suits and legal sanctions against hospital
- Reports from emergency department staff of unavailability or inappropriate responses to telephone calls

* Listed in the sequence in which they present. Developed by the impaired-physician program in Georgia.[180]

that denial and defensiveness prevent early detection, questionnaires such as the CAGE (cutting down, annoyance by criticism, guilty feeling, and eye-openers) and the Michigan Alcohol Screening Test (MAST) may be useful in detecting the problem.[39,48,110] Clearly, recognition and treatment are most important to protect the physician and prevent the development of a serious problem that may jeopardize patient care.

Table 1 lists the problems of the drug- or alcohol-impaired physician in six areas of behavior patterns developed by the impaired-physician program in Georgia.[180] The hospital impaired-physician committee should use and disseminate these or similar lists.

In the usual sequence of events, initially there is a breakdown of family life and relationships, loss of friends, "driving under the influence" infractions, and public intoxication[28] as the problems cited in Table 1 start appearing.[180]

Due process plays an important role here, and basic to the whistleblower's action is proof in the strictest legal sense that there is indeed a problem. This may be difficult because accusation is not tantamount to guilt, and the legal process may be tested by some of these cases.

The Impaired-Physician Committee. Every hospital should have such a physician aid committee made up of perhaps one member of each major department, but especially including an anesthesiologist and a family physician because these are high-risk areas. The committee should not be so large that there is a risk of loss of confidentiality. A limit of seven members has been suggested. The files and monitoring reports should be kept in the strictest confidence. Educational programs should be initiated for the medical staff, hospital personnel, and physician office staff so they will be able to recognize the problem physician.[105]

Intervention with the identified physician should be collegial, often with a friend, and with the realization that the initial confrontation often will be met with denial and a lack of cooperation regarding treatment. A hard line often is required. Once treatment is initiated, a monitoring program should be enforced.

Treatment. Recovery-oriented multidisciplinary treatment programs which have abstinence and early intervention as a goal have found the 12-step program of Alcoholics Anonymous and Narcotics Anonymous to be the most common form of treatment for chemical dependence (Table 2).[14]

A more vigorous control system involves contingency contracting. The physician agrees, in a written contract, that the physician's therapist may mail a license-surrendering letter if a urine sample is positive for the drug of abuse. Probationary privileges can be recovered in some instances, however.[37] Contingency contracting together with long-term urine monitoring offers the highest cure rate for substance abuse.[169]

Fortunately, physicians have a better outcome from treatment for alcohol and substance abuse than the general public. In New Jersey, 73.8% of physicians had no known relapses, and 12.6% had one relapse. A 2-year follow-up on this group showed a recovery rate of 83.8% with no relapses and 13.8% with one relapse.[152] Eighty-three percent of physicians versus 62%

TABLE 2

ELEMENTS OF A MODERN INPATIENT PROGRAM*

- Detoxification from alcohol and drugs
- Monitored abstinence from mood-altering agents
- Treatment of current medical ailments
- Positive health habits in diet, exercise, and sleep
- Participation in supervised group and community therapy
- Diagnostic evaluation and self revelation
- Evaluation and intervention with the family
- Mediation with the employer and authorities
- Introduction to Alcoholics or Narcotics Anonymous
- Short-term limited objective counseling
- Instruction in short-term recovery skills
- Discharge planning and continued aftercare

* Reproduced from Bohigian et al.[14]

of the general population have a good outcome.[130] Regardless of the treatment protocol, duration of treatment seems most important, and one month of in-house treatment with a 2-year monitored follow-up produced the best results. Inpatient treatment is very expensive, however, and may amount to $20,000 for a 30-day stay.[14,69,130] Shore[169] found a 96% improved rate in urine-monitored physicians, but only a 64% improved rate in unmonitored physicians. Involvement with Alcoholics Anonymous was the most successful element in the recovery process.[53] In general, the prognosis is better for those over the age of 40.[29] Interestingly, the drug-addicted physician had a better outcome with fewer relapses than the alcoholic.[69,130]

Impairment due to mental illness unassociated with chemical dependency accounts for between 6% and 20% of cases reported to state physician health programs.[29] Disruptive behavior such as tirades in the operating room, throwing equipment, foul language, obstreperous conduct, abusive treatment of employees or patients, or disruption of meetings must be handled similarly to the alcohol or drug abuser. Courts have held that hospitals have a duty to take action when physicians' conduct disrupts the operation of the hospital, affects the ability of others to get their jobs done, creates a "hostile work environment" for hospital employees or other physicians, or begins to interfere with the physician's own ability to practice competently.[90,105]

Another common problem is sexual harassment, which takes two forms: when job benefits or adverse job consequences are dependent upon sexual favors, and when the environment is made uncomfortable by the fondling, off-color jokes, and sexual overtones of the perpetrator. Under the Civil Rights Act of 1991, victims of sexual harassment may demand jury trials and punitive damages.[105]

Age-related impairments that may be of concern to physicians are: decline in motor ability (particularly for surgeons), decline in short-term memory and learning, altered judgment and decline in intellectual ability, and the development of central nervous system degenerative changes.[79] Aging may be associated with decreased ability to learn and retain new information, memory lapses and lack of recall, social withdrawal, difficulty with change, decreased concentration, and decreased levels of practice and clinical judgment.[108] These considerations are important when one considers that many physicians remain in practice 6 to 7 years beyond the average retirement age of 65.[57] Several or all of the above problems may have to be considered in individual cases.

Psychiatric disease is also problematic. In general, the prognosis for recovery from psychiatric disease is worse than with chemical dependency—78% improvement for addicted physicians vs. 57% for those with psychiatric disorders.[169] The suicide rate among these physicians with psychiatric disorders is 3.5 times greater than in the general population.[10]

An annual review process to assess these and other areas of impairment that is routine, fair, and acceptable to the staff should be a standard hospital function and is now in place in most hospitals. Support groups and counseling should be available. Every state medical society now has a program and committee to evaluate physician impairment and assist physicians with rehabilitation.

Factors Leading Toward Litigation

The increase in the frequency of malpractice suits has raised questions as to whether we are indeed living in a litigious society. Like other aspects of the malpractice question, this question incurs individual bias and preconceived perceptions that are unsupported by the facts.

A 1977 study showed that lawsuits were more common in white-collar, older, educated but unemployed people. There was a greater lawsuit incidence in persons of Jewish faith as compared to Protestant faiths. The study also showed that suits were more common in those dissatisfied with their health care, those who incurred complications, those admitted into a specific department of the hospital, and in instances where a lack of communication between hospital staff and the patient existed.[44] In another study, the best predictors of patients who would later indicate an intent to sue were the number of complications that occurred, the patient satisfaction index, a white-collar job, and being admitted to a specific medical floor.[122] More recent studies, covering larger patient samples, showed that poor patients, the elderly, and uninsured patients were less likely to file claims for malpractice.[24,25] It has been found that the elderly and Medicaid recipients are also less likely to sue.[134,161] A study by the OTA came to similar conclusions,[188] and the U.S. General Accounting Office noted that Medicare beneficiaries were underrepresented in suits.[191]

A study of factors prompting families to sue following perinatal injuries revealed that the initiating factor for 33% of respondents was that they were advised to sue by knowledgeable acquaintances; there was a recognized cover-up in 24%; parents needed money in 24%; there was a realization that the child would have no future in 23%; parents needed information in 20%; and parents decided to seek revenge or protect others from harm in 19%. Over one-third of all families indicated that they were told by medical personnel prior to filing that the care provided had caused their children's injuries. Again, they blamed poor physician-patient communication, saying that doctors would not listen (13%), would not talk openly (32%), attempted to mislead them (48%), or did not warn about long-term neurodevelopmental problems (70%).[71]

A study of 45 plaintiffs' depositions showed four major problem areas that led to the initiation of a suit: deserting the patient or a failure to be available (32%); devaluing patient and/or family views (29%); delivering information poorly (26%); and failing to understand the patient's and/or families' perspective (13%).[7] These problems of communication lead to frustration and a sense of betrayal and may be the primary reason for a suit. This may explain why some suits are initiated in the absence of an actual incident of negligent malpractice. Anger, revenge and vindictiveness are more often the real reasons for the suit. How the physician handles telephone calls, confronts uncertainty, delivers diagnostic information, or confronts patient and/or family grief are issues cited in the study. In 55%, it was apparent that another physician, usually the post-treatment consultant, suggested to the plaintiff that there had been a maloccurrence.[7]

In 80% of suits, the case was initiated by personal contact with a law firm by the plaintiff, and in 25% of these, the law firm contacted specialized in medical malpractice. In 10% to 15%, the attorney contacted the patient.[172]

A more recent study based on the results of 502 responses to unsolicited calls to law firms revealed that the most frequent reason callers gave for contacting the office was television advertising in 78%; poor relationships with doctors prior to the injury were cited in 53%, and other health care providers had recommended the pursuit of a suit in 27%. Twenty-five percent had been involved in other litigation (excluding divorce). The five specialties most often named by callers were obstetrics, family practice, orthopedic surgery, emergency medicine, and general surgery. Failure to diagnose and failure to properly perform a procedure were the acts most frequently claimed. Financial problems in the form of unemployment, lack of health insurance, and outstanding medical bills were present in almost one-half. Of 730 calls received by the law firms, only 3.3% eventually resulted in the filing of lawsuits.[77]

In one study of patients filing a lawsuit, physicians being sued, and physicians not being sued, all of the nonsued physicians felt that unanticipated treatment complications and unavoidable treatment consequences were factors in malpractice claims, while 59% of sued physicians and 70% of suing patients stated that unanticipated complications were factors in their suits, and 46% of sued physicians and 40% of suing patients indicated that unavoidable

treatment consequences played a role. Similarly, 58% of the nonsued physicians gave patients' excessive expectations of medical technology and/or the physicians' skills the highest rating as a factor in malpractice claims, in comparison with only 28% of sued physicians and none of the suing patients. There were two causative factors about which sued and nonsued physicians agreed, but with which patients disagreed. Eighty-three percent of sued and 85% of nonsued physicians felt that patients' desire for financial compensation was an important factor in malpractice claims, while 22% of suing patients felt this way; 60% of patients said it was not a factor at all. Patients themselves reported they sued because of the perception of physician negligence and/or error in 97%, and unexpected complications in 64%.[167]

The perceived risk of being sued is generally much higher than the facts would indicate, and this varies with specialty and location. Low-risk groups of physicians overestimate the risk of being sued by a factor of 3, and high-risk groups by a factor of 1.6. Physicians with cases in which an unintended adverse event occurred estimated a 45% chance of being sued. If there was perceived negligence, this rose to 60%. This is 30 times higher than the actual risk of being sued for negligence. On average, physicians estimate that 19.5 out of 100 of their colleagues will be sued in a given year, approximately three times the actual rate.[89] In Florida, a very litigious state, a study showed that 59% of physicians faced no malpractice claims, 13.4% had any paid claims, and only 7.2% had multiple paid claims.[17]

Is There a Litigious Patient?

There is little in the literature defining the litigious patient. According to one study, the major groups the doctors perceived as being "suit-prone" include the following, in order of frequency:[157]

> Insurance claimants
> Unfamiliar new patients
> Those seeing lawyers prior to seeing the
>   physician
> Back and neck injuries
> Auto accident cases
> Workers' compensation cases
> Patients gullible with lawyer

"Dishonesty, lacking in integrity"
Those previously treated by other doctors
A certain disposition.

In the same study, doctors perceived as the primary reasons that suits were instituted the following:

Patients after money
Unscrupulous lawyers
Lawyers' contingency fees
Publicity about trials
Lawyers seeking out cases
Doctor-patient communication problems
Our "something for nothing" society
Liberalism, permissiveness, intellectual dishonesty
The individual rights movement
A litigious society.

According to Melvin Belli, suit-prone patients include: 1) the "complainers" who find fault with everything and bad-mouth the doctor; 2) the "experts" who write down everything the doctor says or does and attempt to obtain a guarantee of cure; 3) the "malingerers" who miss appointments, do not take their medications, and resist treatment (it would be wise to keep good records on such patients, especially concerning noncompliance, and have a staff member present when giving important instructions); 4) the "cynics" who say "Have you guys cured the common cold yet?" or who chide doctors about their golf game; and 5) the "grievers" or those who are out of work or in debt and who resent the doctor's handsome income. He also warns of the patient who wants "nothing but the best." They must be assured that you are not a miracle worker.[9] This author would add to be cautious about the "take-over" family member who may come in from out of town and establish a hostile atmosphere.

Literature describing the litigious patient may be confusing. Contrary to the usual perceptions, the study of May and Stengel[109] found that patients did not sue because of the physician's lack of communication, his/her failure to involve the patient as a partner, or due to rushing the patient's visit. Instead, only perceived doctor competence and his/her concern differentiated potential suers from nonsuers.

If, as the Harvard study shows, the negligently injured patient rarely sues for malpractice, the question arises as to why so few injured patients file claims. This has not been widely researched but several reasons may be operant: namely, many may fail to recognize negligent care; many may receive adequate health or disability insurance benefits and may not wish to spoil long-standing physician-patient relationships; and others may regard their injuries as minor and consider the small chance of success not worth the cost or they may not like to deal with attorneys. Trial lawyers usually accept only the relatively few cases that have a high probability of a judgment of negligence and an award large enough to defray the high costs of litigation.[99]

Can a Malpractice Suit Lead to Attachment of a Physician's Assets?

Attaching a physician's assets following a malpractice suit verdict is an overriding fear of many physicians. There are several reasons why this is not a valid concern:

1. Verdicts awarding excessive amounts are unusual.

2. Most patients/plaintiffs will settle for the amount of the coverage even if the award exceeds this. It may simply cost too much in time, money, or emotional energy to prolong the process in the hope of receiving a larger award.

3. In general, plaintiff attorneys advise against seeking damages in the form of a physician's personal assets. Among the reasons for this are that it could lead to bad publicity for the attorney and public outcry for state retaliatory legislative action. (Malpractice that is gross or malicious, on the other hand, may be an inducement to seek the highest settlement possible.)

4. Court decisions have recently been inclined to hold insurers liable for excess verdicts. Physicians whose assets were threatened have successfully sued insurers for not protecting them by settling within the policy limits.

5. Fear of loss of assets may lead physicians to seek settlement when the case is one they could probably win.

It has happened, but the odds are all in the physician's favor.[34]

POSSIBLE SOLUTIONS TO THE MALPRACTICE PROBLEM

The National Practitioner Data Bank

The Health Care Quality Improvement Act of 1986 provided for the development of a practitioner data bank which went into effect on September 1, 1990. This national reporting system was designed to be a flagging system offering information of aid to licensing or credentialing authorities about "medical incompetence." The immediate and primary purpose of the program was to prevent the incompetent physician from practicing in one state after being banned in another. It is currently funded entirely by user fees. The law requires that the following be reported: 1) adverse actions taken against practitioners by state medical boards, specifically any revocation, suspension, censure, reprimand, probation, or surrender of a doctor's license; 2) any malpractice payments made on behalf of practitioners; 3) adverse actions on clinical privileges lasting 30 days or more; and 4) adverse actions of professional society memberships. If a practitioner refunds or forgoes a bill because of an unfortunate result, this too must be reported. Once a physician's name is listed in the data bank, it is impossible to remove it except for obvious error. Every reported event is in turn made known to the practitioner, who may appeal.

The information in the bank is available to the doctors themselves, professional societies, state licensing boards, HMOs, and other health care facilities. Every 2 years, hospitals must review any information contained in the Data Bank about their clinical staff before granting new staff appointments. Plaintiff's attorneys, and, in some cases, plaintiffs alone may request this information.[91] Several bills have been introduced into Congress to allow the public direct access to the information in the Data Bank. Information about the number and type of claims paid on behalf of individual physicians as well as specialty groups could be used to influence malpractice actions and legislation.

Of major concern to physicians is the entry of all awards, no matter how small, even if no negligence is proved. In 1994, however, the National Practitioner Data Bank began allowing physicians to submit a 600-character explanatory statement on any report filed.[150] Effective December 1994, physicians who pay malpractice claims out of their own pockets no longer are required to report these claims to the Data Bank. The Data Bank, however, has identified only 300 such cases of the more than 92,000 malpractice payments identified by them as of 1994.

There are some problems yet to be worked out.[46,132] The initial experience of the Data Bank indicates a marked variance in the reporting rate of adverse events from state to state (a low of 7.5% in one state to a high of 40% to 45% in other states) and an absence of conformity in supplying data. Furthermore, as of August 1993, 5,220 doctors were listed as having two liability-related reports each; however, by the Data Bank's own estimates, nearly 1,000 of these were from single incidents improperly recorded twice.

It can be argued that claim frequency is not indicative of competency, nor does it consider the value of the physician to the community.[99,172] Since the bank includes such data, it can be criticized for the same reasons.

Two 1993 reports from the Office of the Inspector General, U.S. Department of Health and Human Services, indicate that data bank information influenced hospital credentialing decisions only 1% of the time and that state boards of licensure were not influenced at all.[175]

Under no-fault and enterprise liability systems (see below) there would have to be a modification of the Data Bank reporting rules in that physician liability is a limited and uncertain factor in these systems.[2]

Of related interest is the recent move, effective in July 1996, by the Massachusetts Medical Society to release physician malpractice profiles to the World Wide Web. It was felt that by providing accurate data in its proper context, by limiting the information to paid claims rather than including open claims, and by excluding "nuisance" suits of less than $75,000, the plan would benefit the public more than the physician would be harmed.[14]

PREVENTION

Risk-management programs emphasize the above problem areas, and preventive actions have been established by various insurance companies, institutions, and legal firms. (Some of these are obligatory.)

The Harvard study identified medication errors as the leading cause of adverse events[20] and, in a large study of closed claims, drug injuries accounted for the highest total expenditure of any type of procedure-related injury.[135] On the other hand, approximately 50% of these adverse drug events are preventable. In one study, preventable excessive dosage of a drug for the patient's weight and calculated renal function accounted for 42% of all adverse drug events.[31] A recent study of the factors related to errors in medication prescribing found that improvement would come about by the standardization of processes, reduction of system complexity, computerization of the drug-prescribing process, improved and refocused prescriber education, and expanded use of the expertise of pharmacists through better integration with the health care system.[94] Many hospitals have computerized their drug management systems.

Another area for prevention involves physicians' staffs. A doctor-patient relationship is established with the first telephone call to the office. The patient must sense a friendly, compassionate, and sympathetic attitude. The staff should be aware of the emergency problems inherent in the practice of the physician and act upon them properly. Most important is the appreciation that all radiology and laboratory reports must be referred to the physician and not filed away. Especially important are abnormal radiograph and biopsy reports. One study showed that 36% of physicians do not always notify patients of abnormal test results.[177] The staff should be aware of the rights of the patient, which include keeping records confidential. Records should be kept of all canceled or missed appointments, and the physician notified. The physician should be made aware of any unusual events and phone calls. Filed information should be recoverable. Secretaries should be made aware that documentation is most important: "If it is not written down (or if it cannot be found), it did not happen." It is helpful if aides wear badges identifying who or what they are. Office personnel and assistants should avoid in any way treating or medically advising patients. They should not refill prescriptions or obtain informed consent. It is also helpful if this advice is spelled out in an office manual. This information should be periodically reviewed with the staff or arrangements made for attendance at risk-management programs.[68]

Alternatives to the Tort System

The determination of competence and causation are often complex issues and may require professional judgment. It has also been suggested that lay juries may react to the skill of the plaintiff attorney and his/her "expert" witnesses.[153] In addition, the present tort system is considered by many to be inefficient, costly, slow, and unable to appropriately compensate the patient or protect the innocent physician. Therefore, various alternatives to a tort system have been proposed.

Alternative Dispute Resolution

Alternative dispute resolution attempts to resolve disputes without litigation and usually involves the presentation of the facts to an impartial body or panel. The most common forms of alternative dispute resolution are arbitration and pretrial screening panels.

Most legislative action on alternative dispute resolution has concerned systems of arbitration. This approach, supported by the AMA and 31 national medical specialty societies, uses experienced decision-makers (rather than a lay jury) to reduce the costs of resolving a dispute, to reduce the costs of resolving small claims, to screen out nonmeritorious suits, and to reduce the anxiety of formal legal proceedings.[120,189] Arbitration panels may be appointed by mutual consent of the injured patient and the defendant provider or by statute. Most arbitration agreements are voluntary but binding. However, there may be a reluctance by any of the parties to relinquish the right to appeal an unacceptable decision. Nonbinding arbitration may only bring out the facts of the case and serve as a rehearsal for a trial. Binding alternative dispute resolution requires a clear and specific agreement between the patient and providers before treatment that they will arbitrate any ensuing malpractice suit. The courts, however, will carefully scrutinize the nature of the original agreement to be sure the patient did not unwittingly give away the right to a jury trial.[195] Fifteen states have malpractice arbitration statutes, but very few medical malpractice cases have been settled by arbitration.

The Kaiser Permanente HMO requires its members in California, Colorado, Hawaii, and Massachusetts to agree to binding arbitration. In this system, claims are more expeditiously processed (19 months vs. 33 months in the court system), costs are substantially reduced, a higher percentage of injured patients are compensated though in more modest amounts, and multimillion dollar verdicts have been eliminated. There has been some difficulty in finding neutral arbitrators.[50] Danzon[42] found that with arbitration, the average award is lower and the plaintiff is more likely to prevail.

Legislation providing for pretrial screening panels has been enacted in about one-half of the states. These panels usually consist of physicians and attorneys who review the merits of each liability claim and offer an opinion regarding the physician's liability. This is nonbinding, but most states permit the findings of these panels to be admitted as evidence although leaving it to the jury to decide how much weight that evidence should be given.[98] These panels have been found to be ineffective in many states. If mandatory, they may be declared unconstitutional by limiting free access to the courts. Where voluntary, they are not used or only delay going to trial.[98]

AMA Proposal

In 1988, the AMA offered the concept of a fault-based administrative process to adjudicate professional liability charges. The cases would be heard before an administrative law judge rather than a jury. It was believed that this would expedite claims, save money, and bring into the decision-making a more experienced arbitrator— the judge. This approach seems to be too pro-defendant to some. It does not truly monitor patient injury, and it creates no ongoing feedback to medical institutions.[14, 165] This proposal is not moving forward at the moment.

No-Fault System

Under a no-fault system, the victims injured during medical care would be compensated without regard to negligence. Most proposals are not, however, pure no-fault in that they identify a specific set of injuries to be compensated. Most no-fault programs would compensate for economic losses only (wage loss, and medical and other expenses) with no payment for pain and suffering. Other collateral sources of remuneration would offset payment.

It is postulated that such a system would more equitably compensate the victims of medical injury, expedite settlement, and reduce costs. The disparity in awards and settlements for comparable injuries would be evened out, and, theoretically at least, there should be a lesser inducement to exaggeration and fraud on the part of the claimant.[164]

Problems inherent in a no-fault system involve the definition of a "compensable injury." The question is what to do about injuries that do not normally occur when patients receive good care. Designated compensable events will have to be defined and categorized, but it is often difficult to distinguish events due to medical intervention and those associated with the natural course of the disease.[182] Borderline or questionable cases can go to litigation. But who is to decide, and on what basis, which case should go to the tort system and which to the no-fault system?

No-fault systems emphasize compensation more than deterrence. Therefore, a concern is that they would not have the deterrent effect on malpractice of the current system. This problem could be overcome by a highly effective quality control system to reduce and minimize physician error.[188] Thus, a consequence of the no-fault system could be the improved detection of careless and incompetent medical treatment.[66]

There might be an increase in cost associated with no-fault proposals. The number of potentially compensable events would increase perhaps 100-fold and outstrip the built-in savings of such a system. Furthermore, savings in litigation expense might be small or nonexistent.[42] Also, claims clearly falling into no-fault systems are probably only a small fraction of current claims. Automatic compensation of obvious negligent action is presently the claim that is usually settled expeditiously out of court with little litigation cost anyway. Those cases where negligence is in doubt would remain in the tort system. The judgment of the New York State

Trial Lawyers Association and the State Bar concerning the findings of the Harvard study was that a no-fault system would remove a deterrent to poor care, reduce compensation to the seriously injured, offer insufficient compensation to victims generally, and cost much more to implement and administer (50% more) than the Harvard study estimates.[123]

It is likely that limitations on coverage would therefore have to be imposed to control costs. This would amount to a "selective no-fault" system. Short-lived disabilities could be excluded. The system could be responsible for only the additional costs which exceeded in-house care of the underlying illness and not for pre-existing medical problems. Payments could be limited to those disabling effects existing after a certain period of time, beyond the time most illnesses would have ceased. A 6-month time period has been suggested which would bring in no-fault after temporary disability benefit plans cease and before Social Security disability benefits for permanent disability take effect.[196]

Another proposal to be considered within the no-fault system is the development of specific categories of medical injuries which are usually avoidable if good care is provided and which would be automatically compensated. These have been called "accelerated compensation events" and would be identified by medical experts using epidemiological tools. This would not be applicable to all events but should provide compensation more quickly and for less administrative cost.[182]

No-fault, in the opinion of some, should function as a secondary payor to direct health care insurance (which covers 80% of medical costs) and disability insurance (which covers 20% of lost wages).[196]

Only in Virginia and Florida are limited no-fault programs now in place, and both were designed to cover only a selected set of severe birth-related neurological injuries. These programs make some sense because this is a major area of malpractice action with high indemnity but often with unclear issues of negligence and of causation. Both states carefully define the circumstances under which no-fault may be instituted. Although in existence for at least 5 years, there are no studies to determine whether these programs have increased the availability of obstetric care or changed the use of any obstetric procedures; however, malpractice insurance for obstetricians is readily available and cheaper in both states.[187]

The Sweden and New Zealand experience with no-fault shows far less legal conflict and administrative difficulty over claims administration than in malpractice litigation in New York.[196] Great Britain has found that escalating damages being awarded in medical negligence cases are beginning to have a serious effect on the ability of the National Health Service to pay for health care, and consideration is now being given to the development of a more economical no-fault system in that country.[66]

No-fault is a social insurance program with all the problems associated with such programs.[41] As discussed, there is no valid information on its likely cost or ultimate benefits. However, in other injury contexts such as workers' compensation, a no-fault program has a lower ratio of administrative to benefit costs than does the tort system. In the tort system, medical malpractice is more expensive than motor-vehicle litigation, in which the determination of fault is easier.[196]

Enterprise Liability

Enterprise liability evolves from the *respondeat superior* doctrine of vicarious liability. Under this proposal, the hospital or organization (e.g., HMO) providing care is responsible for defending the malpractice claims of its physicians. A physician cannot be named in the suit. About 80% of claims arise from events that occur in a hospital, and there is some justification for making hospitals responsible for the actions of their physicians and to encourage hospitals to rigidly enforce quality assurance and risk-management programs. (In recent years, most hospitals have voluntarily upgraded their quality assurance and risk-management programs.) Enterprise liability could reduce the number of defendants and separate claims. It is uniquely adaptable to the increasing shift to managed care. This reform presently exists only in California where university hospitals are liable for the actions of their physicians.[187] Currently, HMOs are increasingly the enterprise being sued and a number of federal trial courts, and two circuit courts of appeal, have found that HMOs are liable for medical malpractice claims under a vicarious liability theory.[126]

Enterprise liability obviously cannot be applied to physicians practicing independently.

Adoption of the English Rule

Under the "English" rule, the losing side in litigation pays the court costs and attorneys' fees for both parties. Indeed, the U.S. is the only major country in which the winner of a lawsuit does not collect fees from the loser.[140] This would undoubtedly reduce frivolous suits, but it seems highly unlikely that the legal climate in this country would ever permit this approach. Florida enacted such a provision in 1980, but it was repealed in 1985 because the doctors who had originally pressed for the reform found that it was very difficult to collect the fees when they won.[195]

The Utah Experiment in Patient Injury Compensation

The Utah Experiment in Patient Injury Compensation (EPIC), funded by a Robert Wood Johnson Foundation grant of $725,000, is evaluating a program to remove malpractice cases from the court system. Compensation would include: "rehabilitation, lost wages, pain and suffering, etc." Patients no longer have to prove that someone else's negligence caused their injury before getting help and claims would be expedited. Only patients with medically caused injuries severe enough to last 2 months or longer would be eligible for automatic compensation. Those whose injuries are less severe would generally be covered by their own health or disability insurance or employment benefits.

Doctors and hospitals would pay liability insurance premiums to compensate injured patients, but only 10%-20 % of the premium dollar would go to administration, in contrast to today's 60% which goes to lawyers' fees and other administrative costs. Administration would be by individual hospitals who would track all patient injuries and pay the injured patient directly. This would give hospitals a strong incentive to maintain high quality care and make improvements where patterns of patient injuries emerge.

For this demonstration project to proceed, state legislation needs to be passed to allow patients treated in those hospitals to be served under the EPIC system.[200]

Reform of the Jury System

In addition to the question of tort reform is the major question of reform of the jury system itself. An informal opinion survey of 1,300 people indicated that 79.8% would like to scrap the jury system entirely. A significant number of those who would like to leave the system as it is were members of a single advocacy group. Some recommend replacing the system with professional jurors instead of judges.[162] The jury system for malpractice is one unique to the U.S. In Canada, malpractice trials are conducted before a judge, not a jury, and this is considered by some to be more reasonable than a jury of people not truly "peers" in terms of understanding of scientific issues. Efforts to introduce the jury system outside the Anglo-American legal orbit have failed. Frequent arguments of those criticizing the jury system in the U.S. are that: lay juries are unable to react knowledgeably to the wealth of data, which is often complex and confusing, presented to them at trial; lay juries respond sympathetically to the injured plaintiff, often with what it believes to be exorbitant and unreasonable awards for pain and suffering; lay juries are partial to claimants over doctors; and lay juries seek large monetary settlements when making decisions.

However, these arguments have all been convincingly refuted by the careful and impressive personal research and analysis of the common literature on the subject by Neil Vidmar.[192] Vidmar pointed out that those making these assumptions failed to recognize the methodological errors of the literature they cite as supportive, ignored the absence of supportive evidence, made decisions on unrepresentative data, and uncritically accepted the scientifically flawed empirical research used to uphold the anecdotal arguments which are cited over and over again by the jury reform enthusiasts and the media. Vidmar also showed that there is no relationship between the severity of the plaintiff's injury and the determination of negligence, refuting the claim that sympathy for injured patients causes jurors to ignore the legal issues bearing on negligence. Furthermore, he cited evidence that even judges in their independent analysis of a case do not vary significantly from the judgment arrived at by the pooled efforts of the jury—contrary to the above arguments as to judicial superiority over lay judgments. It seems that juries do understand the experts and when the jurors are confused with the elements and "facts" of the case, so are the doctors and the judges. It is simply a difficult case for all to understand. The vagaries of the liability or negligence issues are not clear and outcomes not predictable. The cases that end up before a jury are largely a small atypical subset self-selected because of these vagaries.[38,192]

Are panels of physicians in a better position to assess the medical facts than a lay jury? Vidmar cited the study of Taragin et al[183] which spoke to the question of whether independent impartial analysis by physicians of the medical facts of a case would lead to judgments varying from those reached by the jury. His review of 8,231 malpractice cases showed that they did not.[183] A similar study by Sloan et al[18,172] found that panels of physicians examining 187 closed malpractice cases in Florida determined that the liability ratings of the impartial physician panels correlated with the outcomes at trial. An examination of the facts shows that damage awards are proportional to the seriousness of the injury and economic loss, not the perceived ability of defendants to pay.

Is the cry for tort reform a self-serving effort on the part of physicians to protect themselves and place themselves beyond public accountability? And what about the problem of fair compensation for the injured patient? Indeed the Harvard study concluded that since the present system only infrequently compensates injured patients and rarely identifies and holds health care providers responsible for substandard medical care, "the abandonment of malpractice litigation is unlikely unless credible systems and procedures, supported by the public, are instituted to guarantee professional accountability to patients."[99]

Recent Improvements and Trends

The Harvard study is now more than 10 years old. Since that time, there have been alterations in hospital and physician attitudes and awareness regarding malpractice that have significantly changed things for the better. The paternalistic attitude of the past has been tempered by a greater concern for patient needs, and physicians have responded to public demand for more accountability by changes in their attitudes and practice. The Health Care Improvement Act was passed in 1986 and the Patient Self-Determination Act and the Safe Medical Devices Act in 1990. The use of guidelines is burgeoning. Hospitals have improved their quality assurance and risk-management programs, "total quality management" is a constant concern, and more, recently, "continuous quality improvement" programs have been introduced. Proactive approaches have been developed to anticipate and prevent adverse incidents. Working hours of resident physicians have been shortened. There is more awareness of the need for the proper maintenance of equipment. Hospitals have instituted computer analysis of physician activity, established standardized systems, and introduced medication control mechanisms to avoid medication errors. There is an increasing tendency for high-risk surgery and procedures to be performed in centers where experience is great. I see physicians more consciously concerned about limiting their alcohol consumption than they were 10 years ago. Medical licensing boards have significantly responded to the consumer demand for a more vigorous approach to the negligent or impaired physician, although some states are still hampered by budgetary restraints. License revocations, suspensions and other actions rose 58% from 1991 to 1995 according to unpublished data from the National Practitioner Data Bank. The Federation of State Medical Boards noted that the number of physicians facing disciplinary action each year rose 47% during the same period.[186] The number of doctors disciplined for sexual misconduct doubled from 1990 to 1994.[95] The National Practitioner Data Bank should be of assistance in identifying the physicians with unacceptable medical practices. I suspect a review of health care delivery today would yield a far more acceptable report than that produced by the Harvard study of 10 years ago. On the other hand, there is a concern that many present trends encourage cost containment over the best standard of care.

REFERENCES

1. AMA Council on Mental Health: The sick physician: impairment by psychiatric disorders including alcoholism and drug dependence. **JAMA 223:** 684-687, 1973

2. American College of Physicians: Beyond MICRA: new ideas for liability reform. **Ann Intern Med 122:** 466-473, 1995

3. Annas GJ: Medicine, death, and the criminal law. **N Engl J Med 333:**527-530, 1995

4. Ayres JD: 1993 Le Tourneau Award. The use and abuse of medical practice guidelines. **J Legal Med 15:**421-443, 1994

5. Baker MT, Taub HA: Readability of informed consent forms for research in a Veterans Administration Medical Center. **JAMA 250:**2646-2648, 1983

6. Barker DK: The effects of tort reform on medical malpractice insurance markets: an empirical analysis. **J Health Polit Policy Law 17:**143-161, 1992

7. Beckman HB, Markakis KM, Suchman AL, et al: The doctor-patient relationship and malpractice. Lessons from plaintiff depositions. **Arch Intern Med 154:**1365-1370, 1994

8. Bell PA: Legislative intrusions into the common law of medical malpractice: thoughts about the deterrent effect of tort liability. **Syracuse Law Rev 35:** 939-993, 1984

9. Belli M, Carlova J: **Belli: For Your Malpractice Defense.** Oradell, NJ: Medical Economics Books, 1986, pp 35-36

10. Benzer DG: Healing the healer: a primer on physician impairment. **Wisc Med J 90:**70-79, 1991

11. Bierig JR, Hirshfeld EB, Kelly JT, et al: Practice parameters: malpractice liability considerations for physicians. **Legal Med.** 1991

12. Blackett WB: Congress of Neurological Surgeons Tort Reform. **Clin Neurosurg 40:**210-218, 1993

13. Blackmon G, Zeckhauser R: State tort reform legislation: assessing our control of risks, in Schuck PH (ed): **Tort Law and the Public Interest: Competition, Innovation, and Consumer Welfare.** New York, NY: WW Norton & Co, 1991

14. Bohigian GM, Croughan JL, Sanders K: Substance abuse and dependence in physicians: An overview of the effects of alcohol and drug abuse. **Mo Med 91:**233-239, 1994

15. Borzo G: Liability records going on line in Massachusetts. **Am Med News.** July 1996

16. Bovbjerg RR: Medical malpractice: folklore, facts, and the future. **Ann Intern Med 117:**788-791, 1992

17. Bovbjerg RR, Petronis KR: The relationship between physicians' malpractice claims history and later claims. Does the past predict the future? **JAMA 272:**1421-1426, 1994

18. Bovbjerg RR, Sloan FA, Blumstein JF: Valuing life and limb in tort: scheduling "pain and suffering." **Northwest U Law Rev 83:**908-976, 1989

19. Brennan TA: Practice guidelines and malpractice litigation: collision or cohesion? **J Health Polit Policy Law 16:**67-85, 1991

20. Brennan TA, Leape LL, Laird NM, et al: Incidence of adverse events and negligence in hospitalized patients. Results of the Harvard Medical Practice Study I. **N Engl J Med 324:**370-376, 1991

21. Brennan TA, Sox CM, Burstin HR: Relation between negligent adverse events and the outcome of medical-malpractice litigation. **N Engl J Med 335:**1963-1967, 1996

22. Brewster JM: Prevalence of alcohol and other drug problems among physicians. **JAMA 255:**1913-1920, 1986

23. Brickman L: Contingency fees without contingencies: Hamlet without the prince of Denmark? **UCLA Law Rev 37:**29-129, 1989

24. Burstin HR, Johnson WG, Lipsitz SR, et al: Do the poor sue more? A case-control study of malpractice claims and socioeconomic status. **JAMA 270:** 1697-1701, 1993

25. Burstin HR, Lipsitz SR, Brennan TA: Socioeconomic status and risk for substandard medical care. **JAMA 268:**2383-2387, 1992

26. **Business and Health.** Vol 12, No. 3

27. California Medical Association (Mills DH, ed): **Report on the Medical Insurance Feasibility Study.** San Francisco, Calif: Sutter Publications, 1977

28. *Canterbury v Spence*, 464 F2d 772 (CADC Cir 1972)

29. Centrella M: Physician addiction and impairment—current thinking: a review. **J Addict Dis 13:** 91-105, 1994

30. Chassin MR: Standards of care in medicine. **Inquiry 25:**437-453, 1988

31. Classen DC, Pestotnik SL, Evans RS, et al: Adverse drug events in hospitalized patients. Excessive length of stay, extra costs, and attributable mortality. **JAMA 277:**301-306, 1997

32. **Clinical Practice Guidelines, Directions for a New Program.** Institute of Medicine, 1990, pp 109-110

33. Computerized medical records: what you should know. **Medical Assurance Memorandum.** December 1995

34. Cosman MP: Surgical malpractice: the Renaissance and today. **J Fla Med Assoc 78:**505-515, 1991

35. Crane M: Could a malpractice suit wipe out your assets? **Medical Economics.** July 6, 1992, pp 146-153

36. Creasey D: Medical malpractice program: overview. **Robert Wood Johnson Foundation, ABRIDGE.** 1991, p 1

37. Crowley TJ: Contingency contracting treatment of drug-abusing physicians, nurses, and dentists. **Natl Inst Drug Abuse Res Monogr 46:**68-83, 1984

38. Current award trends: **Jury Verdict Research, 1988 Edition.** Solon, Ohio, 1988

39. Cyr MG, Wartman SA: The effectiveness of routing screening questions in the detection of alcoholism. **JAMA 259:**51-54,1988

40. Danzon PM: The frequency and severity of medical malpractice claims: new evidence. **Law Contemp Probl 49:**57-84, 1986

41. Danzon PM: Liability for medical practice. **J Econ Perspect 5:**51-69, 1991

42. Danzon PM: **Medical Malpractice: Theory, Evidence, and Public Policy.** Cambridge, Mass: Harvard University Press, 1985

43. De Ville KA: **Medical Malpractice in Nineteenth Century America: Origins and Legacy.** New York, NY: New York University Press, 1990, p 25

44. Doherty EG, Haven CO: Medical malpractice and negligence. Sociodemographic characteristics of claimants and nonclaimants. **JAMA 238:**1656-1658, 1977

45. Donaldson LJ: Doctors with problems in an NHS

workforce. **Br Med J 308:**1277-1282, 1994

46. Editorial. **Am Med News 37:**30, May 1994

47. Edwards FJ: **Medical Malpractice: Solving the Crisis**. New York, NY: Henry Holt and Co, 1989

48. Ewing JA: Detecting alcoholism. The CAGE questionnaire. **JAMA 252:**1905-1907, 1984

49. Failure to diagnose claims head list of allegations, St Paul finds. **Med Liabil Mon 18(8):**5-6, 1993

50. Felsenthal E: What happens when patients arbitrate rather than litigate? **Wall Street Journal**. Feb 4, 1994, p B11

51. Florin RE: Clinical practice guidelines. **American Association of Neurological Surgeons Bulletin**. Fall 1993, p 5

52. Friendly HJ: Some kind of hearing. **U Pa Law Rev 123:**1267-1317, 1975

53. Galanter M, Talbott D, Gallegos K, et al: Combined Alcoholics Anonymous and professional care for addicted physicians. **Am J Psychiatry 147:**64-68, 1990

54. Garnick DW, Hendricks AM, Brennan TA: Can practice guidelines reduce the number and costs of malpractice claims? **JAMA 266:**2856-2860, 1991

55. Garrison FH: **An Introduction to the History of Medicine**. 4th ed. Philadelphia, Pa: WB Saunders, 1929, p 171

56. Gergen D: America's legal mess. **US News and World Report**. Aug 1991, p 72 (Editorial)

57. Grauer H, Campbell NM: The aging physician and retirement. **Can J Psychiatry 28:**552-554, 1983

58. Grossman SA, Piantadosi S, Covahey C: Are informed consent forms that describe clinical oncology research protocols readable by most patients and their families? **J Clin Oncol 12:**2211-2215, 1994

59. Grudner TM: On the readability of surgical consent forms. **N Engl J Med 302:**900-902, 1980

60. Guthrie D: **A History of Medicine**. London: JB Lippincott, 1946

61. Hamilton FH: Suits for malpractice in surgery: their causes and their remedies. **Papers Read Before the Medico-Legal Society of New York, 1875-1878**. New York, NY: Medico-Legal Society of New York, 1886, p 98

62. Hammerschmidt DE, Keane MA: Institutional review board (IRB) review lacks impact on the readability of consent forms for research. **Am J Med Sci 304:**348-351, 1992

63. Harrington S, Litan RE: Causes of the liability insurance crisis. **Science 239:**737-741, 1988

64. Hartman GW, Hattery RR, Witten DM: Mortality during excretory urography: Mayo Clinic experience. **AJR 139:**919-922, 1982

65. Hatlie MJ: Professional liability: the case for federal reform. **JAMA 263:**584-586, 1990

66. Havard J: "No fault" compensation for medical accidents. **Med Sci Law 32:**187-198, 1992

67. Hensler D, Viana M, Kakalik J, et al: **Trends in Tort Litigation: The Story Behind the Statistics**. Santa Monica, Calif: The RAND Corporation Institute for Civil Justice, 1987

68. Hepler RS: Ophthalmology personnel in risk management. What office personnel need to know to keep you out of trouble. **Ophthalmology 97:**1385-1387, 1990

69. Herrington RE, Benzer DG, Jacobson GR, et al: Treating substance-use disorders among physicians. **JAMA 247:**2253-2257, 1982

70. Herz DA, Looman JE, Lewis SK: Informed consent: is it a myth? **Neurosurgery 30:**453-458, 1992

71. Hickson GB, Clayton EW, Githens PB, et al: Factors that prompted families to file medical malpractice claims following perinatal injuries. **JAMA 267:**1359-1363, 1992

72. Hirshfeld EB: Should practice parameters be the standard of care in malpractice litigation? **JAMA 266:**2886-2891, 1991

73. Holoweiko M: What are your greatest malpractice risks? **Med Economics**. Aug 3, 1992, pp 141-159

74. Holzer JF: The advent of clinical standards for professional liability. **QRB Qual Rev Bull 16:**71-79, 1990

75. Hopper KD, TenHave TR, Hartzel J: Informed consent forms for clinical and research imaging procedures: how much do patients understand? **AJR 164:**493-496, 1995

76. Hughes PH, Brandenburg N, Baldwin DC Jr, et al: Prevalence of substance use among US physicians. **JAMA 267:**2333-2339, 1992

77. Huycke LI, Huycke MM: Characteristics of potential plaintiffs in malpractice litigation. **Ann Intern Med 120:**792-798, 1994

78. Hyams AL, Brandenburg JA, Lipsitz SR, et al: Practice guidelines and malpractice litigation: a two-way street. **Ann Intern Med 122:**450-455, 1995

79. Hyde GL, Miscall BG: **The Impaired Physician: Diagnosis, Treatment and Reentry. Committee of Physicians' Health of the Board of Governors.** Chicago, Ill: American College of Surgeons, 1995, pp 1-32

80. Ibelle B: Median jury verdicts on the rise: medical malpractice skyrockets while product liability plummets. **Lawyers Weekly USA**. Jan 15, 1996, p B8

81. Iglehart JK: The professional liability crisis: the 1986 Duke Private Sector Conference. **N Engl J Med 315:**1105-1107, 1986

82. Imershein AW, Brents AH: The impact of large medical malpractice awards on malpractice awardees. **J Legal Med 13:**33-49, 1992

83. Jacobson PD: Medical malpractice and the tort system. **JAMA 262:**3320-3327, 1989

84. Johnson RP, Connelly JC: Addicted physicians. A closer look. **JAMA 245:**253-257, 1981

85. Kassirer, JP: The use and abuse of practice profiles. **N Engl J Med 330:**634-635, 1994

86. Kinney ED: Malpractice reform in the 1990s: past disappointments, future success? **J Health Polit Policy Law 20:**99-135, 1995

87. Kinney ED, Wilder MM: Medical standard setting in the current malpractice environment: problems and possibilities. **U Calif Davis Law Rev 22:**421-450, 1989

88. Kraushar MF, Steinberg JA: Informed consent. Surrender or salvation? **Arch Ophthalmol 104:**352-355, 1986

89. Lawthers AG, Localio AR, Laird NM, et al: Physicians' perceptions of the risk of being sued. **J Health Polit Policy Law 17:**463-482, 1992

90. *Leach v Jefferson Parish Hospital District No. 2*, 870 F2d 300 (5th Cir 1989)

91. Leaman TL, Saxton JW: **Preventing Malpractice: The Co-Active Solution**. New York, NY: Plenum

Medical Books, 1993

92. Leape LL, Brennan TA, Laird N et al: The nature of adverse events in hospitalized patients. Results of the Harvard Medical Practice Study II. **N Engl J Med 324:**377-384, 1991

93. Leeb D, Bowers DG, Lynch JB: Observations of the myth of "informed consent." **Plast Reconstr Surg 3:** 58, 1976

94. Lesar TS, Briceland L, Stein DS: Factors related to errors in medication prescribing. **JAMA 277:** 312-317, 1997

95. Levy D: Health and behavior: Many 'bad' doctors evade censure. **USA TODAY.** March 29, 1996

96. Lewin-VHI: **Estimating the Costs of Defensive Medicine.** Report Prepared for MMI Companies, Inc, Fairfax, Virginia, Jan 27, 1993

97. Liang MH: From America: cookbook medicine or food for thought: practice guidelines development in the USA. **Ann Rheum Dis 51:**1257-1258, 1992

98. Lobe TE: **Medical Malpractice: A Physician's Guide.** New York, NY: McGraw-Hill, 1995

99. Localio AR, Lawthers AG, Brennan TA, et al: Relation between malpractice claims and adverse events due to negligence. Results of the Harvard medical practice study III. **N Engl J Med 325:**245-251, 1991

100. Louisell DW, Mueller CS: **Federal Evidence.** Rochester NY: The Lawyers Co-Operative Publishing: San Francisco, Calif: Bancroft-Whitney, 1980, Vol 4, p 466

101. Luban D: Speculating on justice: The ethics and jurisprudence of contingency fees, in Parker S, Sampford C (eds): **Legal Ethics and Legal Practice: Contemporary Issues.** Oxford: Clarendon Press, 1995

102. Malpractice costs edged higher in '94. **Modern Healthcare,** Vol 25. July 24, 1995

103. Malpractice plaintiff awards at record high level. **Comment. An MAI Publication.** Charleston, WV, Vol 2, 1996

104. Malpractice: Surgeons seem to think so. **Medical Economics.** Jan 1996, pp 15, 17

105. Mandell WJ: An approach to the impaired physician. **Physician Executive 20:**7-14, 1994

106. Manuel BM: Physician liability: new areas of concern under managed care. **Am Coll Surg Bull 80:** 23-26, 1995

107. Manuel BM: A surgeon's perspective on professional liability. **Am Coll Surg Bull 70:**6-11, 1985

108. Mason SC III: Organic mental disorders and the issue of retirement. **Mich Med 87:**329-334, 1988

109. May ML, Stengel DB: Who sues their doctors? How patients handle medical grievances. **Law Soc Rev 24:** 105-120, 1990

110. Mayfield D, McLeod G, Hall P: The CAGE questionnaire: validation of a new alcoholism screening instrument. **Am J Psychiatry 131:**1121-1123, 1974

111. McAuliffe WE, Rohman M, Breer P, et al: Alcohol use and abuse in random samples of physicians and medical students. **Am J Public Health 81:**177-188, 1991

112. McDonald G: A legal perspective on complications: the American system, in Apuzzo M (ed): **Brain Surgery: Complication Avoidance and Management.** New York, NY: Churchill Livingstone, 1993

113. McLaughlin WH: A look at the Massachusetts malpractice tribunal system. **Am J Law Med 3:**197-207, 1977

114. Meade CD, Howser DM: Consent forms: how to determine and improve their readability. **Oncol Nurs Forum 19:**1523-1528, 1992

115. Medical malpractice: **Report of the Secretary's Commission on Medical Malpractice.** Washington, DC: Government Printing Office, 1973 (DHEW Publication No. (OS) 73-88)

116. Medical malpractice verdicts largest. **Wesgram: Newsletter of the West Virginia Med Assoc.** Vol 7, 1991, p 2

117. Med-mal costs still climbing. **Comment.** An MAI Publication, Charleston, WV, Vol 1, 1995

118. Med-mal suits accounted for the most plaintiff awards in '95. **Comment. An MAI Publication.** Charleston, WV, Vol 2, 1996

119. Meeks JM: Charting medical malpractice claims. **Medical Record: A Medical Professional Liability Report.** Chicago, Ill: CNA Insurance Companies, 1993, pp 1, 3

120. Metzloff TB: Alternative dispute resolution strategies in medical malpractice. **Alaska Law Rev 9:** 429-457, 1992

121. Miller FH: Medical malpractice litigation: do the British have a better remedy? **Am J Law Med 11:** 433-463, 1986

122. Miller RH, Williams PC, Napolitana G, et al: Malpractice: a case-control study of claimants. **J Gen Intern Med 5:**244-248, 1990

123. Millock PJ: The Harvard medical malpractice study and the malpractice debate in New York State. **Legal Med.** 1991, pp 111-125

124. Minnesota Health Rights Act: **Conference Committee Report on HF No. 200. Conference Report.** St Paul, Minn, 1992

125. Mohr JC: The emergence of medical malpractice in America. **Trans Stud Coll Physicians Phila 14:**1-21, 1992

126. Moore NJ: Courts back HMOs in delay of care cases. **Physician Practice Digest.** 1996, pp 53-56

127. Morgan LW, Schwab IR: Informed consent in senile cataract extraction. **Arch Ophthalmol 104:**42-45, 1986

128. Morreim EH: Am I my brother's warden? Responding to the unethical or incompetent colleague. **Hastings Cent Rep 23:**19-27, 1993

129. Morrow GR: How readable are consent forms? **JAMA 244:**56-58, 1980

130. Morse RM, Martin MA, Swenson WM, et al: Prognosis of physicians treated for alcoholism and drug dependence **JAMA 251:**743-746, 1984

131. Morton JR: The Maine demonstration project: using practice parameters as an affirmative defense. **Am Coll Surg Bull 80:**30-33, 1995

132. Mullan F, Politzer RM, Lewis CT, et al: The National Practitioner Data Bank. Report from the first year. **JAMA 268:**73-79, 1992

133. Murgatroyd RJ, Cooper RM: Readability of informed consent forms. **Am J Hosp Pharm 48:** 2651-2652, 1991

134. Mussman MG, Zawistowich L, Weisman CS, et al: Medical malpractice claims filed by Medicaid and non-Medicaid recipients in Maryland. **JAMA 265:** 992-2994, 1991

135. National Association of Insurance Commissioners: **Medical Malpractice Closed Claims, 1975-1978.**

Brookfield, Wisc: National Association of Insurance Commissioners, 1980

136. Newsclips: Managed care pushes hospitals to adopt physician profiling. **Diagnostic Imaging.** March 1995, p 20

137. Northrup G: Statement. **Medical Malpractice Report of the Secretary's Commission of Medical Malpractice 9.** 1973, pp 105-106 (Department of Health, Education, and Welfare)

138. Nye DJ, Gifford DG, Webb BL, et al: The causes of the medical malpractice crisis: an analysis of claims data and insurance company finances. **Georgetown Law J 76:**1495-1561, 1988

139. Ogle PL: Comment: Stripped naked and on parade. **Diag Imaging 16:**5, 1994

140. Olson WK: **The Litigation Explosion: What Happened When America Unleashed the Lawsuit.** New York, NY: Dutton, 1991

141. Orrico KO: Background paper: medical liability reform. **American Association of Neurological Surgeons Bulletin.** Fall 1994, p 18

142. Passineau TL: Workshop on stress at the 1994 International Conference on Physician Health, Ottawa, Canada. **Am Med News 37:**17-21, 1994

143. Pegalis SE, Wachsman HF: **American Law of Medical Malpractice.** 2nd ed. Deerfield, Ill: Clark, Boardman, and Callaghan, 1992

144. Peterson MA: **Civil Juries in the 1980s: Trends in Jury Trials and Verdicts in California and Cook County, Illinois.** Santa Monica. Calif: The RAND Corporation, 1987

145. Physician Insurers Association of America: **Physician Insurers Association of America Data Sharing Reports.** Washington, DC: Physician Insurers Association of America, 1993

146. Posner R: Trends in medical malpractice insurance, 1970-1985. **Law Contemp Probl 49:**37-56, 1986

147. Pozgar GD, Pozgar NS: **Legal Aspects of Health Care Administration.** 6th ed. Gaithersburg, Md: Aspen Publications, 1996

148. Prichard R: **Committee Report. Liability and Compensation Health Care.** Toronto, Can: University of Toronto Press, 1990

149. Priluck IA, Robertson DM, Buettner H: What patients recall of the preoperative discussion after retinal detachment surgery. **Am J Ophthalmol 87:**620-623, 1979

150. Product liability action needed. **Wesgram: Newsletter of the West Virginia State Medical Association.** Vol 10, 1994, p 1

151. **Professional Liability in the '80s, Report I of the American Medical Association Special Task Force on Professional Liability and Insurance.** Chicago, Ill: American Medical Association, October 1985

152. Reading EG: Nine years experience with chemically dependent physicians: the New Jersey experience. **Md Med J 41:**325-329, 1992

153. Relman AS: Changing the malpractice liability system. **N Engl J Med 322:**626-627, 1990

154. Report of the Board of Trustees: **Study of Professional Liability Costs.** Chicago, Ill: American Medical Association, 1983

155. Reynolds RA, Rizzo JA, Gonzalez ML: The cost of medical professional liability. **JAMA 257:**2776-2781, 1987

156. Richman JA: Occupational stress, psychological vul-

157. Ritchey FJ: Physician's perceptions of the suit-prone patient. **Hum Organ 38:**160-168, 1979

158. Robinson G, Merav A: Informed consent: recall by patients tested postoperatively. **Ann Thorac Surg 22:**209-212, 1976

159. Rothwax HJ: **Guilty: The Collapse of Criminal Justice.** New York, NY: Random House, 1996

160. Rozovsky FA: **Consent to Treatment: A Practical Guide.** Boston, Mass: Little, Brown, and Co, 1984

161. Sager M, Voeks S, Drinka P, et al: Do the elderly sue physicians? **Arch Intern Med 150:**1091-1093, 1990

162. Savant VS: Should we change the American jury system? **Parade Publications.** July 30, 1995, p 12

163. Schneidman DS: What surgeons should know about . . . Medical liability reform and the federal government. **Bull Am Coll Surg 80:**9-13, 1995

164. Schwartz DH: Societal responsibility for malpractice. **Milbank Mem Fund Q 54:**469-488, 1976

165. Schwartz WB, Komesar NK: Doctors, damages and deterrence. An economic view of medical malpractice. **N Engl J Med 298:**1282-1289, 1978

166. Shanley MG, Peterson MA: **Posttrial Adjustments to Jury Awards.** Santa Monica, Calif: The RAND Corporation, 1987

167. Shapiro RS, Simpson DE, Lawrence SL, et al: A survey of sued and nonsued physicians and suing patients. **Arch Intern Med 149:**2190-2196, 1989

168. Shehadi WH, Toniolo G: Adverse reactions to contrast media. A report from the Committee on Safety of Contrast Media of the International Society of Radiology. **Radiology 137:**299-302, 1980

169. Shore JH: The Oregon experience with impaired physicians on probation. An eight-year follow-up. **JAMA 257:**2931-2934, 1987

170. Skelly FJ: Coping with being sued. **AMA News.** Nov 7, 1994, p 20

171. Sloan FA, Bovbjerg RR, Githens PB: **Insuring Medical Malpractice.** New York, NY: Oxford University Press, 1991

172. Sloan FA, Githens EW, Clayton EW, et al: **Suing for Medical Malpractice.** Chicago, Ill: University of Chicago Press, 1993

173. Sloan FA, Mergenhagen PM, Bovjberg RR, et al: Effects of tort reforms on the value of closed medical malpractice claims: A microanalysis. **J Health Polit Policy Law 14:**663-689, 1989

174. Sloan FA, Mergenhagen PM, Burfield WB, et al: Medical malpractice experience of physicians: Predictable or haphazard? **JAMA 262:**3291-3297, 1989

175. Smarr LE: Malpractice claims. Does the past predict the future? **JAMA 272:**1453-1454, 1994

176. Smith HW: Legal responsibility for medical malpractice; malpractice claims in the United States and a proposed formula for testing their legal sufficiency. **JAMA 116:**2670-2679, 1941

177. Some physicians inconsistent about abnormal test results. **Wesgram: Newsletter of the West Virginia State Medical Association.** Vol 12, Nov 1, 1996

178. Stephenson J: Trends in malpractice payments. **JAMA 275:**1789, 1996 (Letter)

179. Sugarman SD: Doing away with tort law. **Calif Law Rev 73:**555-664, 1985

180. Talbot GD, Benson EB: Impaired physicians: The

dilemma of identification. **Postgrad Med 68 (6):** 56-64, 1980

181. Talbot GD, Gallegos KV, Wilson PO, et al: The medical association of Georgia's impaired physicians program. Review of the first 1000 physicians: analysis of specialty. **JAMA 257:**2927-2930, 1987

182. Tancredi LR, Bovbjerg RR: Creating outcomes-based systems for quality and malpractice reform: methodology of accelerated-compensation events (ACEs). **Milbank Q 70:**183-216, 1992

183. Taragin MI, Willett LR, Wilczek AP, et al: The influence of standard of care and severity of injury on the resolution of medical malpractice claims. **Ann Intern Med 117:**780-784, 1992

184. Tarnowski KJ, Allen DM, Mayhall C, et al: Readability of pediatric biomedical research informed consent forms. **Pediatrics 85:**58-62, 1990

185. Todd JS: Reform of the health care system and professional liability. **N Engl J Med 329:**1733-1735, 1993

186. **USA TODAY.** Editorial May 22, 1996

187. US Congress, Office of Technology Assessment: **Defensive Medicine and Medical Malpractice.** Washington, DC: US Government Printing Office, 1994

188. US Congress, Office of Technology Assessment: **Do Medicaid and Medicare Patients Sue Physicians More Often Than Other Patients?** Washington, DC: Office of Technology Assessment, 1992

189. US Congress, Office of Technology Assessment: **Impact of Legal Reforms on Medical Malpractice Costs.** Washington, DC: US Government Printing Office, 1993

190. US Department of Health and Human Services, US Public Health Service Agency for Health Care Policy and Research: **Compendium of Selected State Laws Governing Medical Injury Claims.** Washington, DC: US Government Printing Office, 1993 (prepared by SM Spernak)

191. US General Accounting Office: **Medical Malpractice: Characteristics of Claims Closed in 1984.** Washington, DC: US General Accounting Office, 1987

192. Vidmar N: **Medical Malpractice and the American Jury: Confronting the Myths about Jury Incompetence, Deep Pockets, and Outrageous Damage Awards.** Ann Arbor, Mich: The University of Michi-

gan Press, 1995

193. Wachsman HF: **Lethal Medicine: The Epidemic of Medical Malpractice in America.** New York, NY: Henry Holt and Co, 1993

194. Wasted health care dollars. **Consumer Reports.** July 1992, pp 435-448

195. Weiler PC: **Medical Malpractice on Trial.** Cambridge, Mass: Harvard University Press, 1991

196. Weiler PC, Hiatt HH, Newhouse JP, et al: **A Measure of Malpractice: Medical Injury, Malpractice Litigation, and Patient Compensation.** Cambridge, Mass: Harvard University Press, 1993

197. Weiler PC, Newhouse JP, Hiatt HH: Proposal for medical liability reform. **JAMA 267:**2355-2358, 1992

198. Weintraub MI: Expert witness testimony: a time for self-regulation? **J Child Neurol 10:**256-259, 1995

199. Welch HG, Miller ME, Welch WP: Physician profiling: an analysis of inpatient practice patterns in Florida and Oregon. **N Engl J Med 330:**607-612, 1994

200. What to do about malpractice. **Utah Medical Association.** 1996

201. Wilcox DP, Thompson HA: From informed consent to informed refusal. **Tex Med 86:**38-40, 1990

202. Williams SV, Eisenberg JM, Pascale LA, et al: Physicians' perceptions about unnecessary diagnostic testing. **Inquiry 19:**363-370, 1982

203. Wills RV: Why are so many claims settled? Discretion versus valor. **Surgical Rounds.** Nov 1989, pp 90-99

204. Wisconsin malpractice settlement based on MD's inexperience. **Am Med News 40:**21, 1997

205. Wolfram CW: **Modern Legal Ethics.** St Paul, Minn: West Publishing Co, 1986

206. Wright C: Physician addiction to pharmaceuticals: personal history, practice setting, access to drugs, and recovery. **Md Med J 39:**1021-1025, 1990

207. Zuckerman S, Bovbjerg RR, Sloan F, et al: Effects of tort reforms and other factors on medical malpractice insurance premiums. **Inquiry 27:**167-182, 1990

208. Zuckerman S, Norton S, Wadler B, et al: **A State-Based Survey of Malpractice Premiums: Implications for Medicare Physicians Payment Policy.** Washington, DC: The Urban Institute, 1993

CME QUESTIONS

The Physician's Perspective on Medical Law, Volume II

The following questions have been provided to give physicians the option of testing their comprehension of the material provided in *The Physician's Perspective on Medical Law, Volume II*. The test is to be self-scored. Answers may be found in the back of this book. A Continuing Medical Education (CME) certificate will be mailed upon the return of the enclosed test evaluation/feedback card along with a $25 administrative fee. Telephone 847-692-9500 to order additional evaluation/feedback cards or for more information about other CME products from the American Association of Neurological Surgeons.

After reading this book, a physician should be able to:

- understand the basic structure of the legal system and the rules that govern a physician's participation in legal proceedings.
- understand the legal rules that complement the ethical responsibilities of physicians in their relationships with patients.
- recognize the public health issues that cause the greatest problems in our society and understand the opportunity for physicians, as citizens having special expertise, to take an active role in addressing these problems.
- understand the need to protect both the physician and the patient in interactions with the health care and judicial systems.

CHAPTER 13

GUNSHOT INJURIES AND GUN CONTROL

1. Gun ownership is more frequent in:
    (A) large cities.
    (B) black American households.
    (C) the Eastern portion of the United States.
    (D) high-income households.

2. The most common cause of gunshot death is:
    (A) suicide.
    (B) homicide.
    (C) accident.

3. Guns are the:
    (A) first
    (B) second
    (C) third
    (D) fourth
    most common etiology of trauma deaths.

4. Gunshot deaths are most often related to:
    (A) accessibility.
    (B) culture.
    (C) long guns.
    (D) developed countries.

5. Suicide by gunshot:
    (A) is the best method.
    (B) allows control.
    (C) is performed with long guns.
    (D) is not related to the accessibility of guns.

6. Murder is most likely:
    (A) among strangers.
    (B) in the presence of guns.
    (C) if the weapon is a knife.
    (D) all of the above

7. Accidental gunshot deaths:
    (A) often involve alcohol.
    (B) tend to occur outside the house.
    (C) are sometimes not accidents.
    (D) never involve young children.

8. Guns:
    (A) are proven to be helpful in self-defense.
    (B) decrease the risk of injury in a crime.
    (C) have no uses.
    (D) are not dangerous at home.

9. Proven strategies to prevent gun violence include:
    (A) education.
    (B) limiting access.
    (C) regulation by the states.
    (D) public favoring of regulation.

CHAPTER 14

ALCOHOL USE AND THE PHYSICIAN'S ROLE IN TREATMENT

1. Alcohol consumption:
    (A) is pleasurable and anxiety reducing.
    (B) is associated with reinforcement.
    (C) helps prevent cardiovascular problems.
    (D) all of the above

2. With regard to alcoholism, there is:
    (A) an early type associated with antisocial behavior.
    (B) a milder type.
    (C) neither
    (D) both

3. Problems with alcohol include:
    (A) abuse.
    (B) dependence.
    (C) neither
    (D) both

4. Alcohol use is related to:
    (A) one-half of emergency department visits.
    (B) a cost of over $135 billion.
    (C) 20%-40% of hospitalized patients.
    (D) all of the above

5. Alcohol is associated with:
    (A) accidents.
    (B) suicides.
    (C) neither
    (D) both

6. Alcohol can cause:
    (A) acute poisoning.
    (B) chronic organ dysfunction.
    (C) adverse effects in a developing fetus.
    (D) all of the above

7. Prevention of alcohol use can be done through:
    (A) raising the cost of alcohol to con-sumers.
    (B) aggressive enforcement of laws.
    (C) a change in social standards.
    (D) all of the above

8. Alcohol-related domains include:
    (A) a pattern of ingestion.
    (B) dependence upon alcohol.
    (C) associated problems.
    (D) all of the above

9. Treatment of a patient for alcohol abuse requires:
    (A) abstinence from use by the patient.
    (B) control on the part of the patient.
    (C) this is uncertain
    (D) all of the above

10. The physician should:
    (A) not record information regarding a patient's abuse of alcohol.
    (B) record information about a patient's alcohol use in the medical record.
    (C) not be concerned about chain of custody.
    (D) not be concerned about confidentiality.

CHAPTER 15

EFFECTS OF TOBACCO AND CONTROL OF USE

1. Widespread smoking in the United States:
    (A) began in the early 20th century.
    (B) was facilitated by the development of cigarette-making machines.
    (C) was facilitated by use of the safety match.
    (D) all of the above

2. Cigarette smoking was encouraged by:
    (A) the introduction of milder tobacco that was easier to inhale.
    (B) changes in pH that prevent absorption in the oral mucosa.
    (C) both
    (D) neither

3. Cigarette smoking:
    (A) is increasing in use.
    (B) is more common in better educated persons.
    (C) is pleasurable and reduces anxiety.
    (D) increases cognitive performance and suppresses appetite.
    (E) is not addictive.

4. Harm by cigarette smoke is related to the:
    (A) age a person starts smoking.
    (B) number of cigarettes consumed.
    (C) depth of inhalation.
    (D) all of the above

5. Smoking:
    (A) causes 20% of the deaths in the United States.
    (B) costs almost $100 billion/year.
    (C) decreases life expectancy 15 years.
    (D) all of the above

6. Regarding disease, smoking causes:
    (A) cardiovascular disease.
    (B) lung disease.
    (C) 30% of all cancers.
    (D) all of the above

7. Stopping smoking:
   (A) extends a patient's life expectancy.
   (B) immediately returns the patient's risk to baseline.
   (C) may cause excessive weight gain.
   (D) all of the above

8. Regarding pregnant women, smoking causes:
   (A) 5% of prenatal deaths.
   (B) 20% of low birth weight cases.
   (C) 8% of preterm deliveries.
   (D) all of the above

9. The most accurate assessment of the difficulty in stopping smoking is:
   (A) simple.
   (B) impossible.
   (C) difficult.
   (D) useless.

10. Problems that must be faced regarding cigarette smoking include:
    (A) how to prevent people from starting.
    (B) how to help people stop.
    (C) how to protect people from the effects of environmental smoke.
    (D) all of the above

CHAPTER 16

INFECTIOUS DISEASES, PUBLIC HEALTH, AND THE LAW

1. Mandatory serological blood testing for HIV is performed for all of the following *except:*
   (A) armed services recruits.
   (B) marriage license applicants.
   (C) blood donors.
   (D) correctional inmates.
   (E) immigrants to the U.S.

2. The duty of physicians to warn third parties has been invoked in all of the following instances *except*:
   (A) cancer.
   (B) HIV/AIDS.
   (C) tuberculosis.
   (D) smallpox.

3. Transmission of HIV from an infected health care worker to patients has only been documented for:
   (A) a surgeon.
   (B) an anesthesiologist.
   (C) an obstetrician.
   (D) a dentist.

4. A person can be considered to be not "otherwise qualified" under the Americans With Disabilities Act or the Rehabilitation Act of 1973 according to all of the following *except:*
   (A) the nature of the risk.
   (B) the duration of the risk.
   (C) the emotional trauma of the risk.
   (D) the severity of the risk.
   (E) the probability of disease transmission.

5. Epidemiological look-back investigations of HIV-infected workplace exposures are:
   (A) expensive.
   (B) mandatory.
   (C) standard public health practice.
   (D) recommended because of fear of legal liability.

CHAPTER 17

PUBLIC HEALTH ISSUES: RADIATION

1. A patient undergoes a course of radiation treatment in a radiation oncology facility. The cumulative radiation dose delivered is expressed in units of:
   (A) gray.
   (B) sievert.
   (C) roentgen.
   (D) becqueral.

2. Excluding radon, the estimated annual natural environmental radiation exposure per person is approximately:
   (A) 1 mSv.
   (B) 5 mSv.
   (C) 10 mSv.
   (D) 15 mSv.

3. The principal source(s) of environmental radiation are:
   (A) cosmic rays from space.
   (B) terrestrial radionuclides in the south.
   (C) radionuclides in living organisms.
   (D) all of the above

4. The units of rad and rem are often used interchangeably in a medical facility because:
   (A) the biological destructiveness value of the radiation used is unity.
   (B) the units are derived in a similar matter.
   (C) the rad to rem conversion is complex.
   (D) the conversion factor is unity.

5. All but which one of the following are possible harmful effects of radiation:
   (A) solid tumors.
   (B) leukemia.
   (C) loss of hair.
   (D) none of the above

6. The agency that regulates the use of radioactive byproducts is the:
   (A) Nuclear Regulatory Commission (NRC).
   (B) International Commission on Radiological Protection.
   (C) National Council on Radiation Protection and Measurements.
   (D) Committee on the Biological Effects of Ionizing Radiation.

7. What is the annual maximum exposure a visitor can receive while attending a patient receiving radioactive implants?
   (A) 1 mSv
   (B) 5 mSv
   (C) 10 mSv
   (D) 50 mSv

8. Which of the following is *not* true of a misadministration event?
   (A) The referring physician must be informed of the event.
   (B) A written report must be submitted to the NRC within 15 days of the event.
   (C) The NRC must be informed of the event.
   (D) The patient or family member must be informed of the event.

9. Radiation effects may be seen in which procedure(s)?
   (A) cardiac catherization
   (B) balloon angioplasty
   (C) radiation treatment of cancer
   (D) all of the above

10. A gastroenterologist assists the radiation oncologist in the insertion of radioactive sources into the biliary tract under fluoroscopy procedure. What is the annual maximum exposure limit for this gastroenterologist?
    (A) 1 mSv
    (B) 5 mSv
    (C) 10 mSv
    (D) 50 mSv

CHAPTER 19

FOOD AND DRUG ADMINISTRATION: DRUGS AND DEVICES

1. Accurate interpretation of the Food, Drug, and Cosmetic Act requires knowledge of:
   (A) final regulations as they appear in Title 21 of the Code of Federal Regulations.
   (B) Food and Drug Administration (FDA) advisory opinions.
   (C) FDA policy.
   (D) decisions made by federal courts.
   (E) all of the above

2. The Food, Drug, and Cosmetic Act now specifically requires that:
   (A) manufacturers apply for premarket approval before introducing any medical device to the market.
   (B) the FDA assure that there is valid scientific evidence of effectiveness for all drugs and devices.
   (C) the FDA provide reasonable assurance that all drugs and devices are safe and effective.

(D) physicians use drugs only for approved uses.

(E) A, B, and C

3. Federal regulations require that:
   (A) the patient not be charged for an investigational new drug.
   (B) the patient not be charged for an investigational new device.
   (C) insurers not pay for investigational devices.
   (D) A and B

4. Under certain conditions, it is FDA policy to permit implantation of a medical device that has not been legally marketed and that is not covered by an investigational device exemption (IDE) protocol. One necessary condition is that:
   (A) the surgeon obtains permission from the FDA prior to the surgery.
   (B) an IDE is in effect, even though the procedure is not covered by the protocol.
   (C) the manufacturer is notified prior to the surgery.
   (D) there is no reasonable alternative therapy.

CHAPTER 20

ISSUES IN PHYSICIAN LICENSURE

1. Which of the following is *not* one of the traditional reasons asserted in support of licensing physicians?
   (A) Formal licensing helps maintain public confidence in the profession.
   (B) Formal licensing helps improve patient safety.
   (C) Formal licensing protects professional welfare.
   (D) Formal licensing assures government oversight of an otherwise unregulated profession.

2. The earliest colonial licensing laws were drafted primarily to:
   (A) protect patients.
   (B) regulate fees.
   (C) assure that physicians were graduates of colonial medical schools.
   (D) permit governments to identify persons practicing medicine.

3. Which of the following is *not* one of the three universal qualifications for a physician's license?
   (A) good moral and ethical character
   (B) graduation from an approved medical school
   (C) professional liability insurance
   (D) a passing score on the licensing examination

4. Which of the following is a true statement about how the medical schools of the 1990s differ from those of the immediately preceding decades?
   (A) Applicant credentials have improved.
   (B) More lecture hours are included in the curriculum.
   (C) More emphasis is placed on rote learning.
   (D) The number of clinical faculty in medical schools has increased when compared to the number of basic science faculty.

5. Which of the following is *not* a true statement about medical licensing in the United States?
   (A) The U.S. was the first country to stress licensing of physicians.
   (B) A passing score on a national examination is required of all patients who want to obtain a medical license.
   (C) Medical students take the first part of the current medical examination after their second year of medical school.
   (D) The current medical examination stresses problem-solving and is written with descriptions of patient problems that are followed by test questions requiring matching of up to 26 options.

6. Time limits on specialty certification are favored by medical professionals for all but which one of the following reasons?
   (A) Limits help identify impaired physicians.
   (B) Limits promote physician self-improvement by encouraging regular involvement in continuing education.
   (C) Limits prompt the profession to set current standards to assess a quality medical practice.
   (D) Limits prompt collection and maintenance of an expanding body of knowledge in a specialty area.

7. Research seems to indicate that state licensing boards are most effective in identifying and disciplining unqualified or unethical practitioners when all but which one of the following are present?
   (A) adequate funding to support the board's activities
   (B) adequate staff persons to support board activities
   (C) a high degree of physician power on the board
   (D) higher levels of education in the general population

8. A physician whose license is revoked following a medical board's hearing has the right to which one of the following?
   (A) A physician can sue the medical board.
   (B) A physician can get a second hearing.
   (C) A physician must accept the board's decision.
   (D) A physician has a right of appeal to a court.

9. In response to policies that limit a licensed physician's access to patients enrolled in managed care entities, all but which one of the following have occurred?
   (A) Some states have enacted "any willing provider" statutes that guarantee a physician's right to participate if the physician is willing to abide by the managed care entity's operating rules, procedures, and salary structures.
   (B) Some states have statutorily barred all managed care organizations from entering the state.
   (C) The U.S. Congress has considered federal legislation to guarantee fair physician access to managed care organizations.
   (D) Physicians have litigated the right to participate.

10. Physicians participating in a managed care organization should avoid which one of the following activities?
    (A) advocating for a patient when a managed care guideline unfairly restricts treatment for that patient
    (B) participating at a policy level in developing general treatment guidelines for all patients in the managed care organization
    (C) disclosing managed care treatment limitations to patients who may need to seek treatment elsewhere
    (D) entering a contract that creates a conflict of interest for the physician by placing a substantial percentage of physician income at risk when making treatment decisions for patients

CHAPTER 21

ISSUES IN HOSPITAL PRIVILEGES AND PEER REVIEW

1. A formal process for physician peer review in hospitals is required by:
   (A) federal Medicare regulations.
   (B) state hospital licensing bodies.
   (C) the Joint Commission on the Accreditation of Healthcare Organizations.
   (D) the federal Health Care Quality Improvement Act (HCQIA).
   (E) all of the above

2. The National Practitioner Data Bank, which was created by the HCQIA, is a national physician tracking mechanism. Among other things, the HCQIA encourages hospitals to voluntarily report to the Data Bank all peer review decisions that have negatively affected a physician's privi-

leges for longer than 30 days.
(A) true
(B) false

3. A hospital can be held liable for the wrongs committed by a hospital employee, including an employee physician. The name of the legal doctrine that holds the employer liable is *respondeat superior.*
(A) true
(B) false

4. A court also might hold a hospital liable for the wrongs committed by an independent contractor physician if the patient believed the physician to be an agent of the hospital. The plaintiff would rely on which one of the following legal theories?
(A) *res ipsa loquitur.*
(B) ostensible agency.
(C) corporate conspiracy.
(D) *respondeat superior.*

5. Even if the physician did not appear to be an agent of the hospital, a court might find that the hospital was negligent in selecting the physician for privileges or in supervising the physician after awarding privileges. Plaintiffs who sue the physician for malpractice and who also sue the hospital for its independent act of negligence in privileging the physician are utilizing the theory of hospital corporate negligence in holding the hospital liable.
(A) true
(B) false

6. Courts have recognized that the ability to exercise hospital privileges is an important component of the successful physician's practice. Because the Constitutional right to property is implicated when a hospital decides to restrict or deny privileges, courts have demanded that hospitals utilize certain minimum procedures to assure that the physician is treated fairly when a negative privilege decision is made. Thus, when restricting or denying privileges, the hospital must afford the physician his or her constitutional:

(A) due process rights.
(B) free speech rights.
(C) right to have the state appoint an attorney.
(D) right to a jury trial.

7. The HCQIA protects peer review decisions made for quality-of-care reasons. Although some states have their own immunity provisions, the HCQIA provides one kind of immunity that state peer review statutes cannot provide. The additional immunity provided to peer review entities that meet HCQIA guidelines will be available in a case based on which one of the following legal theories?
(A) tortious interference with business relations
(B) breach of state antitrust law
(C) defamation
(D) breach of federal antitrust law

8. "Any willing provider" laws are state statutory laws advocated by many physicians who believe, among other things, that managed care organizations (MCOs) unfairly exclude many good physicians who need to have access to the MCO patients in order to maintain an adequate patient pool.
(A) true
(B) false

CHAPTER 23

MANAGED CARE ORGANIZATIONS

1. The health maintenance organization (HMO) model in which the HMO employs the physicians who render services at HMO-owned or controlled facilities is:
(A) a staff model.
(B) a group model.
(C) an independent practice association.
(D) a direct contract model.
(E) a network model.

2. Health care costs rose during the 1980s at an annual rate of:
   (A) 5%.
   (B) 10%.
   (C) 15%.
   (D) 20%.
   (E) 25%.

3. A health plan may be found directly liable under a theory of:
   (A) *respondent superior.*
   (B) ostensible agency.
   (C) apparent agency.
   (D) breach of contract.

4. The federal law that may pre-empt an action brought by a patient based on state law is:
   (A) ERISA (Employee Retirement Security Act of 1974).
   (B) the Sherman Act.
   (C) the Clayton Act.
   (D) the Federal Trade Commission Act.

5. The method of physician reimbursement unlikely to be found in a managed care plan is:
   (A) salary.
   (B) capitation.
   (C) full fee for service.
   (D) discounted fee for service.

CHAPTER 24

HEALTH INSURANCE, MEDICARE, AND MEDICAID

1. Health insurance is a contract between:
   (A) the insurance company and the health care provider.
   (B) the insurance company and the patient.
   (C) the patient and the health care provider.
   (D) none of the above

2. When a patient has health care insurance, the physician must:
   (A) obtain permission from the insurance company to treat the patient.
   (B) bill the insurance company.
   (C) send medical records to the insurance company.
   (D) treat the patient in an appropriate manner.

3. When a patient has health care insurance, the physician can:
   (A) always send medical information to the insurance company.
   (B) never send medical information to the insurance company.
   (C) send medical information to the insurance company after obtaining patient consent to the release of information.

4. What types of medical records are most sensitive and require specific releases?
   (A) HIV records
   (B) mental health records
   (C) drug or alcohol treatment records
   (D) all of the above

5. Generally, physicians can treat minor patients without parental consent or knowledge for which of the following conditions?
   (A) pregnancy
   (B) drug or alcohol addiction
   (C) venereal disease
   (D) all of the above

6. How long must a physician retain medical records for Medicare patients?
   (A) 2 years
   (B) 5 years
   (C) 10 years

7. What factor is used by Medicare to determine payment amounts for a physician?
   (A) where the physician trained
   (B) how long the physician has been practicing medicine
   (C) the relative value of the service provided
   (D) whether the physician is in solo or group practice
   (E) all of the above

8. Physicians can be terminated from Medicare and/or Medicaid programs if they:
   (A) submit claims for services not performed.
   (B) submit claims for more money than the program pays for that service.
   (C) change locations.
   (D) submit claims for services in excess of the medical needs of the patient.
   (E) A and B
   (F) A and D

9. Medicaid is a:
   (A) federal program.
   (B) state program.
   (C) joint federal and state program.
   (D) private program.

10. Medicare reform:
   (A) was passed in 1996.
   (B) was hotly contested in the U.S. Congress.
   (C) will likely reduce payments to hospitals and physicians.
   (D) will be discussed again by the U.S. Congress.
   (E) all of the above
   (F) B, C, and D

CHAPTER 25

SOCIAL SECURITY DISABILITY: THE ROLE OF THE PHYSICIAN

1. The Social Security Act enacted by the U.S. Congress in 1935 initially provided benefits to:
   (A) wage earners unable to continue to work because of health problems.
   (B) blind persons.
   (C) elderly persons, as a pension plan.
   (D) disabled persons who had minimal or no labor force participation.

2. Disability, as defined by the Social Security Administration (SSA), includes all of the following *except:*
   (A) medical conditions listed by the SSA and published in the Federal Register.
   (B) a severe but treatable medical condition present for 6 months.
   (C) the inability to engage in any substantial gainful activity.
   (D) gainful activity limited by a medically determinable impairment.

3. Physician reports regarding a patient provided to the SSA should contain the following:
   (A) documentation of a response or lack of response to medical treatment.
   (B) medical documentation covering the complete time frame that the condition was present.
   (C) a physician opinion on observation of when and how medical condition(s) affected functioning.
   (D) a medical source statement outlining specific activities the patient can and cannot perform.
   (E) all of the above

4. Since the *Richardson v. Perales* decision in 1971, the treating physician's opinion concerning the patient's ability or inability to work was determined to have less probative value than the consulting physician's opinion.
   (A) true
   (B) false

5. Social Security Disability Insurance benefits are provided to all of the following *except:*
   (A) a nondisabled parent of an entitled child.
   (B) a disabled worker under the age of 65 years.
   (C) a disabled child under the age of 18 years.
   (D) a disabled widow or widower if spouse was covered under Social Security.

CHAPTER 26

WORKER'S COMPENSATION: THE ROLE OF THE PHYSICIAN

1. The physician treating a patient with a work-related injury or illness should consider restricting the patient from work in all of the following situations *except* when:
   (A) re-entry into the work environment is expected to further sensitize the patient to known toxins.
   (B) the patient is unable to ride or drive because of his or her condition.
   (C) the patient is confined to bed rest.
   (D) the patient indicates that "light duty" work is not available.
   (E) the patient is on medication which is causing significant adverse side effects.

2. Physicians participating in the care of patients covered under workers' compensation should be confident in providing professional opinion as to:
   (A) maximum medical improvement.
   (B) causality determination.
   (C) projected and actual return-to-work dates with and without restriction.
   (D) impairment determination and functional capabilities.
   (E) all of the above

3. Russia implemented the first system for scheduled rating and disability based on lost earning capacity.
   (A) true
   (B) false

4. Workers, in general, not covered under some form of workers' compensation system include all of the following *except:*
   (A) maritime workers.
   (B) agricultural workers.
   (C) domestic workers.
   (D) employees of firms with fewer than three employees.

5. Disability is determined based on all of the following factors, whereas impairment is determined by:
   (A) deviation from normal functioning in body part or organ system.
   (B) age.
   (C) education and work experience.
   (D) economic and social environment(s).
   (E) gender.

6. An individual is defined as disabled and protected under the Americans With Disabilities Act except in the case of:
   (A) having a record of impairment.
   (B) being regarded as having an impairment.
   (C) being expected to develop an impairment because of medically accepted risk factors.
   (D) having a mental impairment that substantially limits a major life activity.

CHAPTER 27

MEDICAL MALPRACTICE

1. Negligence, without patient injury:
   (A) is malpractice when intentional or known negligence is present.
   (B) is not malpractice
   (C) is malpractice when there is a proven departure from the standard of care.
   (D) is malpractice when the doctor fails to follow up on the negligence.
   (E) is malpractice when there is a *breach* of the duty to follow the standard of care.

2. Informed consent requires that:
   (A) consent be obtained from the patient by a certified health care worker.
   (B) in emergency situations, consent be obtained by the closest living relative.
   (C) even where the risks are exceedingly remote, consent by a prudent man must be obtained.
   (D) it be confirmed that a meaningful dialogue between physician and patient occurred.

3. Compensable non-economic damages, among other things, consist of which of the following:
   (A) loss of the enjoyment of life

(B) pain and suffering
(C) loss of consortium
(D) none of the above
(E) all of the above

4. The concept of deterrence in the tort system:
   (A) consists of the concept that the tort system in and of itself deters or prevents physician negligence.
   (B) consists of the concept that the tort system deters just compensation of the injured patient.
   (C) is accepted by most legal scholars as an effective tool in preventing physician negligence.
   (D) is negated by the stress and anguish to the physician of a malpractice suit against him or her.

5. In the malpratice arena today:
   (A) the testimony of expert witnesses becomes of secondary importance to the nature of the injury.
   (B) settlement often occurs after the facts are obtained through deposition.
   (C) settlement more often occurs as a result of judicial review.
   (D) settlement is the result of the opposing attorneys sitting down with the judge and making a decision.
   (E) expert witnesses are selected by the judge from a pool of experts available to him or her.

6. The Harvard study:
   (A) is an outdated, poorly conceived and executed study that no longer provides useful data.
   (B) reveals that the most common cause of a malpractice suit is poor communication with the patient in the informed consent process.
   (C) reveals that the largest percentage of adverse events occurred in the emergency department.
   (D) reveals that preventable adverse events were not a realistic problem.
   (E) shows that 98% of all adverse events due to negligence did not result in malpractice claims.

7. Guidelines:
   (A) have become the legal standard for adherence to the standard of care.
   (B) would be a major element in the development of a no-fault malpractice system.
   (C) have proved to be ineffective for anesthesiologists as they relate to monitoring for hypoxia.
   (D) have the problem of the uncertainty of management of some medical problems and rapid outdating.
   (E) have eliminated the need for expert testimony in many cases.

8. The reforms that have had the most significant effect in reducing malpractice costs are:
   (A) limiting attorney contingency fees.
   (B) the use of pretrial screening panels.
   (C) the use of periodic payments.
   (D) caps on intangible (non-economic) damage awards and mandatory collateral source offsets.
   (E) reforms of the tort system.

9. Defensive medicine:
   (A) has probably been over-rated as a significant cause of the high cost of medical care.
   (B) has proved to be a major factor in the performance of unnecessary surgery.
   (C) is considered to be *positive* defensive medicine when it leads to the avoidance of high-risk patients and procedures.
   (D) rarely, if ever, leads to unexpected beneficial effects.
   (E) is hard to evaluate despite the straightforward and readily available facts of the matter.

10. No-fault systems of medical negligence:
    (A) would probably be no more expensive than present systems.
    (B) would be more effective if controls were built in to identify specific compensable events.
    (C) are now in use in several states.
    (D) are social insurance programs without the problems associated with such programs.

INDEX

Volumes I and II

Page numbers for figures and tables are followed by *f* and *t*, respectively.
(1) = entry in Volume I
(2) = entry in Volume II

ANSWERS TO CME QUESTIONS
The Physician's Perspective on Medical Law Volume II

Chapter 13
1. D	2. A	3. B	4. B	5. B
6. B	7. A	8. B	9. B	

Chapter 14
1. D	2. D	3. D	4. D	5. D
6. D	7. D	8. D	9. C	10. B

Chapter 15
1. D	2. C	3. D	4. D	5. D
6. D	7. A	8. D	9. C	10. D

Chapter 16
1. B	2. A	3. D	4. C	5. A

Chapter 17
1. A	2. A	3. D	4. A	5. D
6. A	7. B	8. D	9. D	10. D

Chapter 19
1. E	2. C	3. A	4. D

Chapter 20
1. D	2. B	3. C	4. D	5. A
6. A	7. C	8. D	9. B	10. D

Chapter 21
1. D	2. B	3. A	4. B	5. A
6. A	7. D	8. A		

Chapter 23
1. A	2. B	3. D	4. A	5. C

Chapter 24
1. B	2. D	3. C	4. D	5. D
6. B	7. C	8. F	9. C	10. F

Chapter 25
1. C	2. B	3. E	4. B	5. C

Chapter 26
1. D	2. E	3. A	4. A	5. A
6. C				

Chapter 27
1. B	2. D	3. E	4. A	5. B
6. E	7. D	8. D	9. A	10. B

PREVIOUSLY PUBLISHED BOOKS IN THE
Neurosurgical Topics SERIES

For order information call (847) 692-9500.

Howard H. Kaufman, MD, is Professor and Chairman of the Department of Neurosurgery at West Virginia University School of Medicine. He received a BA from Yale University and an MD from Columbia University. He did his internship in Minnesota, studied a year at the National Hospital for Nervous Diseases in London, spent 2 years at the National Institutes of Health, and then did a residency at Neurological Institute of Columbia University. He was a member of the faculty of the University of Arizona and the University of Texas at Houston before moving to West Virginia. He has been involved with many legal issues, among them brain death and the permanent vegetative state, organ retrieval, and device regulation. He will be developing a national effort on gun safety for organized neurosurgery.

Jeff L. Lewin, JD, is Professor of Law at the Widener University School of Law in Wilmington, Delaware. The son of a psychiatrist and the grandson of a general practitioner, Professor Lewin broke with family tradition to major in Economics at the University of Michigan and receive a JD from Harvard Law School. After several years of law practice, he joined the faculty of the West Virginia University School of Law. Service on that University's Institutional Review Board for the Protection of Human Research Subjects from 1985 to 1990 rekindled his interest in medicolegal issues, and he began collaborating with Dr. Kaufman on a series of projects that culminated in this book. In addition to works on medicolegal issues, Professor Lewin has published articles on such diverse topics as nuisance law, tort law, environmental law and economics, valuation of criminal gains in cost-benefit analysis, and ownership of coalbed methane. The *Maryland Law Review* is publishing his article on the origins of the phrase "reasonable medical certainty," and he currently is exploring the relationship between this phrase and recent developments in evidence and tort law.

This two-volume set is the first contribution to the series for Dr. Kaufman and Mr. Lewin. Dr. Kaufman has been a chapter author in several previous books in the *Neurosurgical Topics Series*.

Publications Office
Lebanon, New Hampshire

Gay Palazzo
Joanne B. Needham
Katherine Mann

Compositor
Barbara Homeyer

Indexer
Sarah Allen Smith

Reference Editor
Kim DeVillers